42.50

The Link between Religion and Health

The Link between Religion and Health

Psychoneuroimmunology and the Faith Factor

EDITED BY

Harold G. Koenig
Harvey Jay Cohen

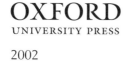
OXFORD
UNIVERSITY PRESS

2002

OXFORD
UNIVERSITY PRESS

Oxford   New York
Athens   Auckland   Bangkok   Bogotá   Buenos Aires   Cape Town
Chennai   Dar es Salaam   Delhi   Florence   Hong Kong   Istanbul   Karachi
Kolkata   Kuala Lumpur   Madrid   Melbourne   Mexico City   Mumbai   Nairobi
Paris   São Paulo   Shanghai   Singapore   Taipei   Tokyo   Toronto   Warsaw

and associated companies in
Berlin   Ibadan

Published by Oxford University Press, Inc.
198 Madison Avenue, New York, New York 10016

Oxford is a registered trademark of Oxford University Press

Library of Congress Cataloging-in-Publication Data
The link between religion and health: psychoneuroimmunology and the faith factor /
edited by Harold G. Koenig and Harvey Jay Cohen.
    p.   cm.
Includes bibliographical references and index.
ISBN-13 978-0-19-514360-7
ISBN 0-19-514360-4
1. Psychoneuroimmunology.   2. Faith—Physiological aspects.   I. Koenig, Harold George.
II. Cohen, Harvey Jay.
QP356.47 .P778   2001
616.07'9—dc21   00-068161

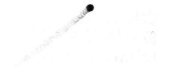

9 8 7 6 5 4 3

Printed in the United States of America
on acid-free paper

To Sir John Templeton

whose vision and generosity made this possible

Foreword

Psychoneuroimmunology and the Faith Factor—what an interesting subtitle and combination of concepts for a book! Psychoneuroimmunology (PNI) is the study of the relationship between the mind, the immune system, and health. Eleven chapters of this book discuss various aspects of PNI. They suggest that when the brain perceives an event as unpleasant or stress evoking, specific areas of the brain are activated, which initiate the release of hormones from nerve terminals in lymphoid tissue, while other hormones associated with the hypothalamic-pituitary-adrenal axis are released into plasma. If the cells that comprise the immune system have receptors for these hormones, the activity of the immune cells may be modified. The summative effect of the multiple hormones that bind to receptors will either increase or decrease the function of a cell. Depending on the biological function of the cells whose function is altered, the activity of the immune system will be modified. The clinical and epidemiological data presented in chapters 5 through 11 suggest that the net effect is decreased immune system function and increased susceptibility to those diseases in which the immune system is related to the disease etiology, pathogenesis, or both.

The obvious intent of this book, as implied by the title, is to suggest that faith may affect the quality of health through pathways being defined by research in the science of PNI. What could be the basis of the relationship? It is unlikely that faith can modify hormone receptors. It is more likely that faith can affect the concentration of hormones released by nerve terminals and produced by the hypothalamic-pituitary-adrenal axis. How? If faith can ameliorate the activation of the brain areas involved with activation of the nerves and release of the hormones associated with altered immune function, a more efficient and effective immune system would result, with decreased development of immune-related disease.

How could faith influence the activity of the brain? Possibly, there are areas of the brain that are activated when individuals invoke their faith-associated belief system or engage in activities that they relate to faith. Activation of these areas may inhibit activation of the stress-responsive brain areas. Possibly, individuals who have high levels of faith interpret events that are potentially high in stress differently than individuals who have low levels of faith—with their belief that God will help them through the difficult time. Possibly, the social relationships that are often associated with sharing one's faith with others may alter an individual's perception of a highly stressful situation, minimizing the activation of stress-related areas of the brain.

Obviously, the mechanisms are not known and can only be speculated upon. As epidemiological data support an association between faith and health, an understanding of the mechanism responsible for the association may provide a means to activate the mechanism through emotional modalities other than those associated with faith. The studies reported in this book suggest that a logical mechanism by which faith can be associated with a better quality of health is through the brain–immune system pathways that are being defined by the discipline of psychoneuroimmunology. The authors hope this book will excite others to pursue studies in this area. The public health impact may be enormous.

Bruce S. Rabin, M.D., Ph.D.
Division of Clinical Immune Pathology
University of Pittsburgh Medical Center
Pittsburgh, Pennsylvania

Contents

Contributors

Warren S. Brown, Ph.D.
Fuller Theological Seminary
180 North Oakland Avenue
Pasadena, CA 91101

Harvey Jay Cohen, M.D.
Director, Center for the Study of
    Aging and Human Development
Duke University Medical Center
Director, Geriatric Research, Educa-
    tion, and Clinical Center
    Durham VA Medical Center
DUMC-3003
Durham, NC 27710

Sheldon Cohen, Ph.D.
Department of Psychology
Carnegie Mellon University
5000 Forbes Avenue
Pittsburgh, PA 15213

Fawzy I. Fawzy, M.D.
Department of Psychiatry and Bio-
    behavioral Science
C8-861 NPI, 760 Westwood Plaza
UCLA, c/o Mail Service, Mail Code
    175919
Los Angeles, CA 90024-1759

Paul J. Griffiths, Ph.D.
University of Chicago
Divinity School
1025-35 E. 58th Street
Chicago, IL 60637

Ronald B. Herberman, M.D.
University of Pittsburgh Cancer
    Institute
201 Kaufmann Building
3471 Fifth Avenue
Pittsburgh, PA 15213-3221

Gail Ironson, M.D., Ph.D.
Department of Psychology
University of Miami
P.O. Box 248185
Coral Gables, FL 33124

Howard L. Kaye, Ph.D.
Department of Sociology
Franklin and Marshall College
119 Deepdate Road
Wayne, PA 19087

Harold G. Koenig, M.D., M.H.Sc.
Departments of Psychiatry and
    Medicine
Duke University Medical Center

Geriatric Research, Education,
   and Clinical Center
   (GRECC), Durham VA
   Medical Center
DUMC-3400
Durham, NC 27710

Bruce S. Rabin, M.D., Ph.D.
Division of Clinical Immune
   Pathology
University of Pittsburgh Medical
   Center
Room 5725, CHP-MT
200 Lothrop Street
Pittsburgh, PA 15213-2582

Neil Schneiderman, Ph.D.
Department of Psychology
Behavioral Medicine Program
University of Miami
P.O. Box 248185
Coral Gables, FL 33124-2070

George F. Solomon, M.D.
Department of Psychiatry and Bio-
   behavioral Science
C8-528 NPI, 740 Westwood Plaza
UCLA, c/o Mail Service, Mail Code
   175919
Los Angeles, CA 90024-1759

David Spiegel, M.D.
Department of Psychiatry and
   Behavioral Sciences
Stanford University School of
   Medicine
401 Quarry Road, 2325
Stanford, CA 94305-5718

Redford B. Williams, M.D.
Department of Psychiatry and
   Behavioral Science
Duke University Medical Center
2212 Elder Street, Box 3926
Durham, NC 27710

We would like to acknowledge the work of science writer James P. Swyers, who assisted the contributors in writing their chapters. His skill and dedication to this project were instrumental in making this book possible.

The Link between
Religion and Health

Introduction

HAROLD G. KOENIG & HARVEY JAY COHEN

On July 12, 1999, twelve of the world's leading psychoneuroimmunologists, theologians, and physicians were brought together at Duke University to review the effects of stress on the immune system and to see how this knowledge might inform us about the religion-health relationship. During the past three decades, hundreds of separate research studies conducted by different investigators studying different populations throughout the world have reported a relationship between religious involvement, better physical health, and greater longevity. Why this connection between religion and physical health exists, however, remains largely a mystery. Because of the close connection between religion and mental health and the increasingly understood connection between mental health and immune functioning, we proposed the possibility that religious involvement might affect physical health through neuroendocrine and immune mechanisms. The Duke conference, entitled Psychoneuroimmunology and the Faith Factor in Human Health, became the first attempt to address this question within the mainstream scientific community.

Who should read this book? Scientists and academic researchers will find here a gold mine of ideas and possible projects, as well as a wealth of information about study methodologies and research instruments. Educators will discover plentiful information to update their students about the newest advances in psychoneuroimmunology (PNI) and to stimulate thinking about how religious beliefs and practices might influence health through known physiological mechanisms. They will also find here thoughtful discussions by eminent theologians and sociologists about the religious and societal implications of such research. Students will learn how the mind, body, and spirit are intimately connected through a host of neurological, endocrine, and immune pathways. The general reader will discover in this book a fascinating exposé of the mind-body relationship—a relationship that may help provide a rational explanation of how devout religious beliefs and practices might affect not only their sense of well-being and quality of life but also their physical health and longevity. Although even the most ardent skeptic may admit the emotional benefits of faith, the physical health ramifications of religious belief, ritual, and community—acting through established physiological pathways—may not have been fully considered. Even if they have pondered these possible health effects of religion, both skeptic and believer may not have thought through the theological and societal implications that such research might have.

This book not only documents the discussions in the Duke conference among this group of highly skeptical scientists but also expands these discussions to include more detailed and thoughtful consideration of the connection between PNI and the religion-health relationship. Several scientists who could not attend the conference nevertheless agreed to work with us to produce chapters on their areas of expertise for this book. The end result is a series of 15 chapters, written by the eminent leaders in the PNI field, that discuss the areas of most active research and consider how research exploring the religion-immunity relationship might be conducted and interpreted.

Chapter 1 reviews research that examines the relationships between religion, mental health, and social support. If there is an association between religious involvement, better mental health, and greater social support, and if mental health and social support contribute to better immune functioning, then perhaps religious practices could also have an impact on immune function. This could help explain recent findings on the relationship between religion and physical health, particularly the rather consistent finding that religious activity is related to greater longevity. While still quite preliminary, a few studies have actually documented the association between religion and immune function, and these are reviewed.

The author of chapter 2 is George Solomon from UCLA, who, together with Robert Ader, helped give birth to the field of psychoneuroimmunology. In his chapter, Solomon reviews the history of the field, highlighting the events that have made this area of study into a highly respected scientific and medical discipline.

In chapter 3, immunologist Bruce Rabin from the University of Pittsburgh describes how psychological stress affects the brain, neuro-

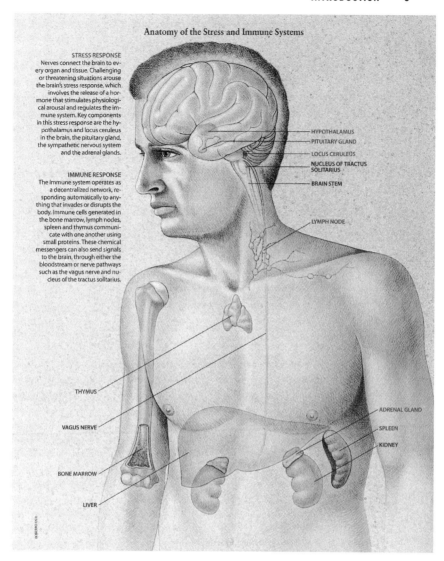

Figure I.1 "Anatomy of the stress and immune systems," by Roberto Osti. From *Scientific American*, special issue vol. 7, no. 1 (1997). Reprinted courtesy of Roberto Osti.

endocrine system, and, ultimately, the cardiovascular and immune systems. A theoretical model is presented that details the effects of stress on the locus ceruleus and sympathetic nervous system, which connect the brain to primary and secondary lymph organs. He outlines how stress affects the hypothalamus, the pituitary, the adrenals, and the hormones

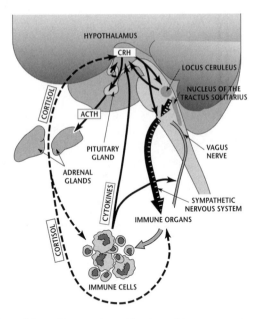

Figure I.2 Adapted from "Interaction of brain and immune system," by Roberto Osti, from *Scientific American*, special issue vol. 7, no. 1 (1997), courtesy of Roberto Osti. The brain and immune system can either stimulate (solid arrows) or inhibit (dotted arrows) each other. Immune cells produce cytokines (chemical signals) that stimulate the hypothalamus through the bloodstream or via nerves elsewhere in the body. The hormone CRH, produced in the hypothalamus, activates the HPA axis. The release of cortisol tunes down the immune system. CRH, acting on the brain stem, stimulates the sympathetic nervous system, which innervates immune organs and regulates inflammatory responses throughout the body. Disruption of these communications in any way leads to greater susceptibility to disease and immune complications.

produced by these glands that ultimately affect cellular immunity, antibody production, and cytokine activity. Rabin discusses how religious beliefs and activity might influence this system by improving coping and increasing support or, alternatively, may simply be a marker for some other factor (genetic or acquired) that is associated with lower stress and greater sociability.

In chapter 4, Ron Herberman describes and discusses natural killer (NK) cells, a type of lymphocyte that may play a critical role in cancer surveillance and containment. As one of the discoverers of the NK cell, Herberman is better qualified than anyone else to review the research that connects psychological and social stress to NK cell activity, which may be a key link to help explain how psychosocial factors influence susceptibility to cancer and affect its course.

In chapter 5, psychiatrists David Spiegel and Fawzy Fawzy describe the effects that social interventions can have on cancer prognosis. These two world-renowned medical scientists at Stanford University and UCLA, respectively, have each led major studies that examined the impact of psychosocial and behavioral interventions on survival in patients with breast cancer and malignant melanoma, respectively. They discuss here in detail these interventions and the immune mechanisms that may be involved in the remarkable effects observed.

In chapter 6, Sheldon Cohen from the University of Pittsburgh discusses his research on psychosocial stress, social support, and susceptibility to infection that has helped to mainstream psychoneuroimmunology into the field of medicine. His review of how social factors may affect immune functioning and disease susceptibility is perhaps the best in the published literature at this time. He goes on to hypothesize that religious factors may influence both psychological and social functioning to a degree that health is significantly affected.

In chapter 7, we further examine the effects of social factors on neuroendocrine and immune function, reviewing the work of Janice Kiecolt-Glaser and her husband, Ronald Glaser, at Ohio State University. These investigators have documented the effects of caregiver stress, marital discord, and even stress during student exams on endocrine and immune functioning. Moreover, in a series of elegant experiments in animals and humans, they have shown how stress—acting through immunological mechanisms—can significantly impair the speed of wound healing (with all the implications that has for recovery from trauma, accidents, and surgery).

In chapter 8, Gail Ironson and Neil Schneiderman at the University of Miami explore the pathogenesis of HIV infection, its treatment, and the various psychosocial factors known to play a role in the progression of HIV to AIDS. They also examine the impact of religious and spiritual beliefs and practices on these psychosocial factors and the implications that this may have for the treatment of HIV/AIDS.

In chapter 9, Redford Williams examines the relationships between hostility and anger, neuroendocrine change, and health outcome. His work has helped to establish how anger and hostile aggression can have devastating cardiovascular effects that shorten survival. Because religious and spiritual traditions emphasize the mastery and control of negative emotions, Williams notes that this may offer opportunities not only for studying the phenomenon of hostility itself but also for understanding the ways that the health-damaging effects of hostility might be thwarted.

In chapter 10, we discuss diseases that result not from a hypoactive immune system but rather from an immune system functioning in an exaggerated or uncontrolled fashion. This is seen in autoimmune diseases such as psoriasis, rheumatoid arthritis, Graves's disease, multiple sclerosis, insulin-dependent diabetes mellitus, lupus erythematosus, inflammatory bowel disease, chronic fatigue syndrome, and a host of other disorders that result when an overactive immune system attacks normal healthy tissue. The work of Esther Sternberg at the NIH and Bruce Rabin at the University of Pittsburgh has helped clarify how stress can affect these diseases and how interventions that reduce stress may help to ameliorate them. In particular, we see how religious beliefs and practices (from Buddhist to Judeo-Christian traditions) may help reduce stress by improving coping and thereby favorably affect the course of these diseases.

In chapter 11, measures of immune function, neuroendocrine function, religion, and spirituality are reviewed and discussed, pointing out the various strengths and weaknesses of different instruments. This chapter is key for researchers and scientists who wish to study the relationship between religion and psychoneuroimmunology. To our knowledge, this is the only source that provides detailed information on both religious and PNI measures, as well as suggestions on which of these measures might best be used to identify relationships.

In chapter 12, eminent theologian Paul Griffiths from the University of Chicago briefly overviews the religious traditions of Buddhism, Hinduism, Taoism, Confucianism, and Shinto, religions adhered to by more than a billion people. He explores the implications that PNI research may have for members of Eastern religious traditions. He also discusses concerns about how information on religion and health may be used and interpreted.

In chapter 13, Warren Brown from Fuller Theological Seminary in Pasadena, California, discusses the implications of PNI research for members of Western religious traditions such as Christianity, Judaism, and Islam, in which God is understood in monotheistic and personal terms. Of particular interest is his discussion of the importance of personal relationship and emotional disclosure as they are expressed in Western religious traditions.

In chapter 14, sociologist Howard Kaye from Franklin and Marshall College discusses the implications for medicine, society, and culture of learning about the biochemical pathways by which spirituality and religious practice exert their influence on health. He discusses important and sometimes difficult questions, including how physicians and health care systems should utilize such information in their care of patients. Kaye draws comparisons with social Darwinism and the eugenics movement of the nineteenth century to make his points. As does Griffiths, he also expresses concern about the utilitarian use of religion to improve health or immune functioning.

In chapter 15, we explore avenues for future research in the area of religion, spirituality, and psychoneuroimmunology. These recommendations come directly from our July conference at Duke and, in particular, from discussions involving the PNI experts and theologians who have written this book. Here we present and prioritize specific research studies that need to be done to advance the field, information that should be useful not only to scientists but also to funding agencies that wish to support this effort.

In these 15 chapters, we have covered an enormous amount of theory and research that will help provide the foundation for future efforts to better understand how the mind, the body, and the spirit are intimately connected. We believe that such research will help validate the importance of treating the whole person in our health care system. It is becoming clearer and clearer that efforts in medicine to treat the biological disease alone will not result in complete healing unless the other aspects of what it means to be human are also considered.

1

The Connection between Psychoneuroimmunology and Religion

HAROLD G. KOENIG

Psychoneuroimmunology is the study of how social and psychological factors affect neuroendocrine and immune functioning. Religion involves beliefs about *the transcendent*, as well as private or communal practices and rituals that reflect devotion or commitment to those beliefs. Why should religion and psychoneuroimmunology be related, and how? This chapter provides a background to help us understand why a connection between these two seemingly disparate topics might exist—and, in fact, makes good sense.

Historical Perspective

Religious beliefs and practices throughout recorded history have been associated with health and healing practices. All early human civilizations (Mesopotamian, Egyptian, Indian, Chinese, Greek, and Roman) dealt with physical illness in religious or spiritual terms (Koenig, McCullough, et al., 2001). Supernatural methods of treatment often involved healing rituals, prayers, incantations, or religious pilgrimages. Until recently, however, it had not been considered that religion might have an impact on physical health through natural mechanisms—that is, via social, psychological, and behavioral pathways. Relatively little attention was paid to the effects of religious beliefs and practices on mental health or social support until the latter half of the twentieth century. Research in this area, however, has been rapidly accumulating. In a recent review of this literature, we discovered that more than 850 studies have examined the relationship

between religious belief or practice and mental health or social functioning (Koenig, McCullough, et al., 2001).

Religion and Coping with Stress

Stress is common in modern society and comes in many forms. These include the stress of interpersonal conflict, unfulfilled expectations, disap-
pointments, job and financial pressure, loss of loved ones or broken relationships, loss of dreams and hopes, and loss of health and independence—
to name just a few. In this book, we will learn that psychosocial stress influences a number of biological processes in the body responsible for
homeostasis—the delicate physiological equilibrium necessary for survival. Religion may be an important way that people cope with stress. As
throughout human history, this continues to be true even today in the
United States, one of the most educated and technologically advanced
countries in the world.

In national surveys asking people to agree or disagree that religion provides personal comfort and support, 78% of Americans of all ages indicate
that the statement is mostly or completely true, and nearly 90% of older
adults do so (Princeton Religion Research Center, 1982, p. 120). A study
of 100 healthy community-dwelling older adults found that religious
methods were the most common form of coping, particularly among
women (nearly two-thirds of whom used religion as their primary coping
strategy during stressful periods) (Koenig, George, & Siegler, 1988). This is
not as true, however, in other parts of the world. According to Rudestam
(1972), approximately 80% of persons in Sweden indicated "none" when
asked about their degree of religiosity (compared to only about 10% of
persons in the United States who give this response). Likewise, Ringdal et
al. (1995) found that nearly half (43–45%) of their cancer patients in Nor-
way did not believe in God or receive comfort from religious beliefs.

In the United States and many other areas of the world, however, most
people report that religious beliefs and activities provide comfort during
stress, especially in the face of acute or chronic medical illness. For example, Kaldjian et al. (1998) reported that 98% of 90 HIV-positive patients at
Yale–New Haven Hospital believed in a loving divine being called "God,"
84% expressed a personal relationship with God, and 82% indicated that
their belief in God helped when they were thinking about death. Such a
finding is not unusual. In fact, more than 40% of medical patients in some

areas of the United States indicate that religion is the *most important factor* that enables them to cope with illness, and an *additional* 50% report that it helps to a moderate or large degree (Koenig, 1998). Only about 10% of patients with medical illness indicate little or no comfort from religion. Other researchers have reported similar findings, particularly among older adults, women, and African Americans (Conway 1985; Manfredi & Pickett, 1987; Swanson & Harter, 1971). To what extent, however, do religious beliefs and practices result in improved coping, better mental health, or greater quality of life?

Religion, Well-Being, and Mental Health

In fact, studies do suggest that religious beliefs and practices contribute to positive emotions such as well-being, life satisfaction, and happiness. In a recent systematic review of the scientific literature that uncovered 100 studies of this relationship, 79% reported a significant positive association between religious involvement and greater well-being (Koenig, McCullough, et al., 2001). Among 10 prospective cohort studies, 9 found that greater religious beliefs or activity predicted greater well-being over time. Thus, the evidence overwhelmingly supports a connection between religious involvement and positive emotions.

Religion, Optimism, and Hope. Optimism is the ability to psychologically distance oneself from negative outcomes. Hope, by contrast, is the ability to set goals, find paths to those goals, and motivate oneself to use those paths. Religious beliefs often provide a worldview that is both optimistic and hopeful, infusing difficult or traumatic life events with purpose and meaning. We identified 14 studies that examined the relationship between religiousness and optimism or hope. Of those studies, 12 found a significant positive correlation and 2 found no association. The research team of Martin Seligman (1998 president of the American Psychological Association, best known for his work on learned helplessness) discovered that persons from fundamentalist Christian groups were more optimistic than persons from liberal religious traditions (Sethi & Seligman, 1993; 1994). These investigators traced greater optimism to the content of hymns and liturgies of fundamentalists, whose themes tended to focus on joy, victory over adversity, and salvation. Studying a random sample of nearly 3,000 older adults, Idler & Kasl (1997) similarly documented an association between religious involvement and optimism that was particularly strong among subjects who were experiencing the stress of physical disability.

Religion, Depression, and Anxiety. If religious involvement fosters hope and an optimistic, meaningful worldview, then one might also expect an inverse relationship with symptoms of depression or anxiety. This could reflect either the prevention or quicker resolution of emotional problems. Many studies appear to bear this out. Examining 850 medically ill older men, Koenig, Cohen, Blazer, et al. (1992) found significantly lower rates of depression among those relying on religious beliefs and practices to cope with the stress of their illnesses. In a follow-up study of 201 of these patients, degree of religious coping at baseline predicted significantly fewer depressive symptoms 6 months later. Conducting a similar study among consecutive patients admitted to Duke University Medical Center (including both men and women this time), Koenig, George, and Peterson (1998) identified 87 depressed patients and followed these patients for nearly 1 year after discharge, carefully tracking the course of the depressive disorder. Rather than studying factors that were protective against depression (as in the 1992 study), investigators examined characteristics of depressed persons that might predict who would recover more quickly from depression. Greater intrinsic religiosity at baseline, measured with a standard 10-item scale, predicted a 70% increase in the speed of remission of depression.

Other investigators have reported similar findings in a variety of populations: Rabins et al. (1990) in caregivers of patients with Alzheimer's disease or end-stage cancer, Miller et al. (1997) in women with recurrent depression and their children, and Braam et al. (1997) in community-dwelling older adults in the Netherlands. In our systematic review referred to earlier, we identified 93 studies that had examined the relationship between religious involvement and depression; we found that 60 of these reported at least one significant correlation between greater religious involvement and less depression (Koenig, McCullough, et al., 2001). Of the remaining 33 studies, 13 reported no association, 4 found greater depression among the more religious, and 16 reported both positive and negative associations with different religious variables. Of particular importance was that 15 of 22 prospective cohort studies found greater religiousness at baseline predicted either less depression or quicker recovery from depression when subjects were reevaluated over time. In addition, of 8 clinical trials conducted using religious interventions, 5 showed that depressed patients who received religious treatments recovered faster than patients receiving only a secular intervention or no treatment. Furthermore, of 68 studies examining the relationship between religion and suicide, 57 (84%) found significantly less suicide or more negative attitudes toward suicide among the more religious.

Similar relationships were found for anxiety symptoms, anxiety disorders, and fears concerning death. We identified 7 clinical trials and 69 observational studies that examined relationships with religious variables. More than half of the observational studies (35 of 69) found significantly less anxiety or fear among the more religious, and 6 of the 7 clinical trials found that religious interventions were more effective for reducing anxiety than secular therapy alone or no treatment.

Religion and Social Support

Religiously involved people consistently report greater social support than do the religiously uninvolved. This applies to both persons attending religious services and those involved in private religious practices like prayer. In our review, 19 of 20 studies found a significant positive association between religious involvement and greater social support (Koenig, McCullough, et al., 2001). Many of the studies involved large random samples of the American population, ranging from 2,956 to 4,522 participants (Bradley, 1995; Ellison & George, 1994; Koenig, Hays, George, et al. 1997; Ortega et al., 1983). More important, support provided by religious sources appears to be more satisfying and more resilient than support from secular resources. This is particularly true for those experiencing declines in physical health and functioning with age, when sources of support often begin to diminish. Continued provision of support from religious sources is bolstered by religious belief systems that emphasize the responsibility to care for and support one another during times of need.

Social Support and Aging. Cutler (1976) conducted a national random survey of 833 elderly persons in the United States to assess voluntary associations. Membership in church-affiliated groups *alone* was a significant predictor of life satisfaction and happiness after covariates and membership in other associations were controlled. About three-quarters of older adults in the sample belonged to one or more voluntary associations: 49% belonged to church-affiliated groups (more than all other associations combined), with the next most common being fraternal groups (18%) and veterans groups (9%). In a random sample of 4,000 community-dwelling older adults, Koenig, Hays, George, et al. (1997) found that frequency of private religious activities (prayer and Bible study) was associated with significantly greater social support after controlling for multiple demographic and health factors, including church attendance.

Social Support and African Americans. Ortega et al. (1983) surveyed a random sample of 4,522 persons in urban, rural, and isolated rural communities in northern Alabama; the sampling method was designed to oversample physically disabled people, elderly people, women, and African-Americans. Using regression models that included multiple controls, investigators found that informal interpersonal contact was the strongest predictor of life satisfaction. Interpersonal contact produced this effect, however, only if friendships had the church as their locus. Investigators concluded that the greater life satisfaction of African-American elderly people in this study was due almost entirely to greater contact with church-related friends; in fact, church-related friendships were more strongly related to life satisfaction than race itself was.

Social Support and Women. Hatch (1991) examined the relationship between religious involvement and social support among 1,439 women participating in the National Survey of Families and Households. Among African-Americans, frequent attendance at religious social events was associated with a lower likelihood of selecting children for help and a greater likelihood of selecting nonrelatives for help. Help received from nonrelatives for both African-Americans and whites was significantly associated with participation in religious social events. Hatch concluded that, especially among older African-American women, greater involvement in religious social activities was associated with greater help given to and provided by nonrelatives and less help involving adult children. As the number of elderly persons grows in countries around the world, and as adult children increasingly face the stress of caring for aging parents, the church may become an increasingly vital resource for relieving this burden (on women, especially).

Quality of Social Support. Ellison and George (1994) surveyed a random sample of 2,956 community-dwelling adults as part of Wave II of the NIMH Epidemiologic Catchment Area (ECA) project, North Carolina site. Using regression analysis to control for other covariates, investigators found that greater church attendance significantly predicted number of non-kin ties, in-person contacts, and telephone calls, as well as amount of instrumental support received. There was also a significant relationship between church attendance and *quality of* social support, even after controlling for other measures of social support. It is clear, then, from multiple studies that religious involvement is a key source of meaningful high-quality support for many Americans, especially older adults, women, and African Americans.

In conclusion, if relationships exist between religion, mental health, and social support, then this provides an important pathway by which religion could influence physical health. This could be largely due to mind-body effects that are now being identified and will be described later in this volume.

Religion, Physical Health, and Mortality

Of particular interest is the relationship between religious involvement and physical health. This relationship is perhaps most evident in studies that examine the effects of religious activities on mortality and survival. Since 1993, 13 published studies have examined the relationship between religious activity and longevity. Twelve of these studies report a significant relationship between greater religious involvement and longer survival.

Jews. Goldbourt et al. (1993), following 10,000 Israeli male civil service workers for 23 years, found that religiously involved Jews were 20% less likely than nonbelievers to die of coronary artery disease (after controlling for multiple risk factors). Kark et al. (1996) conducted a 16-year historical cohort study, comparing survival between members of 11 religious kibbutzim and 11 matched secular kibbutzim in Israel. In this study of 3,900 participants, the likelihood of dying was 93% greater among members of secular than of religious kibbutzim. Even after eliminating social support and other risk factors as confounding variables, members of religious kibbutzim still lived significantly longer than members of secular kibbutzim.

Christians. Oxman et al. (1995), following 232 older adults for 6 months after they had open-heart surgery, found that the likelihood of dying during the follow-up period was three times greater in those receiving no comfort or support from religious faith (a finding independent of other risk factors and social support). In the only one of 13 studies that did not find an effect of religion on survival, Koenig, Larson, et al. (1998) conducted a 9-year follow-up study of 1,010 patients ages 20 to 39 and 65 to 102 years who had been admitted to the general medicine and neurology services of the Durham Veterans Administration Medical Center. Religious coping (degree to which the patient relied on religious faith for comfort and strength) was again examined as a predictor of survival; Cox proportional hazards models were used to control for other predictors of survival. Religious coping was unrelated to survival in both bivariate and multivariate analyses (hazard ratio 1.00, 95% CI 0.99–1.01). Investigators explained this lack of association as being due to persons turning to religion to facilitate coping as illness severity worsened and death approached (thus disguising any impact of religious coping on survival). A more recent study by this research group, however, reported an inverse relationship between private religious activity (prayer and Bible study) and mortality, but only among healthy older adults without physical disability (Helm et al., 2000). They concluded that whereas private religious activity also may prolong the survival of persons with physical illness and disability, this effect can be more easily demonstrated in healthy persons in whom the force of mortality exerted by physical illness is not as great.

Krause (1998) also failed to find an overall association between religious coping and survival, although interactions were again substantial. He examined predictors of mortality over 6 years in a national probability sample of 819 older adults. Self-rated health and functional disability were controlled, along with age, sex, and marital status. Results indicated that religious attendance (organizational religiosity) was inversely related to mortality (odds ratio 0.88, 95% CI 0.79–0.98). Religious coping, however, was not. In fact, there was an overall slight positive relationship with mortality (odds ratio 1.15, 95% CI 1.02–1.29, $p < .05$). However, when the interaction between religious coping and salient roles stress was examined, Krause found that that among those subjects who were experiencing severe stress in areas of life that were important to them, religious coping was associated with lower mortality (odds ratio 0.94, 95% CI 0.88–0.996, $p < .05$). In fact, among less-educated older adults (those with fewer than 10 years of education), stressors in highly valued social roles were associated with a greater than 70% increase in the likelihood of dying for those not relying heavily on their religious faith.

A number of other studies suggest that religious attendance, in particular, is a powerful predictor of survival. Goldman et al. (1995) examined mortality over 6 years in a random national sample of nearly 7,500 persons

age 70 or over (National Health Survey). After controlling for demographics, disability, self-rated health, and medical conditions, not attending
church within the past 2 weeks was associated with an increased probability of dying for both men and women. Expanding that sample to include
15,938 subjects age 55 or older, Rogers (1996) found that 53.7% of persons alive in 1991 had attended church or temple in 1984, compared with
41.1% of those who died during follow-up. This highly significant difference persisted after controlling for multiple social factors, physical health,
and other predictors of survival.

   In one of the best designed studies to date, Strawbridge and colleagues
(1997) followed 5,286 participants in the Alameda County Study for
nearly three decades to examine the effects of religious attendance on survival. At the beginning of the study in 1965, frequent church attenders
typically were women, black, more likely to have close social contacts and
more group memberships, and less likely to smoke cigarettes, consume excessive alcohol, or be depressed, although they also were *more likely* to
have impaired mobility. After adjusting for the usual predictors of survival
at baseline and time-varying covariates during follow-up, frequent religious attendance (once a week or more) was associated with a 23% lower
likelihood of dying during the 28-year period. Investigators also found that
frequent attenders were more likely to stop smoking, increase exercising,
increase social connections, and stay married; none of these factors, however, could explain the lower mortality of churchgoers.

   Likewise, Oman and Reed (1998) reported that religious attendance
was associated with prolonged survival in 1,931 older residents of Marin
County (just north of San Francisco). Frequent attenders, particularly
those who also volunteered time to help others, were significantly less
likely to die during the 5-year follow-up, an effect that persisted after
other predictors of survival were controlled. Interestingly, secular types of
social involvement were not associated as strongly with lower mortality.

   Three other studies that examined large random American samples reported similar findings soon after the Strawbridge and Oman studies from
California were published. Koenig, Hays, Larson, et al. (1999), following
4,000 randomly selected older adults for 6 years, examined the effects of
frequent religious attendance (once per week or more) on survival after
controlling for multiple predictors of survival. Attempting to replicate the
Strawbridge et al. (1997) West Coast study on the East Coast, these investigators used similar control variables and analyzed their data following
Strawbridge's analysis plan. The findings were remarkably similar. After

controlling for multiple physical health, social, and behavioral variables, Koenig, Hays, Larson, et al. found frequent attendance predicted a 28% reduction in mortality (compared with Strawbridge et al.'s 23% reduction). This effect on mortality is equivalent to not smoking versus smoking cigarettes.

In the largest study to date, Hummer and colleagues (1999) followed 21,204 Americans age 18 to 65 over 9 years (National Health Interview Survey) to determine the relationship between religious attendance and mortality. Nonattenders lived to an average age of 55.3 years beyond age 20, compared with 61.9 years for those attending services once a week and 62.9 for more than weekly attenders (7 years longer). Among African Americans, life expectancy beyond age 20 for nonattenders was 46.4 years (living to age 66), compared with 60.1 years (living to age 80) for those attending church more than once a week.

Finally, Glass and colleagues (1999) at Harvard's School of Public Health followed 2,761 men and women participating in the Yale Health and Aging Study (New Haven, Connecticut) over 13 years to examine predictors of survival. Social activities (church attendance; visits to cinema, restaurants, sporting events; day or overnight trips; playing cards, games, bingo; participation in social groups), productive activities (gardening, preparing meals, shopping, unpaid community work, paid community work, and other paid employment), and fitness activities (active sports or swimming, walking, physical exercise) each were associated with longer survival after controlling for age, sex, race, marital status, income, body mass index, smoking, functional disability, and history of cancer, diabetes, smoking, and myocardial infarction. Social activities reduced mortality by 19%, fitness activities by 15%, and productive activities by 23%. Great care was taken to ensure that physical health did not confound this relationship, both by controlling for physical fitness and productive activities and by eliminating from the analysis all those who died during the first 5 years of follow-up (to ensure that nonattenders at the start of the study were not simply too ill or near death to get to services). Church attendance in that study was again an independent predictor of longer survival.

Although these findings are largely the result of observational studies, thereby limiting causal inferences, such consistent and robust findings reported by different research groups around the United States and the world have prompted scientists to try to better understand exactly *how* religion might influence health and extend survival.

Mechanisms of the Religion-Physical Health Relationship

A number of plausible mechanisms exist by which religious involvement *could* affect physical health.

Health Behaviors. Religious involvement has been associated with lower rates of alcoholism, drug use, cigarette smoking, risky sexual activity, failure to wear seat belts, drinking while driving, and other hazardous activities. The fact that health behaviors may explain some of the association between religion and health should not minimize or explain away the importance of religion itself. These health behaviors are "belief-based" behaviors dependent on the religious beliefs of the person; in other words, the reason religious persons drink less alcohol, smoke fewer cigarettes, have sex outside marriage less often, and so on is probably because of their beliefs and personal commitment to those beliefs.

In our review of the literature, we found 138 studies that had examined the relationship between alcohol or drug use or abuse and religiousness (Koenig, McCullough, et al., 2001). Of those studies, 124 (90%) reported significantly lower substance use among the more religious. The vast majority of these studies were conducted in adolescents or college students— young persons just starting out their lives. The fact that religious involvement helps prevent risky health behaviors in adolescents and young adulthood is important because it is at this time in life when such behaviors become established, and young adulthood behaviors are likely to adversely influence health throughout the life span.

We found a similar pattern for cigarette smoking. Of 25 studies that had examined the relationship between religiousness and smoking, 24 found less smoking among the more religious. Again, at least half of the studies were in adolescents or college students. Studies of sexual behaviors and attitudes likewise indicate that religious involvement is inversely related to premarital and extramarital sexual activity and attitudes, number of sexual partners, and likelihood of high-risk sexual practices. Of the 38 quantitative studies located, 37 found more negative attitudes toward nonmarital sex or lower rates of this activity in religious than in nonreligious subjects. Again, almost 85% of these studies were conducted in young adults.

Health Care Practices. Religiously involved persons are also probably more likely to have their medical illnesses diagnosed sooner and treated more effectively. Being part of a religious community increases social support and the likelihood that monitoring for health problems will occur. People in the religious community often check up on members who do not attend services or other religious activities. Similarly, persons who are members of a prayer group or prayer chain, in addition to prayer for healing, will likely receive monitoring and direct help if needed. Consequently, health problems are detected sooner and persons will be encouraged to seek medical attention. Religiously involved people also tend to be more compliant with their medical treatments (Harris et al., 1995; Koenig, George, Cohen, et al., 1998).

Biological Mechanisms That Explain Religion's Health Impact

The rapidly accumulating data on the close relationship between psychosocial functioning and neuroendocrine, immune, and cardiovascular processes provide another possible mechanism by which religion could affect physical health. Psychological stress, depression, and social isolation have all been shown to adversely affect immune function and cardiovascular status. Furthermore, negative health behaviors such as excessive alcohol use, cigarette smoking, and sexually transmitted diseases (including AIDS) have negative influences on immune functioning, blood pressure, and the heart. As already reviewed in this chapter, a huge scientific literature documents a relationship between religious involvement and greater social support, lower stress and anxiety, less depression, and less frequent negative health behaviors such as substance abuse and smoking. Thus, it stands to reason that religious beliefs and behaviors also may have an impact on neuroendocrine, immune, and cardiovascular function.

Religion and Immune Functioning

Again bearing in mind that correlational and not causal data are currently available, how might religious involvement affect immune function? By providing a more positive, optimistic worldview, religion may improve coping with acute or chronic stress, thereby ameliorating the effects that stress has on the immune system. This is likely true for both younger and older adults in times of acute or chronic illness or during the dying process. Religious involvement also may be turned to as a way of coping with stress, rather than relying on negative health behaviors such as cigarette smoking, alcohol use, or drug use (which, as noted here, have negative effects on im-

mune function). Reducing the likelihood of depression and speeding recovery from depression may be another way that religious involvement
could maintain optimum immune functioning. Finally, if religious involvement increases social support and reduces social isolation, this may be another way that religion affects immunity. Thus, numerous psychological,
social, and behavioral pathways exist by which religion could affect neuroendocrine and immune functioning. Let us now review studies that have
examined this possibility.

Because of the fledgling nature of this field, we only have scratched the
surface of what might be a very complex relationship between religion
and immune function. Admittedly, the quality of this research has not
been very great thus far. No investigator groups until recently (2001) have
yet received the type of funding necessary to plan and execute a project
designed specifically to look at the religion–immune system relationship.

To our knowledge, five studies have assessed the association between
some measure of religious activity and immune function. In the first published study, McClelland (1988) found that salivary IgA levels in 70 students watching a religious film (Mother Teresa attending the sick in India)
were significantly higher than in 62 students watching a motivational film
describing German atrocities prior to World War II. Its implications for the
relationship between religion and immune function were unclear, except
that either emotions aroused by viewing the religious film had an acute
stimulatory effect on salivary IgA or that those aroused by viewing the war
film acutely depressed this antibody.

In a second study (the first to examine religious *activity* and immune
function), Koenig, Cohen, George, et al. (1997) measured serum levels of
interleukin-6 (IL-6) and other biological indicators of inflammation in
1,718 participants in the Established Populations for Epidemiologic Studies in the Elderly survey. Religious attendance in 1986, 1989, and 1992
was correlated with IL-6 levels measured in 1992. A significant inverse relationship was found between religious attendance in 1992 and high IL-6
levels in 1992. Subjects who attended religious services were 49% less
likely than nonattenders to have high serum IL-6 levels (>5 pg/ml). When
age, sex, race, education, chronic illness, and physical functioning were
controlled, the effect was reduced from 49% to 42%, but it still remained
significant ($p < .005$). In other analyses, religious attendance in 1986 was
related to $\alpha 2$ globulin ($-.06$, $p < .05$) and number of neutrophils ($-.07$,
$p < .01$), relationships that no longer were significant when other variables
were controlled. Total neutrophil count also was inversely related to

religious attendance in 1989 and 1992, with the 1992 correlation persisting after covariates were controlled ($-.05, p <.05$). All associations were in the expected direction—greater religious attendance predicting more stable immune functioning.

Not long afterward, in a third study, S. Lutgendorf (personal communication, May 1997) at the University of Iowa in Iowa City examined serum IL-6 levels in 55 older adults; there was an inverse correlation between a religious variable (spiritual coping measured by religious items taken from Carver et al.'s COPE scale) and IL-6 levels. After controlling for stress level, a weak inverse correlation remained between religious coping and IL-6 levels (partial $r = -.26, p = .075$)—supporting the previous findings by Koenig, Cohen, George, and colleagues.

In the fourth study, Woods and associates (1999) at the University of Miami surveyed 106 HIV-positive gay men about their religious practices and measured their immune functions. Religious activities, such as prayer, religious attendance, spiritual discussions, and reading religious or spiritual literature, were associated with significantly higher CD4+ counts and CD4+ percentages. Religious coping (such as putting trust in God, seeking God's help, or increasing praying) was related to fewer depressive symptoms as measured by the Beck Depression Inventory ($p <.01$) and less anxiety as measured by the Spielberger Trait Anxiety Inventory ($p = .08$) but not to specific immune markers. These investigators also showed that the association between religious practices and immune function was *not* confounded by disease progression (i.e., as disease worsened and immune function decreased, subjects became less able to participate in religious activities).

A fifth study was conducted by Schaal and colleagues (1998) at Stanford University. These investigators examined correlations between religious involvement and immune function in 112 women with metastatic breast cancer. Importance of religious or spiritual expression was positively correlated with natural killer cell numbers ($r = .19, p = .02$), T-helper cell counts ($r = .16, p = .05$), and total lymphocytes ($r = .15, p = .05$). NK cell activity has been associated with metastatic disease in breast cancer. Religious expression was unrelated to delayed-type hypersensitivity in this study.

Studies also have examined the relationship between religious activities and neuroendocrine function. These are relevant because of the increasingly clear association between neuroendocrine function and immune function. Most of the 11 studies we located on this topic assessed the effects of meditation, with 7 of 9 finding that transcendental medita-tion, mindfulness meditation, and similar practices were associated with lower cortisol or other stress hormones (Koenig, McCullough, et al., 2001). Of the two studies that examined religious activities other than meditation, the first reported that of 30 women awaiting breast biopsies for possible cancer, those who employed prayer and faith to cope tended to have lower cortisol levels than those who did not (Katz et al., 1970). In the second study, Schaal et al. (1998) examined the relationship between cortisol level and religious or spiritual expression in their sample of 112 women with metastatic breast cancer. Evening cortisol levels were signifi-cantly lower among women who scored high on religious expression.

Although this area of research is only in its infancy, and the data do not show causation, the preliminary findings are provocative and consistent with the hypothesis that religious involvement may reduce stress and stress-induced neuroendocrine and immune changes.

Implications of a Religion-Immunity Relationship

If a relationship could be established between religious involvement and immune system function, several questions would need to be addressed. First, is the relationship a causal one? Do religious beliefs and activity buffer the negative effects of stress on immune function by diminishing emotional responses? Alternatively, is there some other factor related to religion (e.g., personality style or affiliative behavior) that also is related to immune function, thereby confounding the relationship? In this latter case, religion may simply be a marker for some other factor that is actually influencing immunity. The gold standard for determining causality is a randomized clinical trial. Randomizing subjects to religious belief/activity or to a control condition without such belief/activity, however, raises ethi-cal concerns. Nevertheless, clinical trials could be designed to avoid these ethical dilemmas. Results from prospective studies, which are easier to de-sign and carry out, may provide at least circumstantial evidence about causality.

Second, if religion does affect immune function, how does it do so? Does religion reduce stress by altering the cognitive appraisal of negative experiences? Does it do so by providing a support system that buffers against stress? Does religion provide a method of coping with stress that is healthier than other behaviors (excessive alcohol use, drug use, or cigarette smoking) that adversely affect immune function?

Third, what aspects of religion—type of belief, personal commitment, private religious activity, public religious activity, and the like—influence immune function? Certain religious activities may enhance immune functioning, whereas others may impair it. Likewise, what component of immune functioning is most likely to be affected by religion—cellular immunity, humoral immunity, cytokine levels, or some other factor? Furthermore, does impairment of the aspect of immune function influenced by religion have any health consequences (e.g., risk of infection, speed of cancer metastasis, or course of AIDs)? Determining specifically which component of religion influences which aspect of immune functioning will be critically important in understanding the religion-health relationship.

If it is determined that one or more aspects of religious involvement influence immune function in a clinically significant way, then interventions that taken advantage of these effects may be developed. Such interventions could be administered to already religious persons to help increase their religiousness (or address their religious or spiritual needs) and thereby affect immune function and health outcomes. Administration of religious interventions to nonreligious persons, however, would not be appropriate unless such persons clearly indicated a desire for such interventions.

If religious involvement is shown to affect immune function, then this may provide a tool that can be used by people to facilitate their own mental and physical well-being. Rather than rely on a health care system that is not always immediately available to meet their needs (and at some future point may be prohibitively expensive), individual and group religious or spiritual practices may be utilized to facilitate immune function and thereby help increase resistance to disease.

In 1998, the total national expenditure for health care was $1.1 trillion. By 2007, that figure is projected to rise to $2.1 trillion (Smith et al., 1998). This astronomical rise in health care costs is occurring *prior to* the most rapid increase in older adults American society has ever known—the aging of baby boomers. That demographic shift will result in more than 70 million older adults by 2040 (nearly double the current number). Given the increasing cost of medical care and the possibility of its reduced availability in the future, religious resources that give people some control over their health may be extremely important in terms of public health. This is particularly true for religious resources that are readily available.

Summary and Conclusions

Religion, medicine, and health care have been closely interconnected throughout most of recorded human history. After the turn of the nineteenth century, however, a wall of separation rose between these two disciplines. But over the past several decades, scientific studies have begun to examine the effects of religious beliefs and practices on mental and physical health. The goal of the studies has been to explain such effects through *natural* mechanisms. The majority of these studies suggest that religious involvement is associated with better mental health, greater social support, and avoidance of negative health behaviors. In addition, studies have found an association between religious involvement, better physical health, and greater longevity. Although a number of possible mechanisms exist for this association, one of the strongest physiological pathways may be rooted in the mind-body relationship.

From the field of psychoneuroimmunology we are learning that what people believe, think, and feel may have a direct impact on neuroendocrine and immune function—systems that play a vital role in warding off disease and speeding recovery from illness. If religious beliefs and practices improve coping with stress, reduce the likelihood of depression or other emotional disorders, and increase social support, then it is possible that such involvement also will reduce the physiological consequences of stress and thereby improve our defenses against diseases. So, at least, the theory goes.

In the subsequent chapters, world-renowned experts in the field of psychoneuroimmunology review their areas of expertise and take a closer look at how to study the relationship between religion and neuroendocrine-immune function. These are exciting times, for we stand at the brink of new discoveries that may unveil explanations for the religion-health relationship—ultimately providing clues that may empower us all and improve public health.

REFERENCES

Braam, A. W., Beekman, A. T. F., Deeg, D. J. H., Smith, J. H., & van Tilburg, W. (1997). Religiosity as a protective or prognostic factor of depression in later life: Results from a community survey in the Netherlands. *Acta Psychiatrica Scandinavia* 96, 199–205.

Bradley, D. E. (1995). Religious involvement and social resources: Evidence from the data set, "Americans' Changing Lives." *Journal for the Scientific Study of Religion* 34, 259–267.

Conway, K. (1985). Coping with the stress of medical problems among black and white elderly. *International Journal of Aging and Human Development* 21, 39–48.

Cutler, S. J. (1976). Membership in different types of voluntary associations and psychological well-being. *Gerontologist* 16, 335–339.

Ellison, C. G., & George, L. K. (1994). Religious involvement, social ties, and social support in a southeastern community. *Journal for the Scientific Study of Religion* 33, 46–61.

Glass, T. A., Mendes de Leon, C., Marottoli, M. A., & Berkman, L. F. (1999). Population based study of social and productive activities as predictors of survival among elderly Americans. *British Medical Journal* 319, 478–485.

Goldbourt, U., Yaari, S., & Medalie, J. H. (1993). Factors predictive of long-term coronary heart disease mortality among 10,059 male Israeli civil servants and municipal employees. *Cardiology* 82, 100–121.

Goldman, N., Korenman, S., & Weinstein, R. (1995). Marital status and health among the elderly. *Social Science and Medicine* 40, 1717–1730.

Harris, R. C., Dew, M. A., Lee, A., Amaya, M., Buches, L., Reetz, D., & Coleman, G. (1995). The role of religion in heart transplant recipients' health and well-being. *Journal of Religion and Health* 34, 17–32.

Hatch, L. R. (1991). Informal support patterns of older African-American and white women. *Research on Aging* 13, 144–170.

Helm, H., Hays, J. C., Flint, E., Koenig, H. G., & Blazer, D. G. (2000). Effects of private religious activity on mortality of elderly disabled and nondisabled adults. *Journal of Gerontology (Medical Sciences)* 55A, M400-M405.

Hummer, R., Rogers, R., Nam, C., & Ellison, C.G. (1999). Religious involvement and U.S. adult mortality. *Demography* 36, 273–285.

Idler, E. L., & Kasl, S. V. (1997). Religion among disabled and nondisabled elderly persons: Cross-sectional patterns in health practices, social activities, and well-being. *Journal of Gerontology* 52B, 300–305.

Kaldjian, L. C., Jekel, J. F., & Friedland, G. (1998). End-of-life decisions in HIV-positive patients: The role of spiritual beliefs. *AIDS* 12, 103–107.

Kark, J. D., Shemi, G., Friedlander, Y., Martin, O., Manor, O., & Blondheim, S. H. (1996). Does religious observance promote health? Mortality in secular vs. religious kibbutzim in Israel. *American Journal of Public Health* 86, 341–346.

Katz, J., Weiner, H., & Gallagher, T. (1970). Stress, distress, and ego defenses. *Archives of General Psychiatry* 23, 131–142.

Koenig, H. G. (1998). Religious beliefs and practices of hospitalized medically ill older adults. *International Journal of Geriatric Psychiatry* 13, 213–224

Koenig, H. G., Cohen, H. J., Blazer, D. G., Pieper, C., Meador, K. G., Shelp, F., Goli, V., & DiPasquale, R. (1992). Religious coping and depression in elderly hospitalized medically ill men. *American Journal of Psychiatry* 149, 1693–1700.

Koenig, H. G., Cohen, H. J., George, L. K., Hays, J. C., Larson, D. B., & Blazer, D. G. (1997). Attendance at religious services, interleukin-6, and other biological indicators of immune function in older adults. *International Journal of Psychiatry in Medicine* 27:233–250.

Koenig, H. G., George, L. K., Cohen, H. J., Hays, J. C., Blazer, D. G., & Larson, D. B. (1998). The relationship between religious activities and cigarette smoking in older adults. *Journal of Gerontology* 53A, M426-M434.

Koenig, H. G., George, L. K., & Peterson, B. L. (1998). Religiosity and remission from depression in medically ill older patients. *American Journal of Psychiatry* 155, 536–542.

Koenig, H. G., George, L. K., & Siegler, I. (1988): The use of religion and other emotion-regulating coping strategies among older adults. *Gerontologist* 28:303–310.

Koenig, H. G., Hays, J. C., George, L. K., Blazer, D. G., Larson, D. B., & Landerman, L. R. (1997). Modeling the cross-sectional relationships between religion, physical health, social support, and depressive symptoms. *American Journal of Geriatric Psychiatry* 5, 131–143.

Koenig, H. G., Hays, J. C., Larson, D. B., George, L. K., Cohen, H. J., McCullough, M., Meador, K., & Blazer, D. G. (1999). Does religious attendance prolong survival? A six-year follow-up study of 3,968 older adults. *Journal of Gerontology* 54A, M370-M377.

Koenig, H. G., Larson, D. B., Hays, J. C., McCullough, M. E., George, L. K., Branch, P. S., Meador, K. G., & Kuchibhatla, M. (1998). Religion and survival of 1010 male veterans hospitalized with medical illness. *Journal of Religion and Health* 37, 15–29.

Koenig, H. G., McCullough, M., & Larson, D. B. (2001). *Handbook of religion and health*. New York: Oxford University Press.

Krause, N. (1998). Stressors in highly valued roles, religious coping, and mortality. *Psychology and Aging* 13, 242–255.

Manfredi, C., & Pickett, M. (1987). Perceived stressful situations and coping strategies utilized by the elderly. *Journal of Community Health Nursing* 4, 99–110.

McClelland, D. C. (1988). The effect of motivational arousal through films on salivary immunoglobulin A. *Psychology and Health* 2, 31–52.

Miller, L., Warner, V., Wickramaratne, P., & Weissman, M. (1997). Religiosity and depression: Ten-year follow-up of depressed mothers and offspring.

Journal of the American Academy of Child and Adolescent Psychiatry 36, 1416–1425.

Oman, D., & Reed, D. (1998). Religion and mortality among the community-dwelling elderly. *American Journal of Public Health* 88, 1469–1475.

Ortega, S. T., Crutchfield, R. D., & Rushing, W. A. (1983). Race differences in elderly personal well-being. *Research on Aging* 5, 101–118.

Oxman, T. E., Freeman, D. H., & Manheimer, E. D. (1995). Lack of social participation or religious strength and comfort as risk factors for death after cardiac surgery in the elderly. *Psychosomatic Medicine* 57, 5–15.

Princeton Religion Research Center (1982). *Religion in America*. Princeton, NJ: Gallup Poll.

Rabins, P. V., Fitting, M. D., Eastham, J., & Zabora, J. (1990b). Emotional adaptation over time in care-givers for chronically ill elderly people. *Age and Ageing* 19, 185–190.

Ringdal, G., Gotestam, K., Kaasa, S., Kvinnslaud, S., & Ringdal, K. (1995). Prognostic factors and survival in a heterogeneous sample of cancer patients. *British Journal of Cancer* 73, 1594–1599.

Rogers, R. G. (1996). The effects of family composition, health, and social support linkages on mortality. *Journal of Health and Social Behavior* 37, 326–338.

Rudestam, K. E. (1972). Demographic factors in suicide in Sweden and the United States. *International Journal of Social Psychiatry* 18, 79–90.

Schaal, M. D., Sephton, S. E., Thoreson, C., Koopman, C., & Spiegel, D. (August 1998). Religious expression and immune competence in women with advanced cancer. Paper presented at the Meeting of the American Psychological Association, San Francisco.

Sethi, S., & Seligman, M. E. P. (1993). Optimism and fundamentalism. *Psychological Science* 4, 256–259.

Sethi, S., & Seligman, M. E. P. (1994). The hope of fundamentalists. *Psychological Science* 5, 58.

Smith, S., Freeland, M., Heffler, S., McKusick, D., & The Health Expenditures Projection Team. (1998). The next ten years of health spending: What does the future hold? *Health Affairs* 17, 128–140.

Strawbridge, W. J., Cohen, R. D., Shema, S. J., & Kaplan, G. A. (1997). Frequent attendance at religious services and mortality over 28 years. *American Journal of Public Health* 87:957–961.

Swanson, W. C., & Harter, C. L. (1971). How do elderly blacks cope in New Orleans? *Aging and Human Development* 2, 210–216.

Woods, T. E., Antoni, M. H., Ironson, G. H., & Kling, D. W. (1999). Religiosity is associated with affective and immune status in symptomatic HIV-infected gay men. *Journal of Psychosomatic Research* 46, 165–176.

2

The Development and History of Psychoneuroimmunology

GEORGE F. SOLOMON

The history of the development of the field of psychoneuroimmunology, or PNI, begins several millennia ago and transcends many cultures. Indeed, long before Robert Ader first coined the term *psychoneuroimmunology* in 1975 to describe the study of the interrelationships among the nervous, endocrine, and immune systems, ancient mystics, philosophers, and healers mused about the impact of one's mental state on physical health and vice versa. Although this chapter cannot nearly do justice to all the people who have contributed to the development of this field, it does attempt to highlight some of the more critical milestones along the way.

Holism in Ancient and Medieval Times

It has been observed since ancient times that the state of mind and beliefs of sick people influence their recovery from illness and that it may even play a role in the *de novo* occurrence of an illness. In the Old Testament of the Bible, for example, Moses states, "Worship the Lord your God, and his blessing will be on your food and water. I will take away sickness from among you. . . . I will give you a full life span" (Exodus 23:25–26, NIV). Reflecting on this passage and Deuteronomy 28:21–22, Browne (2001) notes, "We have not yet learned what to think and how to feel to create health and happiness. Therefore, we create our own illness and unhappiness. When we learn that there are universal laws, which must be obeyed to obtain and keep health and happiness, we have begun our own health and happiness" (p. 1).

Proverbs from a variety of ancient medical systems and cultures intoned similar relationships between mental states and susceptibility to illness. In ancient Ayurvedic medicine dating back almost 4,000 years in India, it commonly was held that certain types of people, based in part on personality, had greater resistance to disease (Shukla et al., 1979). In ancient Greek medicine, Galen (129–ca. 199 CE), the father of experimental physiology, suggested that melancholy (depressed) women were more prone to cancer than sanguine (happy) women. Later, in the Middle Ages, the Jewish rabbi and physician Moses Maimonides, in the third chapter of his *Regimen of Health* (1198), states his concept of "a healthy mind in a healthy body." Here he indicates that the physical well-being of a person is dependent on mental well-being, and vice versa (Gordon, 1958), suggestive (as had been Aristotle before him) of the bidirectional communication between brain and immune system posited by psychoneuroimmunology.

From Holism to Dualism

Beginning in the early seventeenth century in Europe, however, there emerged a purely mechanistic view of vital phenomena that influenced views on medicine for generations to come. William Harvey, the renowned English physician, proposed that the heart is a pump that keeps the blood in closed-loop motion, and French mathematician René Descartes held that the mind and the body were entirely separate, autonomous "machines" (Garrison, 1929).

The mechanical allegory of human biology was taken to the extreme in Italy by Giorgio Baglivi, who was appointed by Pope Clement XI as the chair of medical theory in the Collegio della Sprienza. Baglivi divided the "human machine" into innumerable smaller machines; he likened the teeth to scissors, the chest to a bellows, the stomach to a flask, the viscera and glands to sieves, and the heart and blood vessels to waterworks (Garrison, 1929).

Periodically, an independently thinking scientist or clinician would emerge to challenge this mechanistic paradigm, such as the Transylvanian physician Papai Pariz Ferenc, who said in 1680, "When the parts of the body and its humors are not in harmony, then the mind is unbalanced and melancholy ensues, but on the other hand, a quiet and happy mind makes the whole body healthy" (Ferenc, 1680). For the most part, such views were lost in the chorus of voices who opted to apply newly emerging findings in physics or chemistry to all biological phenomena (Garrison, 1929). "Transduction" of the experiential into the biophysical was difficult to conceptualize scientifically.

Reestablishing the Linkages

It wasn't until the seminal works of Russian surgeon Ivan Pavlov were published in the late nineteenth century that the tide began to shift significantly away from this view of the human body as an amalgam of small machines all working independently. Pavlov showed that dogs could be taught to salivate merely by ringing a bell (a conditioned stimulus) if the bell had earlier been coupled with the dogs' feedings (an unconditioned stimulus) (Pavlov, 1928). Thus, Pavlov demonstrated convincingly that the central nervous system and the digestive system were intricately linked.

Progressing directly from Pavlov's conditioning experiments, in the 1920s Metal'nikov and Chorine at the Pasteur Institute attempted to apply Pavlov's methods to the study of inflammation and immunity. It already had been observed that injecting antigenic material into the peritoneum of guinea pigs elicited a typical immune reaction that includes a nonspecific defense response as well as the formation and secretion of antibodies. Metal'nikov and Chorine (1926) examined the possibility of creating a conditioned response by repeating such injections and associating them with an external stimulus such as warming or scratching of the skin. In a series of experiments, they demonstrated that repeated exposure of guinea pigs to unconditioned stimuli (antigenic material) paired with the conditioned stimuli (warmth or scratching) eventually resulted in the guinea pigs' immune systems' responding to the conditioned stimuli alone. Indeed, although the immune reactions to the conditioned stimuli (CS) were more muted than with the unconditioned stimuli (US), there were still demonstrable increases in polynucleated cells, survival against lethal doses of pathogens, and antibodies as a result of exposure to only CS following US-CS conditioning (Metal'nikov & Chorine, 1926, 1928).

By the early 1940s, Franz Alexander had realized that psychosomatic pathology was the result of the physiological concomitants of conscious or repressed emotions (Alexander & French, 1948), and Hans Selye had discovered that steroid hormones regulate lymphoid organs such as the thymus, lymph nodes, and spleen. Selye and his coworkers also demonstrated that thymic atrophy is mediated by the ACTH-adrenal axis during stress,[1] with glucocorticoids being the final effector molecules; described the anti-inflammatory action of adrenal steroid hormones; and made significant contributions to our understanding of the role of mast cells in various pathological phenomena (Berczi, 1994).

In the 1950s, Andor Szentivanyi decided to use anaphylactic shock in the guinea pig as an animal model for severe asthma attacks in humans, which were sometimes not responsive to adrenaline. It was known at the time that anaphylactic shock in guinea pigs was due to systemic antigen-antibody reactions, and Szentivanyi and his colleagues first reported in 1952 that brain lesions inhibit the anaphylactic reaction in guinea pigs (Filipp et al., 1952).

This sensational finding was followed a few years later by a flurry of studies by Szentivanyi and his colleagues in which they reported, among other things, that (1) lesions of the hypothalamus in preimmunized guinea pigs and rabbits inhibited the anaphylactic reaction elicited by specific antigens, (2) antibody production also was inhibited if the lesions were induced prior to immunization, (3) the reaction of antibodies with specific antigens was not affected by the lesions, (4) lesions inhibited the anaphylactic reaction even when the animals were provided with passively transferred antibodies that elicited lethal shock in normal animals after systemic challenge with the antigen, and (5) lesions inflicted in other areas of the hypothalamus or the central nervous system had no influence on anaphylactic shock or any other immune parameters (Filipp & Szentivanyi, 1958; Szentivanyi & Filipp, 1958; Szentivanyi & Szekely, 1958). In then little noticed Soviet research, Korneva and Khai in 1963 reported that induced lesions in the anterior hypothalamus of rabbits prevented the formation of complement-fixing antibodies and that they led to prolonged retention of antigen in the blood.

Putting the Pieces Together

These lines of evidence, as well as experimental evidence in laboratory animals suggesting that stress could exert effects on viral infections (Rasmussen et al., 1957; Jensen and Rasmussen, 1963), led George Solomon and Rudolph Moos in 1964 to write an integrative article entitled "Emotions, Immunity and Disease." In this article, they posited both experiential and neuroendocrine effects on immunity (Solomon & Moos, 1964). Solomon and Moos had begun to look for potential psychological correlates of the autoimmune disease by comparing 16 female patients who had confirmed rheumatoid arthritis with their closest-aged healthy sisters on 15 personality scales that had been refined from descriptions of people with rheumatoid arthritis. Based on their analysis, Moos and Solomon concluded that arthritics, in comparison with nonarthritic siblings, were (1) more compliant, (2) more likely to have difficulty in expressing anger, (3) more sensitive to the anger of others, (4) more conservative, (5) more self-sacrificing, and (6) more anxious and depressed (Moos & Solomon, 1965a, 1965b). These conclusions were consistent with findings in patients with other autoimmune diseases, such as systemic lupus erythematous (SLE) and thyroiditis (Solomon, 1981).

To determine which was cause and which was effect (personality and distress vs. disease), Solomon and Moos (1965) then examined asymptomatic (as assessed by history, physical examination, and joint x-rays) relatives of patients with rheumatoid arthritis to determine if personality factors played a role in the presence or absence of the characteristic "rheumatoid factor," or anti-immunoglobulin autoantibodies (anti-Ig auto-Abs), found in many patients with rheumatoid arthritis. This study found that those relatives *lacking* the rheumatoid factor were "ordinary folks"—that is, a random population ranging from psychologically healthy to psychiatrically disturbed in a normal distribution curve with most somewhere near the middle. By contrast, those *with* the autoantibody (but who did not have rheumatoid arthritis) were all in excellent emotional shape with no anxiety, depression, or alienation, as well as greater satisfaction in work and personal relationships. Solomon and Moos concluded that psychological well-being was serving a *protective* function in the face of a genetically determined predisposition to an autoimmune disease. This conclusion was based on the fact that asymptomatic persons *with* rheumatoid factor have a greater risk of subsequent development of arthritis than the general population and because the onset of autoimmune disease frequently follows a stressful life event, such as loss of a loved one.

Nevertheless, early findings of a connection between neuroendocrine and immune functions were met with a great deal of skepticism because they were very preliminary and indirect, were poorly designed, or failed to provide important procedural details. Moreover, immunological "doctrine" of the 1960s, strongly influenced by the antibody formation theories of Nobel Prize winner Niels Jerne, held that the immune system was "autonomous" and self-regulatory. No psychologists and few psychiatrists (the latter in relation to schizophrenia) were interested in immunology, and immunologists rarely were interested in psychology. Solomon's (1969) demonstration that stress could reduce both primary and secondary ("booster") antibody response to a novel antigen in rats had little impact on the field. It was with great difficulty that Alfred Amkraut was recruited to Stanford in the late 1960s as the first immunologist in the United States to work exclusively in what was to become PNI. Branislav Jancovic, for whom the Immunology Institute in Belgrade has been named, had preceded Amkraut a bit earlier.

The PNI field gained significant credibility and impetus, however, in the mid-1970s as a result of Ader and Cohen's elegant conditioned immunosuppression experiments. Unaware of Metal'nikov and Chorine's (1926) and other Russian scientists' work almost a half century earlier, Ader and Cohen (1975) paired an immunosuppressive drug (cyclophosphamide) with saccharin (a synthetic sugar) and fed it to rats. By "conditioning" the rats to associate the taste of saccharin with the biological effects of cyclophosphamide, Ader and Cohen demonstrated that the administration of saccharin alone to the rats could produce immunosuppression. Such classical conditioning likely can be mediated only by the central nervous system.

Further evidence that the immune system was "hard-wired" to the central nervous system arose from studies by David and Suzanne Felten and their colleagues. These studies demonstrated that in all lymphoid organs, noradrenergic nerve fibers distribute into specific zones of T cells and macrophages, including entry sites of T and B cells, sites of antigen capture, sites of antigen presentation and lymphocyte activation, and sites of lymphocyte exit. They and others also demonstrated noradrenergic innervation of bone marrow and thymus. (See Felton & Felton, 1988, for a review of this literature.)

Gerard Renoux and colleagues (1983) carried neuroimmunoregulation to the cortex with the discovery of cerebrolaterally differential effects on T-cell maturation and function. The logically essential afferent (immune system to brain) limb of the brain-endocrine-immune axis was shown by changes in corticosterone levels, as well as in firing rates of hypothalamic neurons, after antigenic challenge by Besedovsky et al. (1977).

Although they were doubted at the time, Smith and Blalock (1981) set the stage for the current flood of information about the effects of immune cytokines on the brain and, conversely, the effects of neurohormones, neurotransmitters, and neuropeptides on immunologically competent cells by their discovery that lymphocytes synthesize adrenocorticotropic hormone (ACTH) and the endogenous opioid, β-endorphin. The detection of ACTH and endorphin-like substances in lymphocytes demonstrated that the immune system could produce substances that are (1) related to known polypeptide hormones and (2) capable of signaling the neuroendocrine system. Thus, in reaction to infections, tumors, or chemicals, lymphocytes may be able to signal the brain or other organs and glands to modify the host response(s).

Coming Full Circle

With increasing evidence that "stress" hormones play an important role in immune function, researchers have conducted a number of studies on the effects of a variety of human stressors on immunity, including space flight (Cogli & Tschopp, 1985), bereavement (Bartrop et al., 1977), marital discord (Kiecolt-Glaser, Fisher, et al., 1987), and school examinations (Kiecolt-Glaser, Glaser, et al., 1986), as well as caring for patients with chronic debilitating illnesses such as Alzheimer's disease (Kiecolt-Glaser, Glaser, et al., 1987). In virtually every one of these circumstances, researchers have demonstrated that chronic exposure to such stressors can negatively affect immune functioning.

In recent years, more attention has been given to the immune system "limb" of psychoneuroimmunology. Pro-inflammatory cytokines, such as interleukin-1, have been shown to play multiple roles within the brain, including the generally adaptive induction of "sickness behavior" (sleepiness, anorexia, fatigue), as well as influencing neuroendocrine feedback circuits in immune regulation (see Watkins, 1996, for a review). Indeed, recovery from infection may be aided by "listening" to one's immune system's effects on the brain.

Investigators also recently have turned their attention to the stress-buffering effects of certain beliefs and behaviors and their ultimate impact on immune functioning. In particular, there is growing interest in the experiential aspects of religion (i.e., particularly the spiritual part) and what effects they may have on both mind and body. For example, there is evidence that spiritual practices such as meditation (Infante et al., 1998) and yoga (Schell et al., 1994) can alter the stress response in individuals.

Furthermore, there is evidence that spiritual beliefs and practices can either increase or decrease psychological stress (Genia, 1996), which in turn may affect the production of stress hormones that can affect the activities of the immune system. Certain spiritual beliefs and practices have even been shown significantly to increase the survival time of patients with acquired immune deficiency syndrome (AIDS) (Barroso, 1997; Carson, 1993), as well as bolster the immune systems of the elderly (Koenig et al., 1997). Although the involvement of PNI researchers in this field is only beginning, it offers a rich area for future investigation.

Conclusions

It appears that we have come full circle in recently recognizing that the mind is integrally related to the body and that it is impossible to separate one from the other. Interestingly, this is the very premise of many Eastern religions and systems of medicine. For example, in Ayurvedic medicine, an ancient proverb holds that "the bounds of forces in the body are in harmonious relationship with the environment" (*Charaka Samhita*, English translation, 1949).

In hindsight, if one assumes an adaptive "rationality" to evolutionary processes, it makes sense that the nervous system and the immune system communicate bidirectionally and even might be conceptualized as a single, integrated adaptive-defensive system. Both have a sense of identity, of self and non-self. Both relate the organism to the outside world and assess its components and inhabitants as friendly or harmless or dangerous. Finally, both allow the organism to survive in an often-hostile environment by adaptation and defense.

To do all these things, the two systems possess memory and learn by experience. Both also monitor the inner world and evaluate its makeup as ego-syntonic (acceptable to self) versus dystonic, or as benign self versus malignant non-self, and institute defenses against noxious inner components. Both brain-psyche and immune system make "mistakes" that can lead to illness, even death. When such mistakes occur, relatively innocuous substances or organisms can be perceived by the brain as dangerous (phobias), on the one hand, or by the immune system (allergies) on the other. True self may be not accepted, and depression, even suicide, or autoimmunity, sometimes fatal, analogously, ensue. Both depression and autoimmunity are more common with aging. Recent but not remote memory tends to fail with age, and immunosenescence is characterized by poor primary response to novel antigens and relatively good secondary response to re-called antigens.

Spirituality, as the ancients often noted, may keep the brain-psyche-body in balance, particularly in times of stress, by promoting more adaptive coping styles and positive emotions such as hope and forgiveness. In this re-gard, the Dalai Lama recently (1999) wrote, "I have been able to meet ad-versity with all my resources—mental, physical, and spiritual. . . . Had I been overwhelmed by anxiety and despaired, my health would have been harmed" (p. 1). His Holiness believes that spirituality is concerned with such human qualities as "love and compassion, patience, tolerance, forgive-ness, contentment, a sense of responsibility, a sense of harmony" (p. 22).

NOTE

1. A stressor, which is a demand that places an adaptational requirement on the organism, leads to a "state of stress" ("strain" or "distress") that, in turn, de-pending on external moderators such as social support and on internal mod-erators such as coping ability, leads to no change, to psychosocial growth (thus, the stressor being "eustress" or good stress), or to adverse mental and physical health consequences.

REFERENCES

Ader, R., & Cohen, N. (1975). Behaviorally conditioned immunosuppression. *Psychosomatic Medicine* 37, 333–340.

Alexander, F., & French, T. M. (1948). *Studies in psychosomatic medicine: An approach to the treatment of vegetative disturbances.* New York: Ronald.

Barroso, J. (1997). Social support and long-term survivors of AIDS. *Western Journal of Nursing Research* 19, 554–573.

Bartrop, R. W., Luckhurst, E., Lazarus, L., Kiloh, L. C., & Penny, R. (1977). De-pressed lymphocyte function after bereavement. *Lancet* 1, 834–836.

Berczi, I. (1994). Stress and disease: The contributions of Hans Selye to psy-choneuroimmunology. A personal remembrance. In I. Berczi & J. Szélenyi (Eds.), *Advances in psychoneuroimmunology.* New York: Plenum.

Besedovsky, H., Sorkin, E., Felix, O., & Haas, H. (1977). Hypothalamic changes during immune response. *European Journal of Immunology* 7, 323–325.

Browne, M. (2001). Poster submitted to the American Holistic Medical Associ-ation's twenty-fourth annual meeting, Miami, Florida, May 2001.

Carson, V. B. (1993). Prayer, meditation, exercise, and special diets: Behaviors of the hardy person with HIV/AIDS. *Journal of the Association of Nurses in AIDS Care* 4, 18–28.

Charaka Samhita (English translation, 1949). Jamnagar, India: Gulab Kunwarba Ayurvedic Society.

Cogli, A., & Tschopp, A. (1985). Lymphocyte reactivity during space flight. *Immunology Today* 6, 1–4.

Dalai Lama. (1999). *Ethics for the new millennium.* New York: Riverhead.

Felten, D. L., & Felten, S. Y. (1988). Sympathetic noradrenergic innervation of immune organs. *Brain, Behavior, and Immunity* 2, 293–300.

Ferenc, P. P. (1680). *About the peace and spirit.* Kolozsvar, Transylvania.

Filipp, G., & Szentivanyi, A. (1958). Anaphylaxis and nervous system: Part III. *Annals of Allergy* 16, 306.

Filipp, G., Szentivanyi, A., & Mess, B. (1952). Anaphylaxis and nervous system: Part I. *Acta Medica Hungarica* 2, 163.

Garrison, F. H. (1929). *History of medicine.* 4th ed. Philadelphia: W.B. Saunders.

Genia, V. (1996). I, E, quest, and fundamentalism as predictors of psychological and spiritual well-being. *Journal for the Scientific Study of Religion* 35, 56–64.

Gordon, H. L. (1958). *Moses ben Maimon: The preservation of youth.* Essays on health. New York: Philosophical Library.

Infante, J. R, Peran, F., Martinez, M., Roldan, A., Poyatos, R., Ruiz, C., Samaniego, F., & Garrido, F. (1998). ACTH and beta-endorphin in transcendental meditation. *Physiology and Behavior* 64, 311.

Jensen, M. M., & Rasmussen, A. F. (1963). Stress and susceptibility to viral infection. *Journal of Immunology* 90, 17–20.

Kiecolt-Glaser, J. K., Fisher, L. D., Opgrocki, P., Stout, J. S., Speicher, C. E., & Glaser, R. (1987). Marital quality, marital disruption and immune function. *Psychosomatic Medicine* 49, 13–34.

Kiecolt-Glaser, J. K., Glaser, P., Shuttleworth, E. C., Dyer, C. S., Ogrocki, P., & Speicer, C. E. (1987). Chronic stress and immunity in family caregivers of Alzheimer's disease victims. *Psychosomatic Medicine* 49, 523–530.

Kiecolt-Glaser, J. K., Glaser, R., Strain, E. C., Stout, J. C., Tarr, K. L., Holliday, J. E., & Speicher, C. E. (1986). Modulation of cellular immunity in medical students. *Journal of Behavioral Medicine* 9, 5–21.

Koenig, H. G., Cohen, H. J., George, L. K., Hays, J. C., Larson, D. B., & Blazer, D. G. (1997). Attendance at religious services, interleukin-6, and other biological indicators of immune function in older adults. *International Journal of Psychiatry in Medicine* 27, 233–250.

Korneva, E. A., & Khai, L. M. (1963). The effects of the destruction of areas within the hypothalamus on the process of immunogenesis. *Fiziologiceskii Zhurnal SSSR imeni I. M. Sechenova* 49, 52–62.

Metal'nikov, S., & Chorine, V. (1926). The role of conditioned reflexes in immunity. *Annals of the Pasteur Institute* 40, 893–900.

Metal'nikov, S., & Chorine, V. (1928). The role of conditioned reflexes in the formation of antibodies. *Comptes rendus des seances de la Societé de biologie et de ses filiales* 99, 142–145.

Moos, R. H., & Solomon, G. F. (1965a). Psychologic comparisons between women with rheumatoid arthritis and their non-arthritic sisters. I: Personality test and interview rating data. *Psychosomatic Medicine* 27, 135–149.

Moos, R. H., & Solomon, G. F. (1965b). Psychologic comparisons between women with rheumatoid arthritis and their non-arthritic sisters. II: Content analysis of interviews. *Psychosomatic Medicine* 27, 150–164.

Pavlov, I. P. (1928). *Lectures on conditioned reflexes.* New York: Liveright.

Rasmussen, A. F., Jr., Spence, E. S., & Marsh, J. T. (1957). Increased susceptibility to herpes simplex in mice subjected to avoidance-learning stress or restraint. *Proceedings of the Society for Experimental Biology* 96, 183–189.

Renoux, G., Biziere, K., Renoux, M., & Guillaumen, J. M. (1983). The production of T-cell inducing factors in mice is controlled by brain neocortex. *Scandinavian Journal of Immunology* 17, 45–50.

Schell, F. J., Allolio, B., & Schonecke, O. W. (1994). Physiological and psychological effects of Hatha-Yoga exercise in healthy women. *International Journal of Psychosomatics* 41, 46–52.

Shukla, H. C., Solomon, G. F., & Doshi, R. P. (1979). The relevance of some Ayurvedic (traditional Indian medical) concepts to modern holistic health. *Journal of Holistic Health* 4, 125–131.

Smith, E. M., & Blalock, J. E. (1981). Human lymphocyte production of ACTH and endorphin-like substances associated with leukocyte interferon. *Proceedings of the National Academy of Sciences of the* United States of America 78, 7530–7535.

Solomon, G. F. (1969). Stress and antibody response in rats. *Archives of Allergy and Applied Immunology* 36, 97–104.

Solomon, G. F. (1981). Emotional and personality factors in the onset and course of autoimmune disease, particularly rheumatoid arthritis. In R. A. Ader, D. L. Felten, & N. Cohen (Eds.), *Psychoneuroimmunology.* New York: Academic.

Solomon, G. F., & Moos, R. H. (1964). Emotions, immunity and disease. A speculative theoretical integration. *Archives of General Psychiatry* 11, 657–674.

Solomon, G. F., & Moos, R. H. (1965). The relationship of personality to the presence of rheumatoid factor in asymptomatic relatives of patients with rheumatoid arthritis. *Psychosomatic Medicine* 27, 350–360.

Szentivanyi, A., & Filipp, G. (1958). Anaphylaxis and the nervous system: Part II. *Annals of Allergy* 16, 143.

Szentivanyi, A., & Szekely, J. (1958). Effect of injury to, and electrical stimula-
    tion of, hypothalamic areas on anaphylactic and histamine shock of the
    guinea pig: A preliminary report. *Annals of Allergy* 14, 259.
Watkins, L. R., Maier, S. F., & Groehler, L. E. (1996). Immune activation and the
    role of pro-inflammatory cytokines in inflammation, illness response, and
    pathological pain. *Pain* 63, 284–302.

3

Understanding How Stress Affects the Physical Body

BRUCE S. RABIN

When an individual perceives something in the environment that is considered "stressful," specific regions of his or her brain are activated. As a result, neuronal pathways and hormonal centers release substances that may modify the function of the immune system.

The primary purpose of the immune system is defense against pathogenic microorganisms, with the goal of any immune response being neutralization and elimination of the infectious agents. The immune process involves a host of physiological changes that can be viewed as shifts in the equilibrium of the body, or alterations of *homeostasis*. The immune system works to restore homeostasis by identifying and eliminating internal aberrations (a malignant cell) or external invaders (viruses, bacteria, fungi).

The physiological response to stress also alters homeostasis and often impairs the ability of the immune system to function properly in its attempts to restore homeostasis. Stress may disturb homeostasis through responses to a variety of stimuli such as fear, anxiety, intense exercise, or pain. The stimulus that induces the disturbance of homeostasis is known as a "stressor."

This chapter provides a brief overview of the very complex nature of the brain's response to stress and the potential pathways that may be activated by stress that ultimately may influence immune function. It also briefly discusses potential paradigms by which belief systems may modify or buffer the stress response. However, detailed discussions of these paradigms are to be found in other chapters of this book.

The Pathway of Stress

Figure 3.1 presents a visual overview of the potential pathway(s) by which stress is believed to exert its effects on the immune system. In short:

1. The brain must perceive an event as a stressor. An event termed a *stressor* occurs in the microenvironment of the subject that will develop a physiologic response to the stressor. However, many parameters will qualify what happens in the brain of the subject experiencing the stressor. For example, the following factors can influence whether the brain perceives the event as a stressor: (1) the subject's coping ability (e.g., amount of social support; level of optimism; whether physically fit or sedentary; presence or absence of a sense of humor; belief systems); (2) repetition and other stressors (Is the stressor experienced for the first time or multiple times? Is a stressor being experienced at a time when there are no other stressors, or are there other stressors present?); and (3) the strength of the stressor (How meaningful is the stressor to the subject? Is a single parent told that her child has schizophrenia? Is an individual told that he will have to work late and not be able to go to a movie with friends?).

2. Activated neurons must alter the hormonal milieu of blood and tissue. The response of the brain to the stressor involves activation of neurons in discrete locations. Activation of some neurons will produce alteration of the concentration of hormones in lymphoid tissue, in plasma, and within the parenchyma (the functional part) of various organs. Some of the hormones are released from nerve terminals and others from endocrine tissue and the hypothalamic-pituitary-adrenal axis.

3. The hormones must alter the function of the ability of the body to resist infectious disease, produce autoimmune responses, and possibly prevent malignancy. This area of investigation is still in its infancy. Many parameters will determine the effects on immune system function. For example, the following factors can influence whether the hormones whose concentration is altered by stress can modify immune function: whether the cells of the immune system have receptors for the hormones whose concentration is altered by stress, and whether other cells and tissues, such as neutrophils, become altered by the change in the hormonal environment.

- If the cells of the immune system (CD4 lymphocytes, CD8 lympho-cytes, B lymphocytes, NK lymphocytes) have receptors for the hor-mones whose concentration is altered by stress, the function of the lymphoid cells may change. However, there are balances in the im-mune system. For example, T helper I and II CD4 cells regulate each other's function. Thus, a stressor-induced change in one population of cells may alter the function of other cells. Other concerns include (1) whether the lymphoid cell is naive, a memory cell, or an effector cell; (2) whether the concentration of hormone receptors on a given cell was modified by the concentration of the hormone during the maturation of the cell in the bone marrow; and (3) the response of second messengers to hormone binding.
- Other cells and tissues may also become altered by the change in the hormonal environment. Included are changes in the function of neutrophils, which are essential for removing bacteria from the body, and the concentration of adhesion molecules on endothelial cells and connective tissue, which are essential for directing lym-phoid cells and neutrophils to go where they are needed.

The following sections present a more detailed description of the path-way by which stress may not only impair immune function but also lead to other adverse physical health consequences.

Perception of Stressor by the Central Nervous System

The central nervous system's perception and processing of stressor stimu-lation are immediate. This is evidenced by the rapid appearance in blood of two major neurochemicals, the catecholamines epinephrine and norep-inephrine (Kvetnansky et al., 1993; Pacak et al., 1993). Perhaps the best in-dicator of the immediacy of the central nervous system's response to stress is the rapid increase in heart rate due to stimulation of adrenergic recep-tors by norepinephrine (Manuck et al., 1991).

Activation of Specific Responsive Neurons in the Brain and Release of Neuropeptides

Studies have shown that neurons in areas of both the forebrain and brain stem (the portion of the brain connecting to the spinal cord) are activated in the rat brain after footshock or exposure to a conditioned stimulus.

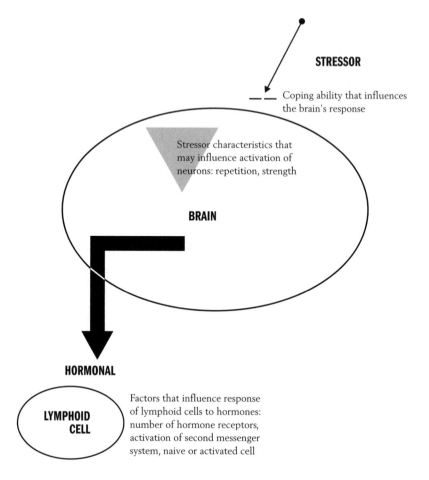

Figure 3.1 Overview of the pathways through which stress may exert an effect on the immune system.

Some brain areas that are activated during stress induce a change in hormone production, sympathetic nervous system activity, or both. Some of the brain-activated changes appear to influence the function of the immune system, whereas other areas activated by stress do not. The following are some of the areas of the rat brain that may be activated by stress.

> *Corticotropin-releasing-hormone–containing neurons in the medial parvicellular division of the hypothalamus*   This area of the hypothalamus contains small "parvicellular" neurons, which secrete several hormones, including corticotropin-releasing hormone (CRH), that

increase or decrease the release of other hormones from the anterior lobe of the pituitary gland (e.g., adrenocorticotropic hormone
[ACTH]). Activation of these neurons is likely to be associated
with stressor-induced immune alteration by increasing the concentration of plasma corticosterone.

Periphery of the posterior magnicellular division of the hypothalamus
These neurons project to the posterior lobe of the pituitary, stimulating of the secretion of oxytocin, an important hormone for lactation and uterine contraction during labor. Stressor-induced activation of oxytocin-containing neurons may stimulate the autonomic
brain nuclei in the brain stem, or they may participate in behavioral
modifications during stress (Watanobe et al., 1995).

Dorsomedial nucleus of the hypothalamus   Axons from these neurons
mainly terminate within various other nuclei in the hypothalamus.
Activation of this area stimulates motility in the intestine and may
regulate fear responses and cardiovascular responses to emotional
stimuli.

Lateral hypothalamus   Communication between the neurons of the
lateral hypothalamus and the immune system has been postulated.
The lateral hypothalamus may participate in the regulation of delayed hypersensitivity, natural killer (NK) cell numbers in the
blood, and NK cell function (Juzwa et al., 1995; Wenner et al.,
1996, 2000; Wrona et al., 1994). Both hunger and thirst are regu-
lated by neurons of the lateral hypothalamus. Whether the hormones responsible for hunger and thirst influence immune function
remains to be determined.

Medial nucleus of the amygdala   Activation of this brain area may be
induced by pain and stimulates the release of ACTH by the pituitary. In this way, it may participate in stressor-induced increases of
glucocorticoids.

Lateral edges of the central nucleus of the amygdala   The function of
this area is unclear, but it may be related to the experience of fear.
Whether there are nerve pathways from this area that participate in
inducing the release of glucocorticoids or neuropeptides has not
been established.

Ventral subdivision of the lateral septal area   Activation is associated
with the development of anxiety.

Dorsomedial nucleus and basal ganglia of the thalamus   This area consists of several groups of cells that connect to sections of the cortex

involved with muscle movement (motor cortex), the perception of sensations (sensory cortex), and cognition (i.e., perceiving, thinking, and memory). The dorsomedial nucleus connects to the frontal lobe of the brain, the hypothalamus, and other areas of the thalamus.

Nucleus of the solitary tract   This brain area is associated with regulation of heart rate.

Noradrenergic neurons of the A5 and A7 areas   Projections from here to the spinal cord may contribute to the activation of postganglionic neurons, which innervate secondary lymphoid tissues.

Locus ceruleus   This accumulation of norepinephrine-containing neurons sends projections to many areas of the brain, including the amygdala, thalamus, hypothalamus, and spinal cord (projecting to sympathetic ganglia and to the adrenal glands). The locus ceruleus is involved in modulating the sensation of pain (Baulmann et al., 2000; Kimura & Nakamura, 1985). Its activation has been shown to suppress lymphocyte function in the spleen and peripheral blood of rats (Caroleo et al., 1993; Rassnick et al., 1994).

Periaqueductal gray   The periaqueductal gray is the part of the brain surrounding the cerebral aqueduct in the midbrain. Injection of morphine into discrete parts of the periaqueductal gray will alter the function of lymphocytes and NK cells (Weber & Pert, 1989). The pathways that induce these changes are not yet known.

Release of Catecholamines by the Sympathetic Nervous System

The postganglionic neurons of the sympathetic nervous system (SNS) innervate a wide variety of vital organs and tissues, fulfilling in part the homeostatic purpose of the autonomic nervous system. It is now well recognized that primary and secondary lymphoid organs and, in particular, the spleen are richly innervated with noradrenergic postganglionic sympathetic fibers (Ackerman et al., 1991; Felten & Felten, 1991).

In addition, it is well established that lymphocytes and monocytes possess β-adrenergic receptors for catecholamines (Felton & Felton, 1991; Fuchs et al., 1988) and that incubation of lymphocytes, monocytes, and NK cells with the SNS–derived catecholamines epinephrine and norepinephrine exerts functional alterations (Roszman & Carlson, 1991), as does in vivo sympathectomy, which ablates peripheral catecholaminergic innervation (Madden & Livnat, 1991).

Infusing catecholamines into humans or experimental animals and measuring the quantitative and functional changes in lymphocytes can provide information regarding the effect of catecholamine elevations on immune function (Crary et al., 1983; De Blasi et al., 1986; van Tits et al., 1990). Epinephrine infusion into humans increases the concentration of CD8 lymphocytes and NK lymphocytes in the blood (Blazar et al., 1986; Kappel et al., 1991). A decreased responsiveness of lymphocytes to mitotic stimulation with nonspecific mitogens also occurs. This may be related to an alteration in the relative distribution of different lymphocyte subsets or to direct effects of epinephrine on second messenger pathways that decrease the ability of lymphocytes to be induced into mitosis. These early studies were unable to consider alterations of the T helper I and II populations as mediators of the altered response to mitogens because this cell population had not yet been identified. In humans who experience an acute laboratory stressor, the same changes are found in the peripheral blood as those changes caused by the injection of epinephrine (Bachen et al., 1992; Manuck et al., 1991; Naliboff et al., 1991; Wang et al., 1998).

To confirm that catecholamines are responsible for the alterations of the peripheral blood lymphocyte populations following a stressor, subjects have been pretreated with an adrenergic receptor antagonist before being exposed to psychological stressors (Bachen et al., 1995). Lymphocyte subsets, natural killer cell function, and the responsiveness of T lymphocytes to stimulation with nonspecific mitogens were compared in specimens obtained before and after the mental stressor in subjects who received an injection of saline or the adrenergic antagonist. Both quantitative and qualitative alterations of the immune system occurred in those subjects who were exposed to the stressor and injected with saline. However, in those subjects who received the adrenergic antagonist, the psychological stressor failed to produce alterations of immune function.

Release of Glucocorticoids by the Hypothalamic-Pituitary-Adrenal Axis

The major end products following activation of the hypothalamic-pituitary-adrenal axis are the adrenal glucocorticosteroids cortisol (in humans) and corticosterone (in rats and mice). Although glucocorticoid release is the result of a complex series of events, the primary factor is corticotropin-releasing factor, a neuropeptide that is stored in the paraventricular nucleus of the brain and released via terminal neuron projections in the median eminence. From there, it travels via a dense capillary network to anterior regions of the pituitary gland, where it stimulates the release of ACTH (Whitnall, 1993).

ACTH then travels through the blood to stimulate cells in the cortex of the adrenal gland, which is located at the top of the kidney, to synthesize and secrete glucocorticoids. In the rat, the rise in plasma corticosterone, a glucocorticoid, becomes evident within a few minutes following exposure to a single footshock but does not peak until around 10 minutes (Shurin et al., 1995). Although quite rapid, the response of the hypothalamic-pituitary-adrenal axis to initial stressor stimulation is relatively slow in comparison to the sympathetic nervous system, which is activated within seconds (Lefkowitz et al., 1990).

Immunological cells have been shown to possess intracytoplasmic receptors for corticosterone (commonly referred to as glucocorticoid receptors [GR]). The two types of glucocorticoid receptors, type I and type II, that vary in their affinity to corticosterone, with type II having a sixfold to tenfold lower affinity (Spencer, Miller, Stein, et al., 1991). Although type I receptors are not detectable in the thymus, type II receptors are much more widespread, being found in the thymus, the spleen, and lymph nodes (Spencer, Miller, Stein, et al., 1991). The presence of these receptors indicates that the immune system is prepared for hypothalamic-pituitary-adrenal activation and the subsequent elevation in circulating corticosterone. Indeed, glucocorticoid receptor occupation is greatest during the peak of the circadian rhythm in plasma corticosterone (Spencer, Miller, Moday, et al., 1993).

Release of Other Hormones That May Modify Immune Function

In addition to the catecholamines, a number of other hormones have been implicated in altering immune homeostasis, including the following.

Endogenous Opioids. A wealth of data, based mostly on in vitro studies, demonstrates that the endogenous opioid peptides (i.e., endorphins, enkephalins, and dynorphins) can modulate immune function (Shavit, 1991; Sibinga & Goldstein, 1988). It has been known for some time that the endogenous opioid system is activated during periods of stress (Shavit, 1991). Because opioid receptors occur on some immune cells, the possibility exists that specific types of immune alterations subsequent to stressor exposure may involve opioid mediation (see Cabot et al., 1996, for description of β-endorphin assay).

In rats, footshock-induced suppression of splenic NK function, but not spleen cell mitogenic activity, can be blocked by pretreatment with naltrexone, an opioid antagonist (Cunnick et al., 1988). By contrast, when a psychological stressor was studied (i.e., a conditioned aversive stimulus), naltrexone attenuated both suppressed NK and mitogenic activities in the spleen (Lysle, Luecken, et al., 1992). This effect is likely due to central opioid activity, because a quaternary form of naltrexone, N-methylnaltrexone, which does not cross the blood-brain barrier, had no influence on the suppressed proliferative and NK activities of spleen cells following exposure to the conditioned aversive stimulus (Lysle, Luecken, et al., 1992).

Substance P. Substance P is a neuropeptide classified as a tachykinin (i.e., it elicits an increased heart rate after it lowers blood pressure). Substance P is found in many areas of the brain, as well as in nerves that project into secondary lymphoid tissues. Receptors for substance P are found on the membranes of both T and B cells, mononuclear phagocytic cells, and mast cells. Substance P is released from sensory nerve fibers and contributes to the induction of localized inflammatory reactions. In this regard, substance P can be said to have pro-inflammatory activity (promoting inflammation), similar to some of the cytokines (IL-l, IL-6, TNF).

Receptors for substance P are present on lymphoid cells, although whether all subpopulations of lymphocytes have substance P receptors remains undetermined (Kaltreider et al., 1997). Substance P receptors are also located on endothelial cells, possibly mediating alterations of adhesion molecules (Tang et al., 1993; see Ku et al., 1998, for a description of the substance P receptor assay).

Neuropeptide Y. Neuropeptide Y is present in the neurons of the central nervous system and in neurons located in tissues throughout the body, including the mucosa. Neuropeptide Y is co-localized in nerve terminals in lymphatic tissues with norepinephrine (see Irwin et al., 1991, for a description of the neuropeptide Y assay). In the rat, neuropeptide Y nerve terminals are located primarily in the macrophage-rich areas of the spleen (Meltzer et al., 1997). Whether antigen-presenting dendritic cells occur in the same location as these neurons has not been determined.

Lymphocytes have receptors for neuropeptide Y, and therefore neuropeptide Y may modulate their function (Petitto et al., 1994). It is likely that macrophages and/or dendritic cells also have neuropeptide Y receptors.

Somatostatin. Somatostatin is released from sensory nerve terminals, many of which terminate in lymphoid follicles of the gastrointestinal tract. Somatostatin also is found in and released from lymphoid cells (Teitelbaum et al., 1996; see Jonsson et al., 1998, for a description of the somatostatin assay).

There are somatostatin receptors on lymphoid cells (Sreedharan et al., 1989), and there may be biological significance for the appearance of somatostatin receptors on activated lymphocytes. For example, the effect of somatostatin on lymphocyte mitosis has been found to be concentration-dependent: low concentrations of somatostatin reduce mitogen-induced mitosis (Payan et al., 1984), but high concentrations of somatostatin enhance it (Pawlikowski et al., 1987).

Furthermore, NK function and immunoglobulin synthesis are decreased by somatostatin (Eglezos et al., 1993; Stanisz et al., 1986). It has not been established whether the decreased immunoglobulin synthesis is due to a direct effect of somatostatin on dendritic cell uptake and processing of antigen (Johannson et al., 1993), a direct effect on B lymphocytes, or mediation by T lymphocytes. However, because somatostatin has been reported to increase cytokine release from both macrophages and T lymphocytes, a direct effect of somatostatin on B lymphocytes or dendritic cells is the more likely possibility (Komorowski & Stepien, 1995; Nio et al., 1993). Other studies indicate that the effect of somatostatin on macrophage function depends on the concentration of somatostatin (Chao et al., 1995).

Vasoactive Intestinal Peptide. Vasoactive intestinal peptide is present in neurons of the central nervous system and in peripheral nerves. Vasoactive intestinal peptide–containing nerves are located in both primary and secondary lymphoid tissues, around blood vessels (thus, the name *vasoactive*), and in the gastrointestinal tract. There are vasoactive intestinal peptide receptors on both T and B lymphocytes (Danek et al., 1983; Johnson et al., 1996; Ottaway & Greenberg, 1984), and binding of this peptide to its receptor on lymphocytes increases cAMP production (O'Dorisio et al., 1985). As would be anticipated in conjunction with increased cAMP levels, vasoactive intestinal peptide decreases the responsiveness of lymphocytes to stimulation with nonspecific mitogens (Ottaway & Greenberg, 1984; see Belenky et al., 1996, for a description of the vasoactive intestinal peptide assay).

Growth Hormone and Insulin-Like Growth Factor. Growth hormone (GH) is synthesized by cells of the anterior lobe of the pituitary and is also produced by lymphocytes and mononuclear phagocytic cells (Hattori et al., 1990; Weigent et al., 1991). GH participates in the regulation of growth of the body, tissue metabolism, and tissue repair. GH may also participate in regulating the growth and function of the immune system (see Bouix et al., 1994, for a description of the GH assay).

Another hormone, insulin-like growth factor (IGF-I), is produced by the liver and other tissues in response to GH, and it interacts with GH to promote the growth-enhancing effects of GH on tissues. IGF-I has autocrine, paracrine, and endocrine activity. IGF-I and GH may not have a complete overlap in regard to the tissues they affect. The various components of the immune system may be affected to different degrees by GH or IGF-I, depending on the presence of receptors for them on lymphoid cells.

Receptors for GH are present on lymphoid cells (Kelly et al., 1991), and GH is a hormone whose concentration is elevated at times of stress. Indeed, both psychological and physical stress increase the production of GH (Flanagan et al., 1997; Gauquelin-Koch et al., 1996; Malarkey et al., 1994).

Likewise, IGF-I receptors are found on various cells of the immune system (Kooijman et al., 1992; Stuart et al., 1991). Binding of IGF-I to its receptor on lymphocytes increases the response of lymphocytes to mitogenic stimulation (Schillaci et al., 1994). IGF-I may also significantly enhance the amount of antibody produced by B lymphocytes (Kimata & Yoshida, 1994).

Prolactin. Prolactin is produced by cells of the anterior pituitary, and its primary function is in lactation, although prolactin receptors are present in many different tissues, including liver, kidney, intestine, and adrenals. In addition to being produced by the pituitary, prolactin is produced by lymphoid cells (Pellegrini et al., 1992), and there are prolactin receptors on lymphoid cells (Russell et al., 1985). Prolactin receptors may be increased on lymphocytes of experimental animals that spontaneously develop autoimmune disease (Berczi, 1993; Gagnerault et al., 1993). Removal of the pituitary in rats is associated with involution of the thymus, which is reversed by treatment with prolactin (Nagy et al., 1983).

The concentration of prolactin increases in plasma at times of stress (Larsen & Mau, 1994; Malarkey et al., 1994) (see Gorman et al., 1992 for a description of the prolactin assay). Therefore, prolactin may contribute to the modulation of immune function both at times of stress and during immune reactions to antigens (when lymphoid cells may release prolactin, which will have an autocrine or a paracrine influence).

Melatonin. Melatonin is produced by the pineal, an endocrine gland located in the brain. The release of melatonin from the pineal is suppressed by light and increased in the dark. Melatonin is associated with sleep induction and sexual maturation. Melatonin receptors have been found on lymphoid cells, which suggests that it may contribute to immune alterations (Garcia-Perganeda et al., 1997; Gonzalez-Haba et al., 1995).

In vivo treatment of animals with melatonin produces an immune-enhancing effect on both cell-mediated immunity and antibody production (Maestroni et al., 1988). The immune-enhancing activity was confined to the secondary immune response. Thus, effector/memory lymphocytes, rather than naive lymphocytes, may be more susceptible to the influence of melatonin. Long-term treatment of mice with melatonin did not alter the function of lymphocytes to nonspecific mitogen, nor did it alter the function of NK cells (Provinciali et al., 1997). Therefore, melatonin may primarily alter the function of effector/memory antigen-specific cells.

Because melatonin concentrations undergo a circadian rhythm and the effect of melatonin on immune function may be indirect and not fully characterized, a precise role for melatonin in stressor-induced immune alteration or in immune regulation has not yet been defined. However, it is likely that melatonin is one of the hormones capable of influencing immune function (see Strassman et al., 1989, for a description of the melatonin assay).

Stress and the Immune System

Stress-induced alteration of the immune system occurs in the secondary lymphoid tissues (spleen, lymph nodes, and mucosa-associated lymphoid tissues), where effector T cells are produced from naive T cells, and T-cell help is provided to B lymphocytes. A stress-related influence on the activation and function of effector lymphocytes in parenchymal tissues is also likely due to stress-induced changes in the hormonal milieu in which the immune system resides. Glucocorticoids and catecholamines are among the principal hormones that contribute to these functional alterations.

It has been shown that subjects who are under stress are more susceptible to upper respiratory viral infection (Cohen et al., 1991) and have a decreased ability to produce antibody to an antigen that they are immunized with (Glaser et al., 1992) (see chapter 7). There are also suggestions from epidemiological studies that individuals who are under stress are at an increased risk for the development of autoimmune disease or the exacerbation of autoimmune disease (see chapter 11).

Thus, it is both logical and important to define the areas of the brain, as well as the hormones and biochemical pathways activated by the hormones, that are associated with regulation of immune function. This knowledge can help develop hypotheses for modulating central nervous system function to prevent stress-induced alterations of immune function that may be increasing susceptibility to disease.

Understanding the interactions within the brain and how the brain facilitates or inhibits stressor-induced suppression of immune function will help in understanding the mechanisms of stressor-induced immune alteration and suggest ways in which it can be prevented. Indeed, although research in this area is just beginning, there is evidence to suggest that the adoption of stress-buffering beliefs and behaviors will have a beneficial effect on health. However, it cannot yet be predicted which specific persons will benefit from such behaviors.

The response of the brain to a stressor is manifested in several ways. Activated neurons increase the intranuclear concentration of proteins such as c-Fos. The hypothalamus produces corticotropin-releasing factor, and the pituitary, ACTH. Postganglionic sympathetic neurons increase heart rate and blood pressure. Plasma concentrations of glucocorticoids and catecholamines increase, bind to appropriate receptors, and produce physiological alterations.

A critical question relates to whether the consequences of stressor-induced activation of the brain must always occur when an individual experiences a stressor. Factors that *may* contribute to the response of the brain to a stressor include:

Perception: whether a person perceives the particular situation as a
    stressor. For example, a physician who is a trauma surgeon will respond differently to maimed individuals in a traffic accident than
    will an individual who has not had exposure to physical trauma.
Habituation: whether the stress-reactive areas of the brain have been
    habituated to repeated activation. For example, animals that engage

in regular exercise respond to a psychological stressor with less immune system alteration than do animals that have not exercised (e.g., Dishman et al., 1995); moreover, the hormonal response to psychological stress in humans (Sothman et al., 1988, 1991) is less in physically fit individuals. If exercise activates the same areas of the brain as does a psychological stressor, the brain areas may habituate to repeated exercise activation and become less responsive to psychological stress. Indeed, repeated stress does attenuate some of the resulting immune alterations (Lysle, Lyte, et al., 1987).

Suppression: whether behaviors that are considered to ameliorate the effects of stress on the immune system do so by activating areas of the brain that suppress activation of the stress-responsive areas. Thus, individuals who are comfortable in social situations and have friends, who are optimistic, who have a sense of humor, and who engage in religious or spiritual practices or beliefs may have developed brain pathways that interfere with immune system and health alterations when those individuals are under stress.

If the suggestions from epidemiological, basic science, and clinical research studies are correct, a variety of diseases are increased in frequency when an individual experiences acute or chronic stress. Some situations may be of minor consequence, such as an upper respiratory infection in a healthy young adult. However, the same infection in a debilitated elderly individual may have serious consequences. Thus, behaviors and belief systems that ameliorate the functional alterations of the immune system that occur subsequent to the perception of a stressor may have important implications for preventive medicine. This is the topic of the next section.

Religion and Spirituality as Potential Stress-Buffering Beliefs and Behaviors

There is little question that the practice of religious principles and belief in the teachings of a religion can have a beneficial influence on health. For example, there is decreased atherosclerotic heart disease, emphysema, and cirrhosis of the liver in individuals who regularly attend church services (Comstock & Partridge, 1972), and overall mortality has been found to be significantly lower for those who regularly attend religious services than for those who do not (Levin, 1994; Strawbridge et al., 1997). Hypertension also is significantly lower among those who attend church services frequently (Levin & Vanderpool, 1989).

Many of the beneficial effects of religion on health may be due to their influences on lifestyles. In fact, those who are more (as compared with less) active in their attendance at religious services appear to follow better health-promoting behaviors and have more social interactions and stable marriages (Levin, 1994; Strawbridge et al., 1997). Obviously, these are behaviors that are capable of contributing to good health. However, not all studies have found a relationship between the frequency of church attendance and social support, even when there was a relationship between church attendance and health (Koenig et al., 1997a). Similarly, not all studies have found increased longevity and health with increased religious participation (Blazer & Palmore, 1976; Simons & West, 1985). Therefore, it is possible that the teachings and practices of various religions may inhibit the stressor-induced activation of those areas of the brain that modify immune function. Indeed, activities such as church attendance may provide a mental state that is associated with a hormonal environment that facilitates greater resistance to the development of infectious disease (see chapters 1 and 7).

It may be that participation in activities centered around a religious structure induce "relaxation" and, thereby, reduce sympathetic nervous system activity, thus enhancing immune function. An association between techniques that are believed to induce mental relaxation and reduced SNS activity, however, is not firmly established. At least one study has found that in subjects who were trained to relax, there was a greater increase in physical stressor–induced plasma norepinephrine than in control (non-relaxed) subjects (Hoffman et al., 1982). This finding was interpreted as indicating that more catecholamine stimulation was required for a stressor to produce an increase in heart rate and blood pressure in the relaxation-trained group, suggesting that there was less responsiveness to catecholamines in this group. The hormonal response to the psychological stressor was not evaluated, however.

A similar finding of higher plasma catecholamine concentrations in subjects trained in transcendental meditation than in untrained subjects has been reported (Cooper et al., 1985). The effect of a psychological stressor on altering catecholamine concentrations was not determined. Another report suggested that transcendental meditation, which is a Hindu-derived relaxation method, can lower systolic blood pressure (Wallace et al., 1983). Unfortunately, the transcendental meditation practitioners were not compared with a group of control persons who were carefully matched for age and medical conditions.

Additional evidence for the involvement of religious and spiritual activities in moderating the effects of stress on the immune system comes from the study of interleukin-6 (IL-6), which is produced by several different cell types, one of which is the macrophage. Synthesis of IL-6 is induced when macrophages ingest bacteria. Thus, an increased plasma concentration of IL-6 may indicate the presence of an infection and an inflammatory response to limit the spread of the infection. IL-6 was measured in the plasma of older individuals who either regularly attended church services or did not regularly attend church services (Koenig et al., 1997b). An elevated plasma concentration of IL-6 was present in the plasma of significantly fewer churchgoing individuals than individuals who did not attend church regularly. This may be interpreted as meaning that there were fewer infectious diseases or inflammatory processes present in the churchgoing subjects. Alternatively, as IL-6 has been reported to increase in plasma during stress (Zhou et al., 1993), the church-attending subjects may have had less of a response to stress than did the other subjects.

It also is possible that religious and spiritual beliefs and practices may promote health by increasing satisfaction with life and personal happiness and decreasing one's negative thoughts and emotions associated with traumatic and stressful life events (Ellison, 1991). Religion may do this indirectly through social support. For example, research shows that individuals who engage in more social interactions through marriage, close friends, religious participation, and group associations have lower mortality rates than those of individuals without such interactions (Berkman & Syme, 1979; Schoenbach et al., 1986).

The perception of social support may be more important than actual social support (Blazer, 1982). The importance of perception may indicate that a positive perception of the environment can influence the mind to influence the hormonal milieu of the body. (See chapters 1 and 7 for a more detailed discussion of social interactions and health and the role that religion may play in promoting social interactions.)

The positive effect of religious beliefs on health also may be due, at least in part, to the "placebo response." There is considerable evidence that belief in the effectiveness of a treatment will enhance one's chances of having a meaningful therapeutic response (Lupoarello et al., 1970; Roberts, 1995).

It is possible that religious beliefs may promote an optimistic attitude (i.e., the tendency to expect positive outcomes in the future).

Conclusions

Although many questions remain regarding the relationship of stress to immune function, it is apparent that information from the central nervous system (brain) to the immune system is transmitted through several pathways, inducing changes in immune function that are either short- or long-lived. Identifying these pathways has been made easier by the wealth of data available on how stress activates the hypothalamic-pituitary-adrenal axis, the sympathetic nervous system, and the endocrine system. Because all three systems are active shortly after stressor exposure, it is likely that their combined influence on immune activity reflects the modulation of the function of the various components of the immune system.

Hence, to the same extent that our knowledge of stressor-induced immune modulation is limited to knowing merely that it does happen, our knowledge of how it happens is similarly confined to knowing that the HPA axis, catecholamines, and endogenous opioids and other neuropeptides are all involved. What is currently lacking is more detailed information about the stress conditions under which each of these factors predominates over the others; the specific leukocyte targets that each of these factors interacts with; the nature of the cellular alteration induced by the stressor-activated mediator(s); and whether the neural mediators act additively, synergistically, or in opposition to each other.

Although still speculative at this point, it is possible that the beliefs and behaviors associated with religious and spiritual pursuits may contribute to buffering the alteration of immune function by stress. In this regard, it is likely that the most important host factor is believing that the activity that one is using as a stress buffer will work. Individuals may respond differently to belief systems, however, and their responses may be influenced by factors as diverse as their in utero environments and the happiness of their marriages. It is important to emphasize that generalization must be avoided when discussing behaviors that will buffer the effect of stress on the immune system and health. However, this appears to be a field that is rich with possibilities for investigation.

REFERENCES

Ackerman, K. D., Bellinger, D. L., Felten, S. Y., & Felten, D. L. (1991). Ontogeny and senescence of noradrenergic innervation of the rodent thymus and spleen. In R. Ader, D. L. Felten, & N. Cohen (Eds.), *Psychoneuroimmunology*, 2nd ed. New York: Academic.

Bachen, B. A., Manuck, S. B., Cohen, S., Muldoon, M. F., Raibel, R., Herbert, T. B., & Rabin, B. S. (1995). Adrenergic blockade ameliorates cellular immune responses to mental stress in humans. *Psychosomatic Medicine* 57, 366–372.

Bachen, B. A., Manuck, S. B., Marsiand, A. L., Cohen, S., Malkoff, S. B., Muldoon, M. F., & Rabin, B. S. (1992). Lymphocyte subsets and cellular immune responses to a brief experimental stressor. *Psychosomatic Medicine* 54, 673–679.

Baulmann, J., Spitznagel, H., Herdegen, T., Unger, T., & Culman, J. (2000). Tachykinin receptor inhibition and c-Fos expression in the rat brain following formalin-induced pain. *Neuroscience* 95, 813–820.

Belenky, M., Wagner, S., Yarom, Y., Matzner, H., Cohen, S., & Castel, M. (1996). The suprachiasmatic nucleus in stationary organotypic culture. *Neuroscience* 70, 127–143.

Berczi, I. (1993). The role of prolactin in the pathogenesis of autoimmune disease. *Endocrine Pathology* 4, 178–195.

Berkman, L. F., & Syme, S. L. (1979). Social networks, host resistance, and mortality: A nine-year follow-up study of Alameda County residents. *American Journal of Epidemiology* 109, 186–204.

Blazar, B. A., Rodrick, M. L., O'Mahony, J. B., Wood, J. J., Bessey, P.Q., Wilmore, D.W., & Mannick, J. A. (1986). Suppression of natural killer-cell function in humans following thermal and traumatic injury. *Journal of Clinical Immunology* 6, 26–36.

Blazer, D., & Palmore, E. (1976). Religion and aging in a longitudinal panel. *Gerontologist* 16, 82–85.

Blazer, D. G. (1982). Social support and mortality in an elderly community population. *American Journal of Epidemiology* 115, 684–694.

Bouix, O., Brun, J. F., Fedou, C., Raynaud, E., Kerdelhue, B., Lenoir, V., & Orsetti, A. (1994). Plasma beta-endorphin, corticotrophin and growth hormone responses to exercise in pubertal and prepubertal children. *Hormone and Metabolic Research* 26, 195–199.

Cabot, P. J., Carter, L., Gaiddon, C., Zhang, Q., Schafer, M., Loeffler, J. P., & Stein, S. (1996). Immune cell-derived β-endorphin. *Journal of Clinical Investigation* 100, 142–148.

Caroleo, M. C., Pulvirenti, L., Arbitrio, M., Lopilato, R., & Nistico, G. (1993). Evidence that CRH microinfused into the locus coeruleus decreases cell-mediated immune response in rats. *Functional Neurology* 8, 271–277.

Chao, T. C., Cheng, H. P., & Walter, R. I. (1995). Somatostatin and macrophage function: Modulation of hydrogen peroxide, nitric oxide and tumor necrosis factor release. *Regulatory Peptides* 58, 1–10.

Cohen, S., Tyrrell, D. A. I., & Smith, A. P. (1991). Psychological stress and suscep-tibility to the common cold. *New England Journal of Medicine* 325, 606–612.

Comstock, G. W. & Partridge, K. B. (1972). Church attendance and health. *Journal of Chronic Disease*, 25, 665–672.

Cooper, R., Joffe, B. I., Lamprey, J. M., Botha, A., Shires, R., Baker, S. G., & Sef-tel, H. C. (1985). Hormonal and biochemical responses to transcendental meditation. *Postgraduate Medical Journal* 61, 301–304.

Crary, B., Hauser, S. L., Borysenko, M., Kutz, I., Hoban, C., Ault, K. A., Weiner, H. L., & Benson, H. (1983). Epinephrine induced changes in the distribution of lymphocyte subsets in peripheral blood of humans. *Journal of Immunology* 131, 1178–1181.

Cunnick, J. E., Lysle, D. T., Armfield, A., & Rabin, B. S. (1988). Shock-induced modulation of lymphocyte responsiveness and natural killer cell activity: Differential mechanisms of induction. *Brain, Behavior, and Immunity* 2, 102–113.

Danek, A., O'Dorisio, M. S., O'Dorisio, T. M., & George, J. M. (1983). Specific binding sites for vasoactive intestinal polypeptide on nonadherent peripheral blood lymphocytes. *Journal of Immunology* 131, 1173–1177.

De Blasi, A., Maisel, A. S., Feldman, R. D., Ziegler, M. G., Fratelli, M., DiLallo, M., Smith, D. A., Lai, C.Y., and Motulsky, H. J. (1986). In vivo regulation of beta-adrenergic receptors on human mononuclear leukocytes: Assessment of receptor number, location, and function after posture change, exercise, and isoproterenol infusion. *Journal of Clinical Endocrinology and Metabolism* 63, 847–853.

Dishman, R. K., Warren, J. M., Youngstedt, S. D., Yoo, H., Bunnell, B. N., Mougey, E. H., Meyerhoff, J. L., Jaso-Friedman, L., & Evans, D. L. (1995). Activity—wheel running—attenuates suppression of natural killer cell activ-ity after footshock. *Journal of Applied Physiology* 78, 1547–1554.

Eglezos, A., Andrews, P. V., & Helme, R. D. (1993). In vivo inhibition of the rat primary antibody response to antigenic stimulation by somatostatin. *Immunology and Cell Biology* 71, 125–129.

Ellison, C. G. (1991). Religious involvement and subjective well-being. *Journal of Health and Social Behavior* 32, 80–99.

Felten, S. Y., & Felten, D. L. (1991). Innervation of lymphoid tissue. In Ader, R., Felten, D. L., & Cohen, N. (Eds.), *Psychoneuroimmunology*, 2nd ed. New York: Academic.

Flanagan, D. E., Taylor, M. C., Parfitt, V., Mardell, R., Wood, P. J., & Leatherdale, B. A. (1997). Urinary growth hormone following exercise to assess growth hormone production in adults. *Clinical Endocrinology* 46, 425–429.

Fuchs, B. A., Albright, J. W., & Albright, J. F. (1988). Adrenergic receptors on murine lymphocytes: Density varies with cell maturity and lymphocyte subtype and is decreased after antigen administration. *Cell Immunology* 114, 231–245.

Gagnerault, M. C., Touraine, P., Savino, W., Kelly, P. A., & Dardeene, M. (1993). Expression of prolactin receptors in murine lymphoid cells in normal and autoimmune situations. *Journal of Immunology* 150, 5673–5681.

Garcia-Perganeda, A., Pozo, D., Guerrero, J. M., & Calvo, J. R. (1997). Signal transduction for melatonin in human lymphocytes: Involvement of a pertussis toxin-sensitive G protein. *Journal of Immunology* 159, 3774–3781.

Gauquelin-Koch, G., Blanquie, J. P., Viso, M., Florence, G., Milhaud, C., & Gharib, C. (1996). Hormonal response to restraint in rhesus monkeys. *Journal of Medical Primatology* 25, 387–396.

Glaser, R., Kiecolt-Glaser, J., Bonneau, R., Malarkey, W., Kennedy, S., & Hughes, J. (1992). Stress-induced modulation of the immune response to recombinant hepatitis B vaccine. *Psychosomatic Medicine* 54, 22–29.

Gonzalez-Haba, M. G., Gaarcia-Maurino, S., Calvo, J. R., Goberna, R., & Guerrero, J. M. (1995). High-affinity binding of melatonin by human circulating T lymphocytes (CD4+). *FASEB Journal* 9, 1331–1335.

Gorman, J. M., Warne, P. A., Begg, M. D., Cooper, T. B., Novacenko, H., Williams, J. B., Rabkin, J., Stern, Y., & Ehrhardt, A. A. (1992). Serum prolactin levels in homosexual and bisexual men with HIV infection. *American Journal of Psychiatry* 149, 367–370.

Hattori, N., Shimatsu, A., Sugita, M., Kumagai, S., & Imura, H. (1990). Immunoreactive growth hormone(GH) secretion by human lymphocytes. Augmented release by exogenous GH. *Biochemical and Biophysical Research Communication* 168, 396–401.

Hoffman, J. W., Benson, H., Arns, P. A., Stainbrook, G. L., Landsberg, L., Young, J. B., & Gill, A. (1982). Reduced sympathetic nervous system responsivity associated with the relaxation response. *Science* 215, 190–192.

Irwin, M., Brown, M., Patterson, T., Hauger, R., Mascovich, A., &Grant, I. (1991). Neuropeptide Y and natural killer cell activity: Findings in depression and Alzheimer caregiver stress. *FASEB Journal* 5, 3100–3107.

Johannson, O., Hilliges, M., & Wang, L. (1993). Somatostatin like immunoreactivity is found in dendritic guard cells of human sweat glands. *Peptides* 14, 401–403.

Johnson, M. C., McCormack, R. J., Delgado, M., Martinez, C., & Ganea, D. (1996). Murine T lymphocytes express vasoactive intestinal receptor 1 (VIP R1) mRNA. *Journal of Neuroimmunology* 68, 109–119.

Jonsson, B. H., Uvnas-Moberg, K., Theorell, T., & Gotthard, R. (1998). Gastrin, cholecystokinin, and somatostatin in a laboratory experiment of patients with functional dyspepsia. *Psychosomatic Medicine* 60, 331–337.

Juzwa, W., Gnacinska, G., Rawicz-Zegrzda, I., & Kaczmarek, J. (1995). Modulation of cellular immunity by a lesion of the lateral hypothalamic area (LHA) in rats. *Experimental and Toxicologic Pathology* 47, 403–408.

Kaltreider, H. B., Ichikawa, S., Byrd, P. K., Ingram, D. A., Kishiyama, J. L., Sreedharan, S. P., Warnock, M. L., Beck, J. M., & Goetzel, E. J. (1997). Upregulation of neuropeptides and neuropeptide receptors in a murine model of immune inflammation in lung parenchyma. *American Journal of Respiratory Cell and Molecular Biology* 16, 133–144.

Kappel, M., Tvede, N., Galbo, H., Haahr, P. M., Kjaer, M., Linstow, M., Klarlund, K., & Pedersen, B. K. (1991). Evidence that the effect of physical exercise on NK cell activity is mediated by epinephrine. *Journal of Applied Physiology* 70, 2530–2434.

Kelly, P. A., Djiane, J., Postel-Vinay, M. C., & Edery, M. (1991). The prolactin/growth hormone receptor family. *Endocrine Reviews* 12, 235–251.

Kimata, H., & Yoshida, A. (1994). The effect of growth hormone and insulin-like growth factor-I on immunoglobulin production by and growth of human B cells. *Journal of Clinical Endocrinology and Metabolism* 78, 635–641.

Kimura, F., & Nakamura, S. (1985). Locus coeruleus neurons in the neonatal rat: Electrical activity and responses to sensory stimulation. *Brain Research* 355, 301–305.

Koenig, H. G., Cohen, H. J., George, L. K., Hays, J. C., Larson, D. B., & Blazer, D. G. (1997). Attendance at religious services, interleukin-6, and other biological parameters of immune function in older adults. *International Journal of Psychiatry in Medicine* 27, 233–250.

Koenig, H. G., Hays, J. C., George, L. K., Blazer, D. G., Larson, D. B., & Landerman, L. R. (1997). Modeling the cross-sectional relationships between religion, physical health, social support, and depressive symptoms. *American Journal of Geriatric Psychiatry* 5, 131–144.

Komorowski, J., & Stepien, H. (1995). Somatostatin (SRIF) stimulates the release of interleukin-6 from human peripheral blood monocytes (PBM) in vitro. *Neuropeptides* 29, 77–81.

Kooijman, R., Williams, M., DeHaas, C. J., Rijkers, G. T., Schuurmans, A. L., Van Buul-Offers, S. C., Heijnen, C. J., & Zegers, B. J. (1992). Expression of type-I insulin-like growth factor receptors on human peripheral blood mononuclear cells. *Endocrinology* 131, 2244–2250.

Ku, Y. H., Tan, L., Li, L. S., & Ding, X. (1998). Role of corticotropin-releasing factor and substance P in pressor responses of nuclei controlling emotion and stress. *Peptides* 19, 677–682.

Kvetnansky, R., Fukuhara, K., Pacak, K., Cizza, G., Goldstein, D. S., & Kopin, L. I. (1993). Endogenous glucocorticoids restrain catecholamine synthesis and release at rest and during immobilization stress in rats. *Endocrinology* 133, 1411–1419.

Larsen, P. J., & Mau, S. E. (1994). Effect of acute stress on the expression of hypothalamic messenger ribonucleic acids encoding the endogenous opioid precursors preproenkephalin a and proopiomelanocortin. *Peptides* 15, 783–790.

Lefkowitz, R. J., Hoffman, B. B., & Taylor, P. (1990). Neurohumoral transmission: The autonomic and somic nervous systems. In A. G. Gilman, T. W. Rall, A. S. Nies, & P. Taylor (Eds.), *The pharmacological basis of therapeutics*, 8th ed. New York: Pergamon.

Levin, J. S. (1994). Religion and health: Is there an association, is it valid, and is it causal? *Social Science and Medicine* 38, 1475–1482.

Levin, J. S., & Vanderpool, H. Y. (1989). Is religion therapeutically significant for hypertension? *Social Science and Medicine* 29, 69–78.

Lupoarello, T., Leist, N., Lourie, C. H., & Sweet, P. (1970). The interaction of psychologic stimuli and pharmacologic agents on airway reactivity in asthmatic subjects. *Psychosomatic Medicine* 32, 509–513.

Lysle, D. T., Luecken, U., & Maslonek, K. A. (1992). Modulation of immune status by a conditioned aversive stimulus: Evidence for the involvement of endogenous opioids. *Brain, Behavior, and Immunity* 6, 179–188.

Lysle, D. T., Lyte, M., Fowler, H., & Rabin, B. (1987). Shock-induced modulation of lymphocyte reactivity: Suppression, habituation, and recovery. *Life Sciences* 41, 1805–1814.

Madden, K. S., & Livnat, S. (1991). Catecholamine action and immunologic reactivity. In R. Ader, D. L. Felten, & N. Cohen (Eds.), *Psychoneuroimmunology*, 2nd ed. New York: Academic.

Maestroni, G. J. M., Conti, A., & Pierpaoli, W. (1988). Pineal melatonin, its fundamental immunoregulatory role in aging and cancer. *Annals of the New York Academy of Sciences* 521, 140–148.

Malarkey, W. B., Kiecolt-Glaser, J. K., Pear,l D., & Glaser, R. (1994). Hostile behavior during marital conflict alters pituitary and adrenal hormones. *Psychosomatic Medicine* 56, 41–51.

Manuck, S. B., Cohen, S., Rabin, B. S., Muldoon, M. F., & Bachen, E. A. (1991). Individual differences in cellular immune responses to stress. *Psychological Science* 2, 1–5.

Meltzer, J. C., Grimm, P. C., Greenberg, A. H., & Nance, D. M. (1997). Enhanced immunohistochemical detection of autonomic nerve fibers, cytokines, and inducible nitric oxide synthase by light and fluorescent microscopy in rat spleen. *Journal of Histochemistry and Cytochemistry* 45, 599–610.

Nagy, E., Berczi, I., Wren, G., Asa, L., & Kovacs, K. (1983). Immunomodulation by bromocryptine. *Immunopharmacology* 6, 231.

Naliboff, B. D., Benton, D., Solomon, G. E., Morley, J. E., Fahey, J. L., Bloom, E. T., Makinodan, T., & Gilmore, S. L. (1991). Immunological changes in young and old adults during brief laboratory stress. *Psychosomatic Medicine* 53, 121–132.

Nio, D. A., Moylan, R. N., & Roche, J. K. (1993). Modulation of T lymphocyte function by neuropeptides. Evidence for their role as local immunoregulatory elements. *Journal of Immunology* 150, 5281–5288.

O'Dorisio, M. S., Wood, C. L., Wenger, G. D., & Vassalo, L. M. (1985). Cyclic AMP-dependent protein kinase in Molt 4b lymphoblasts: Identification by photoaffinity labeling and activation in intact cells by vasoactive intestinal polypeptide (VIP) and peptide histadine isoleucine (PHI). *Journal of Immunology* 134, 4078–4086.

Ottaway, C. A., & Greenberg, G. R. (1984). Interaction of vasoactive intestinal peptide with mouse lymphocytes: Specific binding and the modulation of mitogen responses. *Journal of Immunology* 132, 417–423.

Pacak, K., Kvetnansky, R., Palkovits, M., Fukuhara, K., Yadid, G., Kopin, I. L., & Goldstein, D. S. (1993). Adrenalectomy augments in vivo release of norepinephrine in the paraventricular nucleus during immobilization stress. *Endocrinology* 133, 1404–1410.

Pawlikowski, M., Stepien, H., Kunert, J., Zelazowski, P., & Schally, A. V. (1987). Immunomodulatory activity of somatostatin. *Annals of the New York Academy of Sciences* 496, 233–239.

Payan, D. G., Hess, C. A., & Goetzl, E. J. (1984). Inhibition by somatostatin of the proliferation of T lymphocytes and Molt–4 lymphoblasts. *Cellular Immunology* 84, 433–438.

Pellegrini, I., Lebrun, J. J., Ali, S., & Kelly, P. A. (1992). Expression of prolactin and its receptor in human lymphoid cells. *Molecular Endocrinology* 6, 1023–1031.

Petitto, J. M., Huang, Z., & McCarthy, D. B. (1994). Molecular cloning of NPY-Y1 receptor cDNA from rat splenic lymphocytes: Evidence of low levels of mRNA expression and NPY binding sites. *Journal of Neuroimmunology* 54, 81–86.

Provinciali, M., DiStefano, U., Bulian, D., Stronati, S., & Fabris, N. (1997). Long-term melatonin supplementation does not recover the impairment of natural killer cell activity and lymphocyte proliferation in aging mice. *Life Sciences* 61, 857–864.

Rassnick, S., Sved, A. F., & Rabin, B. S. (1994). Locus coeruleus stimulation by corticotropin-releasing hormone suppresses in vitro cellular immune responses. *Journal of Neurosciences* 14, 6033–6040.

Roberts, A. H. (1995). The powerful placebo revisited: Magnitude of nonspecific effects. *Mind/Body Medicine* 1, 35–43.

Roszman, T. L., & Carlson, S. L. (1991). Neurotransmitters and molecular signaling in the immune response. In R. Ader, D. L. Felten, & N. Cohen (Eds.), *Psychoneuroimmunology*, 2nd ed. New York: Academic.

Russell, D. H., Kibler, R., Matrisian, L., Larson, D. F., Poulos, B., & Magun, B. E. (1985). Prolactin receptors on human T and B lymphocytes: Antagonism of prolactin binding by cyclosporine. *Journal of Immunology* 134, 3027–3031.

Schillaci, R., Ribaudo, C. M., Rondinone, C. M., & Roldan, A. (1994). Role of insulin-like growth factor-I on the kinetics of human lymphocyte stimulation in serum free culture medium. *Immunology and Cell Biology* 72, 300–305.

Schoenbach, V. J., Kaplan, B. H., Fredman, L., & Kleinbaum, D. G. (1986). Social ties and mortality in Evans County, Georgia. *American Journal of Epidemiology* 123, 577–591.

Shavit, Y. (1991). Stress-induced immune modulation in animals: Opiates and endogenous opioid peptides. In R. Ader, D. L. Felten, & N. Cohen (Eds.), *Psychoneuroimmunology*, 2nd ed. New York: Academic.

Shurin, M. R., Kusnecov, A. W., Riechman, S. E., & Rabin, B. S. (1995). Effect of a conditioned aversive stimulus on the immune response in three strains of rats. *Psychoneuroendocrinology* 20, 837–849.

Sibinga, N. E. S., & Goldstein, A. (1988). Opioid peptides and opioid receptors in cells of the immune system. *Annual Review of Immunology* 6, 219–249.

Simons, R. L., & West, G. E. (1985). Life changes, coping resources, and health among the elderly. *Journal of Psychiatric Treatment and Evaluation* 4, 403–408.

Sothman, M. S., Gustafson, A. B., Garthwaite, T. L., Horn, T. S., & Hart, B. A. (1988). Cardiovascular fitness and selected adrenal hormone responses to cognitive stress. *Endocrine Research* 14, 59–69.

Sothman, M. S., Horn T. S., & Hart, B. A. (1991). Plasma catacholamine response to acute physiological stress in humans: Relation to aerobic exercise and fitness training. *Medicine and Science in Sports and Exercise* 23, 860–867.

Spencer, R. L., Miller, A. H., Moday, H., Stein, M., & McEwen, B. S. (1993). Diurnal differences in basal and acute stress levels of type I and type II adrenal steroid receptor activation in neural and immune tissues. *Endocrinology* 133, 1941–1950.

Spencer, R. L., Miller, A. H., Stein, M., & McEwen, B. S. (1991). Corticosterone regulation of type I and type II adrenal steroid receptors in brain, pituitary, and immune tissue. *Brain Research* 549, 236–246.

Sreedharan, S. R., Kodama, K. T., Peterson, K. E., & Goetzl, E. J. (1989). Distinct subsets of somatostatin receptors in cultures human lymphocytes. *Journal of Biological Chemistry* 264, 949–952.

Stanisz, A. M., Befus, D., & Bienenstock, I. (1986). Differential effects of vasoactive intestinal peptide, substance P, and somatostatin on immunoglobulin synthesis and proliferation by lymphocytes from Peyer's patches, mesenteric lymph nodes, and spleen. *Journal of Immunology* 136, 152–156.

Strassman, R. J., Appenzeller, O., Lewy, A. J., Qualls, C. R., & Peake, G. T. (1989). Increase in plasma melatonin, beta-endorphin, and cortisol after a

28.5-mile mountain race: Relationship to performance and lack of effect of naltrexone. *Journal of Clinical Endocrinology and Metabolism* 69, 540–545.

Strawbridge, W. J., Cohen, R. D., Shema, S. J., & Kaplan, G. A. (1997). Frequent attendance at religious services and mortality over 28 years. *American Journal of Public Health* 87, 957–961.

Stuart, C. A., Meehan, R. T., Neale, L. S., Cintron, N. M., & Furlanetto, R. W. (1991). Insulin-like growth factor-I binds selectively to human peripheral blood monocytes and B lymphocytes. *Journal of Clinical Endocrinology* 72, 1117–1122.

Tang, S. C., Fend, F., Muller, L., Braunsteiner, H., & Wiedermann, C. J. (1993). High-affinity substance P binding sites of neurokinin-1 receptor type autoradiographically associated with vascular sinuses and high endothelial venules of human lymphoid tissues. *Laboratory Investigation* 69, 86–93.

Teitelbaum, D. H., DelValle, J., Reyas, B., Post, L., Gupta, A., Mosely, R. L., & Merion, R. (1996). Intestinal intraepithelial lymphocytes influence the production of somatostatin. *Surgery* 120, 227–232.

Van Tits, L. J. H., Michel, M. C., Wilde, H., Rappel, M., Eigler, F. W., Soleman, A., & Brodde, O. E. (1990). Catecholamines increase lymphocyte beta–2-adrenergic receptors via a beta–2-adrenergic, spleen dependent process. *American Journal of Physiology* 258, 191–201.

Wallace, P. K., Silver, J., Mills, P. J., Dillbeck, M. C., & Wagoner, D. E. (1983). Systolic blood pressure and long-term practice of transcendental meditation and TM-Sidhi program: Effects of TM on systolic blood pressure. *Psychosomatic Medicine* 45, 41–46.

Wang, T., Delahanty, D. L., Dougall, A. L., & Baum, A. (1998). Responses of natural killer cell activity to acute laboratory stressors in healthy men at different times of day. *Health Psychology* 17, 428–435.

Watanobe, H., Sasaki, S., & Takebe, K. (1995). Involvement of oxytocin and cholecystokinin-8 in interleukin-1 beta-induced adrenocorticotropin secretion in the rat. *Neuroimmunomodulation* 2, 88–91.

Weber, R. J., & Pert, A. (1989). The periaqueductal gray matter mediates opiate-induced immunosuppression. *Science* 245, 188–190.

Weigent, D. A., Riley, J. E., Galin, F. S., LeBoeuf, R. D., & Blalock, J. E. (1991). Detection of growth hormone and growth hormone-releasing hormone-related messenger RNA in rat leukocytes by the polymerase chain reaction. *Proceedings of the Society for Experimental Biology and Medicine* 198, 643–648.

Wenner, M., Kawamura, N., Ishikawa, T., & Matsuda, Y. (2000). Reward linked to increased natural killer cell activity in rats. *Neuroimmunomodulation* 7, 1–5.

Wenner, M., Kawamura, N., Miyazawa, H., Ago, Y., Ishikawa, T., & Yamamoto, H. (1996). Acute electrical stimulation of lateral hypothalamus increases natural killer cell activity in rats. *Journal of Neuroimmunology* 67, 67–70.

Whitnall, M. H. (1993). Regulation of the hypothalamic corticotropin-releasing hormone neurosecretory system. *Progress in Neurobiology* 40, 573–629.

Wrona, D., Jurkowski, M. K., Trojniar, W., Staszewska, M., & Tokarski, J. (1994). Electrolytic lesions of the lateral hypothalamus influence peripheral blood NK cytotoxicity in rats. *Journal of Neuroimmunology* 55, 45–54.

Zhou, D., Kusnecov, A. W., Shurin, M. R., DePaoli, M., & Rabin, B. S. (1993). Exposure to physical and psychological stressors elevates plasma interleukin 6: Relationship to the activation of hypothalamic-pituitary-adrenal axis. *Endocrinology* 133, 2523–2530.

4

Stress, Natural Killer Cells, and Cancer

RONALD B. HERBERMAN

It is now fairly well established that the way individuals cope with stress may affect the development and progression of infections and diseases, including cancer. Of particular interest to researchers attempting to better understand the potential immunological mechanisms that may mediate the influences of the central nervous system on host defenses against cancer and other diseases are *natural killer* (NK) cells.

NK cells are a third subtype of lymphocytes, besides B and T cells, that mediate immune responses against a variety of intracellular pathogens, including tumor cells and a wide variety of infectious microbes (Whiteside & Herberman, 1994). They are called "natural" killers because, unlike cytotoxic T cells, they do not need to recognize a specific antigen before swinging into action. Rather, NK cells have innate cytolytic activity and are stimulated to broader and higher levels of activity by *cytokines*,[1] which are low-molecular-weight proteins that are released by other immune cells (as well as other cells in the body) in response to infectious agents, such as bacteria, viruses, fungi, and parasites (Rabin, 1999, p. 64). When stimulated by cytokines, NK cells have an enhanced ability to selectively seek out and kill[2] target cells that fail to express "self" MHC class I molecules.

This important "immunosurveillance" property, combined with the relative ease with which NK cell activity can be measured (see chapter 11), have made them a major focus of research on the effects of stress on susceptibility to a number of viral illnesses (e.g., AIDs, hepatitis) and cancers.

This chapter provides a brief overview of the effects of stress on NK cell activity, as well as cancer progression. It then discusses research on the relationship between psychosocial factors and NK cell activity and the implications of this research for the study of the relationship between religion and PNI.

Effects of Stress on NK Cell Activity

Research has shown that emotional stress is often followed by increased susceptibility to infections (Cohen et al., 1991, 1993) as well as tumor progression (Levy, Herberman, Maluish, et al., 1985). Because NK cells play a major role in the immediate immune response to both infection and cancer, there has been intense scientific interest in the role of stress on NK cell activity. For the most part, these studies, which often use short-term (acute) psychological and physical stressors, have shown that NK cell activity is reduced by stress, although to different degrees in various experimental subjects.

Acute Stress and NK Activity

Short-lasting episodes of, or acute, stress have been shown to significantly decrease NK cell activity in both laboratory animals and humans. For example, Zalcman and colleagues (1991) exposed three strains of mice (C57BL/6J, C3H/HeJ, and BALB/cByJ) to the stress of "uncontrollable" electrical footshock and measured their NK cell activity at 0.5, 24, and 48 hours later. This study found that the stress of not being able to control the footshock caused all of the mice to have reductions of NK activity. However, the time until the appearance and disappearance of changes in the mice's NK cell activity varied across strains. Indeed, whereas NK cell activity was markedly reduced in C57BL/6J mice during the whole 0.5- to 48-hour follow-up time period, a reduction in NK cell activity was delayed in the C3H/HeJ mice until 24 to 48 hours following the footshock. Then again, in BALB/cByJ mice, NK activity was significantly reduced 24 hours after footshock, but in contrast to the other strains, NK activity returned to control levels within 48 hours of the stressor exposure.

In a similar study using a different stressor, Simpson and Hoffman-Goetz (1990) trained male C3H mice to run on a treadmill for 10 weeks, while a control group was not trained to run. At the end of the training program, half of the mice from each group (trained and untrained) were sacrificed and the other half were exercised to exhaustion. The researchers measured splenic catecholamine concentrations, splenic NK cell activity against tumor targets, and frequency of asialo GM1-positive (a selectively exposed glycolipid on the murine cell surface) NK splenocytes. Exhaustive exercise in both trained and untrained mice reduced the in vitro killing of tumor targets by splenic NK cells relative to killing by splenocytes from mice that did not undergo the acute exercise bout. The frequency of asialo GM1-positive splenocytes was also reduced in the exhaustively exercised animals.

In contrast, training alone, without the additional stress of exhaustive exercise, reduced the frequency of asialo GM1-positive splenocytes relative to control mice (no training). However, moderate training did not compromise NK cell cytolytic activity against the tumor targets. Splenic epinephrine concentrations in the exhaustively exercised animals were elevated threefold to fivefold above the concentrations observed in trained and sedentary mice. According to the researchers, these results suggest that a single acute episode of exhaustive exercise reduces the capacity of splenic NK cells to kill tumor targets in vitro, whereas moderate training enhances splenic NK cell cytolytic activity, on a per cell basis, against tumor targets.

In human studies, researchers have shown that acute stress similarly reduces NK activity. For example, Schedlowski, Jacobs, and colleagues (1993) studied 45 first-time parachutists by continuously measuring their blood plasma concentrations of cortisol and catecholamines from 2 hours before to 1 hour after jumping out of an airplane. The researchers also measured lymphocyte subsets, NK cell activity, and antibody-dependent cellular cytotoxicity (ADCC, which is mediated by NK cells) 2 hours before, immediately after, and 1 hour after jumping.

This study found a "significant" increase in sympathetic-adrenal hormones during (adrenaline, noradrenaline) and shortly after (cortisol) jumping. There also was an increase in lymphocyte subsets and the "functional" capacity of NK cells immediately after jumping. However, 1 hour after jumping, there was a significant decrease in NK activity below starting values (i.e., 2 hours before jumping). These NK activity changes were significantly correlated to plasma concentrations of noradrenaline. Based on these results, the investigators concluded that quick mobilization of NK cells is a "major" mechanism for this effective adaptation of the immune system to stress situations.

Chronic Stress and NK Activity

Although the studies described previously suggest that NK activity is significantly reduced by acute stress, there are only a few studies on the effects of long-term, or chronic, stress on NK activity. Nevertheless, the studies that do exist indicate that chronic stress, similar to acute stress, is detrimental to NK activity.

In one study, for example, Locke et al. (1984) examined the relationships between self-reported "life change stress," psychiatric symptoms (e.g., depression), and NK activity among 114 healthy undergraduate volunteers. Although the correlation between life change stress and NK activity was not significant, subjects reporting few adverse psychiatric problems in the face of significant amounts of life change stress had significantly higher NK activity than did those who were experiencing high levels of both psychiatric problems and life change stress. Furthermore, self-reported psychiatric symptoms were found to inversely correlate with NK activity, suggesting that psychiatric problems, such as anxiety and depression, may negatively affect immunity.

Anxiety and NK Activity

Ongoing or trait anxiety, which is a manifestation of chronic stress, has been found to be associated with dysregulation of the autonomic nervous system (Antoni et al., 1990), which may extend to the immune system. Indeed, worry, an aspect of anxiety in which potential problems are anticipated and enumerated in an attempt to control the future (Andrews & Borkovec, 1988; Minor & Gold, 1985), has been shown to negatively affect NK activity. For example, Segerstrom and colleagues (1998) took blood samples of 47 hospital employees at three follow-up points after the Northridge earthquake in California in 1994. The investigators also administered an assessment scale that measured the subjects' trait worry. This study found that participants who scored above the median on trait worry had fewer NK cells than participants with worry scores below the median, as well as fewer NK cells than control subjects (individuals who had not been exposed to the earthquake). In addition, this observed effect of worry on NK cells was not mediated by intrusive thoughts, avoidance, anxious mood, or health behavior. According to the investigators, these results suggest that worry may have a detrimental effect on the regulation of

NK cells during stress, and this effect may be due to differences in auto-nomic responsiveness associated with worry.

Depression and NK Activity

Although depression is not always directly associated with lower NK ac-tivity, the two often co-occur (Irwin, 1999; Irwin et al 1987). Birmaher and colleagues (1994), for example, found in a study of depressed adoles-cents that increases in adverse life events were associated with low NK ac-tivity, independent of the diagnoses of depression and socioeconomic sta-tus. Furthermore, Hall and colleagues (1998) examined the sleep patterns of 29 individuals seeking treatment for bereavement-related depression and found that a greater frequency of intrusive thoughts and avoidance be-haviors was associated with more time spent awake and lower numbers of NK cells. This study also found that more time spent awake during non-rapid-eye-movement sleep (NREM-1) was significantly associated with lower NK cell numbers. However, this statistically significant relationship between symptoms of depression-related intrusion and avoidance and NK cell number was no longer significant when time spent awake during NREM-1 was entered into the regression equation.

Stress and Cytokine Production

Research suggests that acute psychological stress reduces NK activity via its profound effects on cytokine production. Sonnenfeld and colleagues (1992) found, for example, that the stress induced by mild electric foot-shock in rodents decreased interferon gamma (IFN-γ) production by splenocytes, decreased the expression of cell surface MHC class II mole-cules, and reduced NK activity. Furthermore, when Dobbin et al. (1991) assessed the cytokine profile of medical students during an examination period, they found that, immediately after the examination, there was marked elevation of IL-1β and a concomitant decrease in IFN-γ. This ob-served "downregulation" of IFN-γ is biologically significant because this cytokine enhances the expression of both MHC class I and class II mole-cules (Mobus et al., 1993). Consequently, inhibited expression of IFN-γ has the potential to inhibit the expression of MHC class I and class II anti-gen presentation to the T cells.

Brambilla et al. (1994) found elevated IL-1β in psychiatric patients suffering from panic disorder—a recurring anxiety state that is accompanied by marked physiological symptoms. Given that IL-1β is elevated in stress and such states as panic disorder, it is theoretically possible that in these conditions IL-1β may induce production of TNF-α (Abraham, 1991). Although the relative expression of TNF-α does not appear to have been examined experimentally in relation to psychiatric disorders, it has been studied in relation to stress. Arck et al. (1995) found that stress promotes secretion of TNF-α. In this study, pregnant mice were subjected to ultrasonic stress, which resulted in elevated TNF-α and fetal resorption at 5.5 days. Increased production of TNF-α also has been found in peritoneal macrophages of mice subjected to cold water stress (Zhu et al., 1996) and systemically in mice subjected to the stress of sleep deprivation (Yamaso et al., 1992).

Acute psychological stress also induces a significant elevation of β-endorphin (Schedlowski, Huge, et al., 1995). Elevated β-endorphin has been detected in anxious and frustrated adolescent women (Gerra et al., 1992), and Darko, Risch, and colleagues (1992) found elevated concentrations of β-endorphin in clinically depressed patients who also displayed symptoms of severe anxiety, phobias, and obsessive-compulsive disorder. The co-occurrence of elevated β-endorphin and IL-1β in stress-related disorders may be due to the fact that β-endorphin regulates IL-β and IL-2 production, whereas IL-β also upregulates β-endorphin binding in brain tissue (Carr, 1991).

The observation that stress, anxiety, and depression coincide with elevated β-endorphin is noteworthy because Darko, Irwin, et al. (1992) have demonstrated that low concentrations of β-endorphin enhance NK activity in vivo. Thus, elevated β-endorphin levels may well reduce NK activity in vivo. It is also noteworthy that reduced NK activity (Nakazaki, 1992; Zanker & Kroczek, 1991) and elevated β-endorphin secretion have been found in patients with various malignant tumors (Kita et al., 1992; Pasi et al., 1991; Xu et al., 1993).

In summary, the research shows that acute stress reduces NK activity. In particular, if the acute stressors become prolonged, or chronic, they can lead to anxiety and worry. Additionally, when acute stress is repeated over and over again, it can become chronic, and these chronic stressors can result in major disruptions in one's life, inducing anxiety, chronic worry, and potentially depression, leading directly and indirectly (e.g., through sleep deprivation) to suppression of NK activity. These studies also suggest that stress reduces NK activity by increasing TNF-α and IL-1β production, decreasing IFN-γ production, inhibiting MHC class I and II molecule expression, and increasing β-endorphin secretion. Each of these stress-induced pathways is likely to exert an additive effect on NK activity, which would increase susceptibility to infections and cancer under such psychological conditions (as discussed later in this chapter).

Stress, NK Activity, and Cancer Progression

Studies have shown not only that NK cells have potent antitumor reactivity but also that they play a major role in the immune system's defense against the spread, or metastasis, of tumor cells from the original tissue or organ to other tissues or organs in the body (Whiteside & Herberman, 1994). A number of studies in laboratory animals have demonstrated that environmental stimuli—including stress or drugs such as alcohol or morphine—that suppress NK activity also cause an increase in cancer metastasis (Ben-Eliyahu et al., 1991; Ishihara et al., 1999; Page et al., 1994; Wu & Pruett, 1999).

For example, a study with rats conducted by Ben-Eliyahu et al. (1991) found that increased stress coincides with reduced NK activity, as well as with tumor progression. In this study, the acute stress was a heavy weight attached to the tail of a rat that was trying to swim. The effect of the additional stress on the rats' nervous systems decreased NK activity and caused a corresponding twofold increase in lung metastases.

In a more recent study, Volpe and colleagues (1999) pretreated mice with either of two types of anti-NK cell neutralizing antibodies and one type of anti-T-cell neutralizing antibodies 1 day prior to giving them an injection of tumor cells. Mice treated with either of the anti-NK neutralizing antibodies (anti-AsGM1 or anti-NK1.1) developed a "massive increase" in the number of hepatic tumor foci and decreased survival, compared with the control treated mice. Furthermore, although tumor cells were unable to colonize the liver of athymic nude mice (which have high levels of NK activity), pretreatment with anti-AsGM1 antibody abolished this resistance to metastases. Pretreatment with anti-T-cell (anti-Thy1.2) antibodies resulted in a significant decrease in the number of hepatic tumor foci, however, suggesting that T cells were not directly involved in resistance to tumor metastases.

In human studies, researchers have found a significant inverse correlation between levels of NK cell activity around the time of cancer diagnosis and the risk of developing disease recurrence or metastasis after the initial treatment of the cancer (Pross & Lotzova, 1993; Schantz & Ordonez, 1991). However, to date, these attempts to exploit this knowledge in clinical trials have proven unsatisfactory.

Although IL-2-activated NK cells have been used to treat nude mice with metastatic human cancer and have eliminated most, but not all, metastases and significantly prolonged survival (Okada et al., 1996), several analogous human clinical trials have shown benefit in only a small proportion of patients. Trials that have attempted to treat cancer by the upregulation of NK activity by using biological response modifiers also thus far have had only limited success (Whiteside et al., 1998).

To date, however, human clinical trials employing IL-2-activated NK cells have been confined largely to patients with advanced metastatic disease. It is quite likely that tumor-induced immunosuppression interferes with or limits the potential benefits of therapy using biological response modifiers (Lai et al., 1996) and that substantial levels of NK cell activation sufficient for metastasis elimination have seldom been achieved in these clinical trials.

Thus, research suggests that stress may affect the course of cancer by decreasing NK activity. In animal studies, even acute stress increased tumor spread by decreasing NK activity, and other factors that can cause short-term NK activity reduction can induce cancer metastasis. Although research on using IL-2-activated NK cells to treat cancer in animals is promising, trials in humans have not been as successful. For this reason, research has also focused on psychosocial factors that may help protect against the negative consequences of stress on NK activity, especially in cancer. This is the topic of the next section.

Psychosocial Factors and NK Activity

In the mid-1980s, Levy, Herberman, Maluish, and colleagues (1985) investigated the predictive power of NK activity and selected psychological and demographic factors on breast cancer status. This study found that NK activity reliably predicted the status of cancer spread to the axillary lymph nodes. Additionally, patients who had low levels of NK activity were rated as well adjusted to their illness, whereas patients who had higher NK activity appeared to be maladjusted or distressed. This seems counterintuitive, because one would assume that the well-adjusted patients would have higher levels of NK activity. This can be explained, however, by the observation in a later study by the same group (Levy, Herberman, Lippman, & d'Angelo, 1987) that patients rated as well adjusted reported lower family support and were more likely to give responses that were listless and apathetic. Therefore, the authors concluded that at early stages of the illness, appearing adjusted may reflect passive stoicism at a time when more active types of coping strategies might be more appropriate (Levy, Herberman, Lippman, & d'Angelo, 1987).

In several follow-up studies of women with breast cancer, Levy, Herberman, Whiteside, and colleagues (1990) found that a significant amount of NK activity variance could be explained by five variables. Specifically, higher NK activity could be predicted by (1) the perception of high-quality emotional support from a spouse or intimate other, (2) perceived social support from the patient's physician, (3) estrogen receptor-negative tumor status, (4) having an excisional biopsy as surgical treatment, and (5) actively seeking social support as a major coping strategy. In addition, the perceived quality of support accounted for a significant amount of NK activity variance (Levy, Herberman, Lee, et al., 1990).

In another study of 90 women with recently diagnosed stage I or stage II breast cancer, Levy, Herberman, Lippman, d'Angelo, and Lee (1991) showed that NK activity was a strong predictor of disease outcome when the outcome variable was defined as recurrence versus nonrecurrence of disease. Indeed, higher NK activity at follow-up predicted disease-free survival over the follow-up period. However, when the disease outcome variable was operationally defined as "time to recurrent disease," psychosocial factors were more strongly predictive of the rate of disease progression for those who had a recurrence, whereas NK cell activity was seemingly less relevant in this latter case.

These findings underscore the potential importance of social support in affecting NK activity and have led to a burgeoning field of research attempting to find psychosocial interventions that may help bolster NK activity, particularly in cancer patients. A number of studies of psychosocial interventions as complementary approaches to managing cancer patients suggest that such approaches can delay the recurrence of cancer, as well as increase survival times (see chapter 5).

Implications for the Study of Religion

A number of studies have established that religion provides many individuals with a greater sense of social support (see chapter 7), as well as improved coping skills (Bienenfeld et al., 1997; Koenig et al., 1998; Krause, 1998). Thus, the social support and coping aspects of religion provide a fertile ground for studying the link between religion and PNI.

For example, studies of psychological interventions that provided enhanced coping skills and social support in patients with breast cancer have shown that such interventions increase survival (Spiegel et al., 1989). Additionally, NK cell function has been shown to increase in patients with malignancy who have undergone psychological intervention programs designed to produce relaxation and greater ability to cope with the diagnosis of malignancy (Fawzy et al., 1990, 1993; Gruber et al., 1988). These studies also have demonstrated that increases in NK function, as a result of these interventions, correlated with a lower level of depression and anxiety. (See chapter 6 for a more detailed discussion of this literature.)

Because a major aspect of religious activities involves social support and coping skills and research shows that interventions that increase an individual's perception of social support enhance their ability to cope with stress, it is likely that religious activities may have an effect on NK activity, as well as on resistance to cancer progression. With the exception of Schaal and colleagues (1998; see chapter 1), very little research has directly addressed this topic.

NOTES

1. Cytokines are typically designated as IL (interleukin), IFN (interferon), TGF (transforming growth factor), or TNF (tumor necrosis factor), followed by a number (e.g., IL-6) or Greek letter (e.g., IFN-α), or both (e.g., IL-1β).
2. NK cells kill through two mechanisms. Similar to cytotoxic T cells, NK cells kill on contact. NK cells also contribute to the immune attack on virally infected and cancer cells by secreting high levels of influential lymphokines that activate other immune cells.

REFERENCES

Abraham, E. (1991). Effects of stress on cytokine production. *Methods and Achievements in Experimental Pathology* 14, 45–62.

Andrews, V., & Borkovec, T. D. (1988). The differential effects of inductions of worry, somatic anxiety, and depression on emotional experience. *Journal of Behavior Therapy and Experimental Psychiatry* 19, 21–26.

Antoni, M. H., August, S., LaPerriere, A., Baggett, H. L., Klimas, N., Ironson, G., Schneiderman, N., & Fletcher, M. A. (1990). Psychological and neuroendocrine measures related to functional immune changes in anticipation of HIV-1 serostatus notification. *Psychosomatic Medicine* 52, 496–510.

Arck, P. C., Merali, F. S., Manuel, J., Chaouat, G., & Clark, D. A. (1995). Stress-triggered abortion: Inhibition of protective suppression and promotion of tumor necrosis factor-alpha (TNF-alpha) release as a mechanism triggering resorptions in mice. *American Journal of Reproductive Immunology* 33, 74–80.

Ben-Eliyahu, S., Yirmiya, R., Liebeskind, J. C., Taylor, A. N., & Gale, R. P. (1991). Stress increases metastatic spread of a mammary tumor in rats: Evidence for mediation by the immune system. *Brain, Behavior, and Immunity* 5, 193–205.

Bienenfeld, D., Koenig, H. G., Larson, D. B., & Sherrill, K. A. (1997). Psychosocial predictors of mental health in a population of elderly women: Test of an explanatory model. *American Journal of Geriatric Psychiatry* 5, 43–53.

Birmaher, B., Rabin, B. S., Garcia, M. R., Jain, U., Whiteside, T. L., Williamson, D. E., al-Shabbout, M., Nelson, B. C., Dahl, R. E., & Ryan, N. D. (1994). Cellular immunity in depressed, conduct disorder, and normal adolescents: Role of adverse life events. *Journal of the American Academy of Child and Adolescent Psychiatry* 33, 671–678.

Brambilla, F., Bellodi, L., Perna, G., Bertani, A., Panerai, A., & Sacerdote, P. (1994). Plasma interleukin-1 beta concentrations in panic disorder. *Psychiatry Research* 54, 135–142.

Carr, D. J. (1991). The role of endogenous opioids and their receptors in the immune system. *Proceedings of the Society for Experimental Biology and Medicine* 198, 710–720.

Cohen, S., Tyrrell, D. A. J, & Smith, A. P. (1991). Psychological stress and susceptibility to the common cold. *New England Journal of Medicine* 325, 606–612.

Cohen, S., Tyrrell, D. A. J., & Smith A. P. (1993). Negative life events, perceived stress, negative affect, and susceptibility to the common cold. *Journal of Personality and Social Psychology* 64, 131–140.

Darko, D. F., Irwin, M. R., Risch, S. C., & Gillin, J. C. (1992). Plasma beta endorphin and natural killer cell activity in major depression: A preliminary study. *Psychiatry Research* 43, 111–119.

Darko, D. F., Risch, S. C., Gillin, J. C., & Goishan, S. (1992). Association of beta-endorphin with specific clinical symptoms of depression. *American Journal of Psychiatry* 149, 1162–1167.

Dobbin, I. P., Harth, M., McCain, G. A., Martin, R. A., & Cousin, K. (1991). Cytokine production and lymphocyte transformation during stress. *Brain, Behavior, and Immunity* 5, 339–348.

Fawzy, F. I., Fawzy, N. W., Hyun, C. S., Elashoff, R., Guthrie, D., Fahey, J. L., & Morton, D. L. (1993). Malignant melanoma: Effects of an early structured psychiatric intervention, coping, and affective state on recurrence and survival 6 years later. *Archives of General Psychiatry* 50, 681–689.

Fawzy, F. I., Kemeny, M. E., Fawzy, N. W., Elashoff, R., Morton, D., Cousins, N., & Fahey, J. L. (1990). A structured psychiatric intervention for cancer patients, II: Changes over time in immunological measures. *Archives of General Psychiatry* 47, 729–735.

Gerra, G., Volpi, R., Delsignore, R., Caccavari, R., Gagiotti, M. T., Montani, G., Maninetti, L., Chiodera, P., & Coiro, V. (1992). ACTH and beta-endorphin responses to physical exercise in adolescent women tested for anxiety and frustration. *Psychiatry Research* 41, 179–186.

Gruber, B. L., Hall, N. R., Hersh, S. P., & Dubois, P. (1988). Immune system and psychological changes in metastatic cancer patients using relaxation and guided imagery: A pilot study. *Scandinavian Journal of Behavior Therapy* 17, 25–46.

Hall, M., Baum, A., Buysse, D. J., Prigerson, H. G., Kupfer, D. J., & Reynolds, C. F. (1998). Sleep as a mediator of the stress-immune relationship. *Psychosomatic Medicine* 60, 48–51.

Irwin, M. (1999). Immune correlates of depression. *Advances in Experimental Medicine and Biology* 461, 1–24.

Irwin, M., Daniels, M., Bloom, E. T., Smith, T. L., & Weiner, H. (1987). Life events, depressive symptoms, and immune function. *American Journal of Psychiatry* 144, 437–441.

Ishihara, Y., Matsunaga, K., Iijima, H., Fujii, T., Oguchi, Y., & Kagawa, J. (1999). Time-dependent effects of stressor application on metastasis of tumor cells in the lung and its regulation by an immunomodulator in mice. *Psychoneuroendocrinology* 24, 713–726.

Kita, T., Kikuchi, Y., Oomori, K., & Nagata, I. (1992). Effects of opioid peptides on the tumoricidal activity of spleen cells from nude mice with or without tumors. *Cancer Detection and Prevention* 16, 211–214.

Koenig, H. G., Pargament, K. I., & Nielson, J. (1998). Religious coping and health status in medically ill hospitalized older adults. *Journal of Nervous and Mental Disease* 186, 513–521.

Krause, N. (1998). Stressors in highly valued roles, religious coping, and mortality. *Psychology and Aging* 13, 242–255.

Lai, P., Rabinowich, H., Crowley-Nowick, P. A., Bell, M. C., Mantovani, G., & Whiteside, T. L. (1996). Alterations in expression and function of signal-transducing proteins in tumor-associated T and natural killer cells in patients with ovarian carcinoma. *Clinical Cancer Research* 2, 161–173.

Levy, S. M, Herberman, R. B., Lee, J., Whiteside, T., Kirkwood, J., & McFeeley, S. (1990). Estrogen receptor concentration and social factors as predictors of natural killer cell activity in early-stage breast cancer patients: Confirmation of a model. *Natural Immunity and Cell Growth Regulation* 9, 313–324.

Levy, S., Herberman, R., Lippman, M., & D'Angelo, T. (1987). Correlation of stress factors with sustained suppression of natural killer cell activity and predictive prognosis in patients with breast cancer. *Journal of Clinical Oncology* 5, 348–353.

Levy, S. M, Herberman, R. B., Lippman, M., D'Angelo, T., & Lee, J. (1991). Immunological and psychosocial predictors of disease recurrence in patients with early-stage breast cancer. *Behavioral Medicine* 17, 67–75.

Levy, S. M, Herberman, R. B., Maluish, A. M., Schlien, B., & Lippman, M. (1985). Prognostic risk assessment in primary breast cancer by behavioral and immunological parameters. *Health Psychology* 4, 99–113.

Levy, S. M, Herberman, R. B., Whiteside, T., Sanzo, K., Lee, J., & Kirkwood, J. (1990). Perceived social support and tumor estrogen/progesterone receptor status as predictors of natural killer cell activity in breast cancer patients. *Psychosomatic Medicine* 52, 73–85.

Locke, S. E., Kraus, L., Leserman, J., Hurst, M. W., Heisel, J. S., & Williams, R. M. (1984). Life change stress, psychiatric symptoms, and natural killer cell activity. *Psychosomatic Medicine* 46, 441–453.

Minor, S. W., & Gold, S. R. (1985). Worry and emotionality components of test anxiety. *Journal of Personality Assessment* 49, 82–85.

Mobus, V. I., Asphal, W., Knapstein, P. G, & Kreienberg, R. (1993). Effects of interferon gamma on the proliferation and modulation of cell-surface structures of human ovarian carcinoma cell lines. *Journal of Cancer Research and Clinical Oncology* 120, 27–34.

Nakazaki, H. (1992). Preoperative and postoperative cytokines in patients with cancer. *Cancer* 70, 709–713.

Okada, K., Nannmark, U., Vujanovic, N. L., Watkins, S., Basse, P., Herberman, R. B., & Whiteside, T. L. (1996). Elimination of established liver metastases by human interleukin-2-activated natural killer cells after locoregional or systemic adoptive transfer. *Cancer Research* 56, 1599–1608.

Page, G. G., Ben-Eliyahu, S., & Liebeskind, J. C. (1994). The role of LGL/NK cells in surgery-induced promotion of metastasis and its attenuation by morphine. *Brain, Behavior, and Immunity* 8, 241–250.

Pasi, A., Amsler, U., & Messiha, F. S. (1991). Beta-endorphin-like immunoreactivity: Assessment of blood levels in patients with tumors of different origin. *Journal of Medicine* 22, 327–337.

Pross, H. F, & Lotzova, E. (1993). Role of natural killer cells in cancer. *Natural Immunity* 12, 279–292.

Rabin, B. S. (1999). *Stress, immune function, and health: The connection.* New York: Wiley.

Schaal, M. D., Sephton, S. E., Thoreson, C., Koopman, C., & Spiegel, D. (August 1998). Religious expression and immune competence in women with advanced cancer. Paper presented at the meeting of the American Psychological Association, San Francisco.

Schantz, S. P., & Ordonez, N. G. (1991). Quantitation of natural killer cell function and risk of metastatic poorly differentiated head and neck cancer. *Natural Immunity and Cell Growth Regulation* 10, 278–288.

Schedlowski, M., Huge, T., Richter, S., Tewes, U., Schmidt, R. E., & Wagner, T. O. (1995). Beta-endorphin, but not substance-P, is increased by acute stress in humans. *Psychoneuroendocrinology* 20, 103–110.

Schedlowski, M., Jacobs, R., Stratmann, G., Richter, S., Hadicke, A., Tewes, U., Wagner, T. O., & Schmidt, R. E. (1993). Changes of natural killer cells during acute psychological stress. *Journal of Clinical Immunology* 13, 119–126.

Segerstrom, S. C., Solomon, G. F., Kemeny, M. E, & Fahey, J. L. (1998). Relationship of worry to immune sequelae of the Northridge earthquake. *Journal of Behavioral Medicine* 21, 433–450.

Simpson, J. R., & Hoffman-Goetz, L. (1990). Exercise stress and murine natural killer cell function. *Proceedings of the Society for Experimental Biology and Medicine* 195, 129–135.

Sonnenfeld, G., Cunnick, J. E., Arnifield, A. V., Wood, P. G., & Rabin, B. S. (1992). Stress-induced alterations in interferon production and class II histocompatibility antigen expression. *Brain, Behavior, and Immunity* 6, 170–178.

Spiegel, D., Bloom, J. R., Kraemer, H. C., & Gottheil, E. (1989). Effect of psychosocial treatment on survival of patients with metastatic breast cancer. Lancet 2, no. 8668, 888–891.

Volpe, C. M., Mehta, N., Kim, U., Hordines, J., Doerr, R. J., & Cohen, S. A. (1999). AsGM1+ NK cells prevent metastasis of invading LD-MCA–38 tumor cells in the nude mouse. *Journal of Surgical Research* 84, 157–161.

Whiteside, T. L., & Herberman, R. B. (1994). Role of human natural killer cells in health and disease. *Clinical and Diagnostic Laboratory Immunology* 1, 125–133.

Whiteside, T. L., Vujanovic, N. L., & Herberman, R. B. (1998). Natural killer cells and tumor therapy. *Current Topics in Microbiology and Immunology* 230, 221–244.

Wu, W. J., & Pruett, S. B. (1999). Ethanol decreases host resistance to pulmonary metastases in a mouse model: Role of natural killer cells and the ethanol-induced stress response. *International Journal of Cancer* 82, 886–892.

Xu, C. T., Pan, B. R., & Wang, Y. M. (1993). Study on the peptides of serum and gastric juice in patients with gastric cancer. *Chung Hua I Hsueh Tsa Chih* (Taipei) 52, 32–35.

Yamaso, K., Shimada, Y., Sakaizumi, M., Soma, G., & Mizuno, D. (1992). Activation of the systemic production of tumor necrosis factor after exposure to acute stress. *European Cytokine Network* 3, 391–398.

Zalcman, S., Irwin, J., & Anisman, H. (1991). Stressor-induced alterations of natural killer cell activity and central catecholamines in mice. *Pharmacology, Biochemisty and Behavior* 39, 361–366.

Zanker, K. S., & Kroczek, R. (1991). Looking along the track of the psychoneuroimmunologic axis for missing links in cancer progression. *Journal of Sports Medicine* 12, S58-S62.

Zhu, G. F., Chancellor-Freeland, C., Berman, A. S., Kage, R., Leeman, S. E., Beller, D. I., Black, P. H. (1996). Endogenous substance P mediates cold water stress-induced increase in interleukin-6 secretion from peritoneal macrophages. *Journal of Neuroscience* 16, 3745–3752.

5

Psychosocial Interventions and Prognosis in Cancer

DAVID SPIEGEL & FAWZY I. FAWZY

Over the last 20 years, research in psycho-oncology has progressed through several important phases to provide clinicians with a framework for understanding and treating the psychological needs of cancer patients. In the initial phase, researchers used observations of the types of distress experienced by cancer patients to develop effective interventions to help with these problems. During this same period, there was growing evidence that both psychological and social factors play roles in the progression of cancer and survival time with cancer. Indeed, by the late 1980s and early 1990s, evidence emerged suggesting that certain negative psychological states can enhance the progression of cancer, whereas social connections and social support may slow its progression. More recently, studies have been conducted to identify mediating immune and endocrine mechanisms for these effects.

This chapter explores the impact of psychosocial variables on cancer recurrence and survival, as well as the evidence that psychosocial interventions can be used to affect the clinical course of this illness. It also examines the evidence that religion and spirituality, as elements of psychosocial support, have a role to play in the support, treatment, and prognosis of cancer patients.

Psychosocial Variables and Cancer Recurrence and Survival

During the late 1970s and early 1980s, descriptive studies began appearing in the literature, documenting both positive and negative psychological reactions of cancer patients (Holland, 1980). These studies also drew attention to the prevalence of psychiatric disorders, such as depression and anxiety, among this group (Derogatis et al., 1983). Most psychiatric disorders appeared to be the result of difficulties in adjusting to the diagnosis of cancer (Derogatis et al., 1983).

At about the same time, other studies suggested that the ability to successfully adjust to a cancer diagnosis could play a role in slowing the progression and/or increasing survival of cancer. For example, Greer et al. (1979) conducted a prospective 5-year study of 69 female patients with early-stage breast cancer and assessed their psychological responses to the diagnosis of cancer 3 months postoperatively. They found that women's psychological responses were related to their clinical outcome 5 years after their operation and that recurrence-free survival was significantly more common among patients who had initially reacted to cancer by denial or who had a "fighting spirit." In contrast, cancer recurrence was more common among women who had responded with stoic acceptance of their diagnosis or feelings of helplessness and hopelessness.

These early findings have been partially corroborated by a more recent study by Greer and colleagues (Watson et al., 1999) among a group of almost 600 early-stage breast cancer patients who were followed up for at least 5 years. This study reported a significantly increased risk of death from all causes in women with a high score on the depression subscale of the Hospital Anxiety and Depression Scale. Furthermore, there was a significantly increased risk of relapse or death at 5 years among women with high scores on the helplessness and hopelessness category of the Mental Adjustment to Cancer Scale, compared with those with a low score in this category. However, contrary to their earlier findings, the investigators found no significant effect of "fighting spirit" on relapse. This research team concluded that, for 5-year event-free survival, a high helplessness/ hopelessness score has a moderate but detrimental effect and a high score for depression is linked to a significantly reduced chance of survival. They noted, however, that this result was based on a relatively small number of patients and should be interpreted with caution.

Another important finding among early studies of psychosocial variables and cancer demonstrated that stress and mood disturbance also may have an adverse effect on disease outcome in cancer patients. Ramirez and colleagues (1989), for example, conducted a retrospective comparison of 50 recently relapsed breast cancer patients (i.e., their cancers were again active and growing) and 50 control patients who were in remission.

Subjects were matched for original diagnosis and disease status. This study found that relapsed patients had suffered significantly more severe adverse life events, but not minor ones. In fact, the frequency of severe adverse life events, such as family deaths or job loss, among the relapsed patients yielded an increased relative risk of relapse of 5.67 compared with nonrecurrent breast cancer patients.

Contradictory to the Ramirez finding, however, in a study involving a larger sample and a prospective design, Barraclough and colleagues (1992) found no relationship between severe life events and risk of relapse in a prospective study involving 204 women with breast cancer. However, consistent with the Ramirez study, Geyer (1991) found that among 97 women who presented with a breast lump for diagnosis, severe life events were significantly more common among those who later were confirmed to have a malignancy. Thus, two of three studies found a significant association between increased severe life stress and cancer relapse.

Social Support and Cancer

Social support also has been found to play a role in cancer progression and survival. Goodwin, Hunt, and colleagues (1987) found that cancer patients who were married had significantly better survival than unmarried patients. More recently, Reynolds and Kaplan (1990) found that women who were socially isolated had a substantially elevated risk for dying of cancer. In fact, those women in the study who had few social contacts and felt isolated had an almost fivefold increase in relative risk for mortality from hormone-related cancers and an almost twofold increase in incidence of smoking-related cancers. Men with few social connections had significantly poorer cancer survival rates as well.

The finding that marital status plays a role in cancer survival is supported by a more recent study by Maunsell and colleagues (1995), who examined the relationship between social support and mortality among 224 women with newly diagnosed breast cancer. This study found that married women had a relative death rate of 0.86 (i.e., a 14% reduced rate) compared with unmarried women over a 7-year follow-up. Furthermore, compared with women who had no confidants in the few months after surgery, those women who did have confidants had a relative death rate of 0.55 (a 45% reduced rate), and it was even lower among those who had more than one confidant. Thus, the availability of social support proved to be a robust predictor of subsequent mortality.

In addition to marriage, research suggests that other types of social support may play a role in protecting patients with cancer. For example, in a study involving 133 patients diagnosed with primary intraductal breast cancer, of whom 26 had died at 4-year follow-up and 38 had a recurrence, Hislop et al. (1987) and Waxler-Morrison and colleagues (1991) found that 6 of 11 measures of social relationships were significantly associated with longer survival. These six measures were (1) marital status; (2) support from friends; (3) contact with friends; (4) total support from friends, relatives, and neighbors; (5) employment status; and (6) social network size. In particular, expressive social activities and social support, not merely extroversion, were related to longer survival time. In other words, it was the quality, not the quantity, of social interactions that predicted longer survival time.

In a similar study, Ell and colleagues (1992) examined relationships between social support and survival following a diagnosis of breast, colorectal, or lung cancer. When the analysis was conducted, 74 of 294 patients had died, and the majority of the deceased subjects (57%) had been diagnosed with breast cancer. Emotional support appeared to have a protective influence in regard to survival for patients with earlier stages of disease, especially women with breast cancer. There was no effect with more advanced disease or among the smaller number of patients with lung or colorectal cancer.

This literature, therefore, suggests that the presence of social support, via marriage or close friendship, frequent daily contact with others, or the presence of confidants who can provide emotional support, reduces mortality risk from cancer.

Psychosocial Interventions for Cancer

Building upon such descriptive studies, subsequent research has focused on developing psychosocial "interventions" that might improve both psychological and physiological outcomes for cancer patients. Many of these interventions have four primary objectives: (1) to decrease feelings of alienation among patients by getting them to talk with others in a similar situation (e.g., support groups); (2) to reduce their anxiety about treatments, disease progression, and death; (3) to assist them in clarifying misperceptions and misinformation; and (4) to lessen their feelings of isolation, helplessness, and being neglected by others (Holland, 1982; Spiegel & Classen, 2000).

In one of the earliest published outcome studies in this field, Spiegel, Bloom, and Yalom (1981) conducted a randomized trial of supportive-expressive group therapy for women with metastatic breast cancer. Specifically, 50 of 86 women were randomly assigned to weekly support groups (the other 36 served as controls), which emphasized building strong supportive bonds, encouraging emotional expression, dealing directly with fears of dying and death, and reordering life priorities. The support group also helped the women to improve their relationships with family and friends, to enhance communication and shared problem solving with physicians, and to learn self-hypnosis for pain control. At 10-year follow-up (Spiegel, Bloom, Kraemer, et al, 1989), there was a statistically significant survival advantage—an average of 18 months—for women in the group therapy condition compared with the controls. Although there was no difference in median survival, by 48 months after the study had begun, all of the control patients had died, and a third of the group therapy patients were still alive.

Two other randomized trials also found a positive effect of psychosocial support on the rate of cancer progression. In the first trial, Richardson and colleagues (1990) reported on a home visiting and educational intervention, using a randomized, prospective design, among lymphoma and leukemia patients. Those patients who received the intervention adhered more strictly to their medical treatment, as measured by their usage of their prescribed medication (allopurinol). However, even when this difference in medication compliance was controlled for, the intervention patients lived significantly longer than controls. Similarly, in the second trial, Fawzy, Fawzy, and colleagues (1993) found a survival advantage among 40 patients with malignant melanoma who had been randomly assigned to just 6 weeks of intensive group psychotherapy, compared with 40 control patients who did not receive group psychotherapy. In addition to increased survival, those who received the intervention had lower rates of cancer recurrence than controls. This study also found, at 6-month follow-up, higher α-interferon-augmented NK cell activity among intervention patients than in controls. This difference did not predict recurrence or survival, however, although baseline NK cell activity did predict recurrence.

By contrast, several studies have looked for but failed to find any relationship between a psychosocial intervention and cancer survival. In one study, Gellert and colleagues (1993) compared subjects enrolled in the Exceptional Cancer Patient Program developed by Bernard Siegel (1986) with a matched sample of cancer patients who had undergone routine care. In this study, 102 cancer patients who took part in the Exceptional Cancer Patient Program were matched to 34 patients selected from local hospital tumor registries who had not participated. Patients were diagnosed between 1971 and 1980 and were followed until 1991. Program participants were matched to nonparticipants 3:1 on the basis of race, age at histological diagnosis (±2 years), stage of disease (localized, regional involvement, or distant), surgery (positive or negative history), and sequence of the malignancy (single primary cancer, primary cancer with one subsequent cancer, or secondary cancer with at least one previous cancer; Gellert et al., 1993). This study found no statistically significant relationship between cancer program participation and survival. Thus, it confirmed an earlier report from the same group (Morgenstern et al., 1984) showing that when time from initial diagnosis to study entry was controlled, there were no differences between treatment and control conditions.

Similarly, Linn et al. (1982) studied the effects of counseling on quality of life, level of physical functioning, and survival time in 120 men diagnosed with a range of cancer types, including lung, pancreatic, leukemia, and lymphoma. The aim of the counseling was to establish close relationships with the patients and their families. This closeness fostered open communication, which allowed the patients to experience greater trust in their counselors. The therapist helped the participants find meaning in their lives, share their feelings, plan for those they would leave behind at the time of their deaths, adopt a realistic view of their prognosis, and yet maintain a sense of hope. Most important, the therapist was intended to be a supportive presence, listening to the patient and serving as an understanding confidant. Members of the family would also take part in the counseling sessions when the patient chose.

At the conclusion of the study, however, no difference in survival between treatment and control groups was found. Functional status was also not affected, but quality of life did show a significant improvement for the treatment group. Linn et al. (1982) initially had hypothesized that if patients' quality of life improved, their physical functioning would also improve, thereby resulting in increased survival time. However, their subjects' disease had progressed to the point where, as the researchers said, any psychosocial intervention likely would have little or no effect on the body. In addition, there was a high attrition rate throughout this study due to patient death, and, consistent with the initial prognosis, virtually the entire sample died within the initial year of the study. This reduced the likelihood that any intervention would have an effect on survival time.

Ilnyckyj et al. (1994) conducted a randomized, prospective group psychotherapy trial in which 127 mixed-diagnosis (e.g., breast, lymphoma, colon, and ovarian) cancer patients were assigned to either a control group ($n = 31$) or one of three treatment groups: (1) a group ($n = 31$) that was professionally led, (2) a group ($n = 30$) that was professionally led for the first 3 months and then self-led for the remaining 3 months, and (3) a group ($n = 35$) that was self-led for the entire 6 months. An additional group of 21 patients was later admitted to the program and assigned to the unled group for the last 3 months of the intervention.

The groups that had professional leadership were run by a social worker with experience in facilitating groups. However, the social workers were not told to structure the groups by applying any specific therapeutic model; rather, they were encouraged to give information and be supportive. For the group without professional leadership, a social worker attended the first meeting to instruct them on logistics and to let them know that they could do anything they wanted during their meetings. All treatment groups met weekly for 60 minutes for 6 months. The psychological instruments that the researchers used measured depression, anxiety, and locus of control. These measures were administered prior to randomization and at regular intervals throughout the study.

This study did not produce any positive psychological or survival benefit. Ilnyckyj and colleagues postulated a number of possible explanations for such negative findings, including the heterogeneous composition of the groups (i.e., they had different types of cancer), the qualifications of the group leaders, the absence of the teaching of pain management techniques, and the high attrition rate (only 55% of the original 127 participants completed the study). They noted that the highest attrition rate was in the group without professional leadership. They also noted that those who withdrew from the study had a poorer prognosis and disease status, as well as more advanced disease progression. The high attrition in the unled groups, thus, may indicate that those participants were the most dissatisfied with the intervention.

Finally, Cunningham et al. (1998) conducted a study to examine the effects of a psychosocial intervention on mood, quality of life, and survival time among metastatic breast cancer patients. All 66 participants in this study received routine oncological care. However, the women were randomized to receive either an additional psychosocial intervention ($n = 30$) or no additional treatment ($n = 36$). The intervention consisted of three components: (1) 35 weekly group therapy sessions with the option to continue for an addition 15 sessions; (2) a 20-week, cognitive-behavioral homework assignment; and (3) an intensive workshop focused on coping skills, to be held over the course of one weekend.

Cunningham and colleagues found no effect of the intervention on either survival or psychosocial factors, with the exception of an increase in anxious preoccupation and a decrease in helplessness over time among the intervention group compared with the control group. However, a post hoc analysis showed that those study participants who attended outside support groups and/or the intervention provided by the investigators had a significantly longer survival time than all other participants. This study had a number of drawbacks, however, including a small sample, a brief and complex intervention, lack of psychological benefit, and sample selection issues that make it difficult to draw conclusions from it (Spiegel & Kraemer, 1999).

Thus, among investigations of a relationship between psychosocial interventions and cancer prognosis, three randomized, prospective studies found a survival difference favoring cancer patients given psychosocial treatment over controls, and one matching and three randomized studies did not show such a difference. Clearly, more research is needed, but these initial studies suggest a possible modulating effect of psychotherapeutic treatment on the course of cancer, as well as patient adjustment to it. Four major replication efforts are currently under way, testing the effect of supportive and/or expressive group therapy on the progression of metastatic breast cancer (Goodwin, Leszcz, et al., 1996; Spiegel, Sephton, et al., 1998; Kissane et al., 1998; Spiegel, Morrow, et al., 1999). Outcome results are expected in 2001–2002.

Psychosocial Interventions and Immune Status

The relationship between cancer growth and immune function is somewhat unclear. For example, it is not yet known whether observed changes in serum immune measures are caused by or are a result of changes in disease status. Some evidence suggests that tumor cells may evade and subvert immune mechanisms for their own survival. Thus, more severe tumors may be associated with greater suppression of immune mechanisms (Fawzy, Kemeny, et al., 1990; Sapolsky & Donnelly, 1985; Somers & Guillou, 1994; Spiegel, Sephton, et al., 1998).

Nevertheless, numerous immune mechanisms are likely to combat tumor growth, multiplication, and metastasis (Souberbielle & Dalgleish, 1994), and research in animals as well as humans suggests that immunosuppression may be a factor in the rate of disease progression (Bergsma, 1994; Sapolsky & Donnelly, 1985; Whiteside & Herberman, 1995). For example, there is now a general consensus that T cell–mediated immunity is of critical importance for rejection of solid tumors. Indeed, histological examination of breast tumors has revealed the presence of lymphocytes, suggesting immune influences on breast tumor growth. Furthermore, NK cells, although thought to have evolved mainly as antiviral cells, also appear to play an important role in tumor surveillance (Souberbielle & Dalgleish, 1994). These lymphocytes are able to kill tumor cells of many different types when tested either in vitro or in animal studies (Herberman, 1985; Trinchieri, 1989; Whiteside & Herberman, 1995; see chapter 4 in this volume for more details).

Several studies have found that psychosocial interventions can affect immune status in cancer patients. For example, Gruber et al. (1988) studied the effect of behavioral training (imagery and relaxation) on the immune systems of 10 adult patients with metastatic cancer. This study found that both immune and emotional changes paralleled the use of relaxation and imagery. Indeed, compared with their own baseline data, several measures of the subjects' immune system function were found to be significantly elevated over the course of 1 year. An examination of the subjects' psychological states also revealed increased aggression and greater internal locus of control as a result of the intervention.

In a follow-up study, Gruber et al. (1993) randomly assigned 13 patients with breast cancer either to an immediate-treatment group that received relaxation training, guided imagery, and biofeedback training or to a delayed-treatment control group. Pretreatment and posttreatment measures included blood samples, psychological testing, and a computerized psychophysiological stress evaluation. The results showed that the only psychological difference between pretreatment and posttreatment was in anxiety levels, which were reduced shortly after each group began the intervention. Nevertheless, several immune system parameters, including NK cell activity, mixed lymphocyte responsiveness, and the number of pe-

ripheral blood lymphocytes, were significantly improved and directly correlated with the behavioral interventions.

Stress, Endocrine Function, and Cancer Progression

Having a life-threatening illness such as cancer is a serious chronic stressor, and recent literature indicates that the hormones associated with the
stress response may mediate the progression of cancer. For example,
research suggests that chronic stress is associated with abnormalities of
cortisol, which can have a variety of adverse health effects (McEwen,
1998). Sephton and colleagues (2000) recently showed that loss of the
normal diurnal variation in cortisol (i.e., high in the morning, low in
the afternoon and evening) predicts earlier mortality from breast cancer
years later. Indeed, the loss of this normal cortisol variation was associated
with poorer marital status, poor sleep, and lower NK cell numbers and
cytotoxicity.

Another recent report demonstrates that a mutation in prostate cancer
cells renders them susceptible to growth stimulation by cortisol, which activates androgen receptors in the tumor (Zhao et al., 2000). Surgical stress
also has been shown to be immunosuppressive among breast cancer patients (Andersen et al., 1998). Thus, even minor variations in the way the
body responds to stress could have major negative health effects.

There is also some evidence that psychosocial treatment may ameliorate some of the body's stress response. Cruess and colleagues (2000), for
example, demonstrated that a cognitive-behavioral stress-management intervention reduced mean serum cortisol levels among women with early-
stage breast cancer. Thus, improving the response to stress may potentially
mediate the effect of psychosocial support on cancer progression.

Religion, Spirituality, and Cancer

Victor Frankl (1976/1959) said that "people can endure almost any 'what'
if they have a 'why,'" and there is evidence that a search for "why," or
meaning, is a critical aspect of people's adjustment to cancer (Spiegel,
1998; Yalom, 1980). Effective psychotherapies for cancer patients often
address existential issues, which include not only fear of dying and death,

but reexamining core issues of meaning in life in the context of the threat to survival (Spiegel & Glafkides, 1983).

Studies show that people diagnosed with cancer often turn to religion, among other factors, as a means of coping with and adjusting to their diagnosis (Jenkins & Pargament, 1988; Spilka et al., 1993). Indeed, Carver and colleagues (1993) assessed styles of coping among 59 recently diagnosed breast cancer patients and found that acceptance, positive reframing, and use of religion were the most common coping reactions, whereas denial and behavioral disengagement were the least common reactions. Furthermore, in a small study of a group of 41 mostly elderly, male patients with a wide variety of cancers, Wagner and colleagues (1995) found that two coping strategies in particular were related to a better quality of life in this group: (1) suppression of competing activities and (2) using religious practices.

A number of studies also have found significant relationships between religiousness and measures of adjustment, symptom management, or both in cancer patients. Strong religious beliefs have been related to decreased levels of pain, anxiety, hostility, and social isolation, as well as higher levels of life satisfaction in cancer patients (Acklin et al., 1983; Gibbs & Acterberg-Lawliss, 1978; Kaczorowski, 1989; Yates et al., 1981). In addition, related concepts, such as spiritual well-being, hope, and optimism, have been found to be related to better adjustment in cancer patients (Halstead & Fernsler, 1994; Jenkins & Pargament, 1995).

Fehring et al. (1997) conducted a study to determine the relationships among spiritual well-being, religiosity, hope, depression, and other mood states in 100 elderly people coping with cancer. This study also examined whether differences in hope, depression, and other mood states distinguished individuals with high intrinsic[1] religiosity and high spiritual well-being from those who scored lower on these two characteristics. The investigators found a consistent positive correlation among intrinsic religiosity, spiritual well-being, hope, and other *positive* mood states. In contrast, there was a consistent negative correlation between intrinsic religiosity and depression and other *negative* mood states. Analysis of variance indicated that significantly higher levels of hope and positive mood existed in patients with high levels of intrinsic religiosity and spiritual well-being. Based on these findings, the authors concluded that "intrinsic religiosity and spiritual well-being are associated with hope and positive mood states in elderly people coping with cancer."

Kaczorowski (1989) also found a consistent "inverse relationship" between better spiritual well-being and state-trait anxiety in 114 adults who had been diagnosed with cancer. Furthermore, this inverse relationship between higher levels of spiritual well-being and lower levels of anxiety in cancer patients held regardless of influences of gender, age, marital status, diagnosis, group participation, and length of time since diagnosis. According to Kaczorowski, this finding "supports the theory that persons with high levels of spiritual well-being have lower levels of anxiety."

Then again, not all research studies have found religion and spirituality to be related to better coping with and adjustment to cancer. Rifkin et al. (1999) recently tested the hypothesis that religious variables, such as a person's belief that his or her illness was God's will, would predict psychosocial adjustment in 50 patients who were predominantly Catholic Hispanic women attending a medical oncology clinic. The patients in this study were free from mental disorders, cognitive impairment, and severe pain and were not undergoing intensive chemotherapy. Using the Psychosocial Adjustment to Illness Scale as the outcome measure, the authors found few associations with religious variables, but many to clinical variables.

Thus, all religious and spiritual beliefs and practices may not be equal when it comes to facilitating adjustment in cancer patients. Some religious and spiritual factors (e.g., intrinsic religiosity, spiritual well-being) may facilitate adjustment and coping, whereas others (e.g., extrinsic religiosity) may inhibit adjustment and coping, and yet others may have little effect. Indeed, a recent literature review by Creagan (1997) that looked at the evidence for using psychosocial and spiritual factors in the management of cancer found that the literature is inconsistent and beset with major methodological problems. Nevertheless, Creagan concluded that a "social support system and an element of spirituality and religion seem to be the most consistent predictors of quality of life and possible survival among patients with advanced malignant disease."

Thus, the available evidence suggests that many religious and spiritual beliefs and practices may contribute to answering the "why" questions that cancer patients ask, as well as give them greater access to social support. In addition, having cancer may spur a search for meaning through religion and spirituality that can lead to emotional growth rather than decline (Spiegel, Bloom, & Yalom, 1981; Yalom, 1980). No studies have yet been done on the impact of religion and spirituality on clinical prognosis or long-term survival. However, based on findings that religion and spirituality can have an impact on coping and adjustment to cancer, may provide access to enhanced social support, and can reduce anxiety and, hence, stress, it is entirely possible that there will be some clinical benefit as well.

Conclusions

There is growing evidence that psychosocial factors play a role in cancer prognosis and that psychosocial interventions can be used effectively as adjunct therapies in the treatment of cancer patients. Although a number of questions remain as to whether religion and spirituality improve adjustment to cancer or influence survival time, there is some evidence to suggest that they do. People choose religious and spiritual support for a variety of important personal, family, and social reasons. Such recourse is important whether or not it can be shown to improve measures of coping or reduce disease progression. Nonetheless, there seems to be a convergence of evidence that factors involved in religious and spiritual belief, including meaning, purpose and hope in life, and social support, may have beneficial effects on how well and even how long people live with cancer.

NOTE

1. *Intrinsic religiosity* reflects a deep commitment to one's faith, which is reflected in an integration of religious beliefs and practices into one's life. In contrast, *extrinsic religiosity* is essentially utilitarian and involves the use of religion to reinforce one's social status or to justify one's way of life.

REFERENCES

Acklin, M. W., Brown, E. C., & Mauger, P. A. (1983). The role of religious values in coping with cancer. *Journal of Religion and Health* 22, 322–333.

Andersen, B. L., Farrar, W. B., Golden-Kreutz, D., Kutz, L. A., MacCallum, R., Courtney, M. E., & Glaser, R. (1998). Stress and immune responses after surgical treatment for regional breast cancer. *Journal of the National Cancer Institute* 90, 30–36.

Barraclough, J., Pinder, P., Cruddas, M., Osmond, C., Taylor, I., & Perry, M. (1992). Life events and breast cancer prognosis. *British Medical Journal* 304, 1078–1081.

Bergsma, J. (1994). Illness, the mind, and the body: Cancer and immunology: An introduction. *Theoretical Medicine* 15, 337–347.

Carver, C. S., Pozo, C., Harris, S. D., Noriega, V., Scheier, M. F., Robinson, D. S., Ketcham, A. S., Moffat, F. L. Jr., & Clark, K. C. (1993). How coping mediates the effect of optimism on distress: A study of women with early stage breast cancer. *Journal of Personality and Social Psychology* 65, 375–390.

Creagan, E. T. (1997). Attitude and disposition: Do they make a difference in cancer survival? *Mayo Clinic Proceedings* 72, 160–164.

Cruess, D. G., Antoni, M. H., McGregor, B. A., Kilbourn, K. M., Boyers, A. E., Alferi, S. M., Carver, C. S., & Kumar, M. (2000). Cognitive-behavioral stress management reduces serum cortisol by enhancing benefit finding among women being treated for early stage breast cancer. *Psychosomatic Medicine* 62, 304–308.

Cunningham, A. J., Edmonds, C. V. I., Jenkins, G. P., Pollack, H., Lockwood, G. A., & Warr, D. (1998). A randomized controlled trial of the effects of group psychological therapy on survival in women with metastatic breast cancer. *Psycho-Oncology* 7, 508–517.

Derogatis, L. R., Morrow, G. R., Fetting, J., Penman, D., Piasetsky, S., Schmale, A. M., Henrichs, M., & Carnicke, C. L., Jr. (1983) The prevalence of psychiatric disorders among cancer patients. *Journal of the American Medical Association* 249, 751–757.

Ell, K., Nishimoto, R., Mediansky, L., Mantell, J., & Harnovitch, M. (1992) Social relations, social support and survival among patients with cancer. *Journal of Psychosomatic Research* 36, 531–541.

Fawzy, F. I., Fawzy, N. W., Hyun, C. S., Elashoff, R., Guthrie, D., Fahey, J. L., & Morton, D. L. (1993). Malignant melanoma. Effects of an early structured psychiatric intervention, coping, and affective state on recurrence and survival 6 years later. *Archives of General Psychiatry* 50, 681–689.

Fawzy, F. I., Kemeny, M. E., Fawzy, N. W., Elashoff, R., Morton, D., Cousins, N., & Fahey, J. L. (1990). A structured psychiatric intervention for cancer patients. II. Changes over time in immunological measures. *Archives of General Psychiatry* 47, 729–735.

Fehring, R. J., Miller, J. R., & Shaw, C. I. (1997). Spiritual well-being, religiosity, hope, depression, and other mood states in elderly people coping with cancer. *Oncology Nursing Forum* 24, 663–671.

Frankl, V. E. (1976/1959). *Man's search for meaning*. New York: Pocket.

Gellert, G. A., Maxwell, R. M., & Siegel, B. S. (1993). Survival of breast cancer patients receiving adjunctive psychosocial support therapy: A 10-year follow-up study. *Journal of Clinical Oncology* 11, 66–69.

Geyer, S. (1991). Life events prior to manifestation of breast cancer: A limited prospective study covering eight years before diagnosis. *Journal of Psychosomatic Research* 35, 355–363.

Gibbs, H. W., & Achterberg-Lawliss, J. (1978). Spiritual values and death anxiety: Implications for counseling with terminal cancer patients. *Journal of Counseling Psychology* 25, 563–569.

Goodwin, J. S., Hunt, W. C., Key, C. R., & Samet, J. M. (1987). The effect of marital status on stage, treatment, and survival of cancer patients. *Journal of the American Medical Association* 258, 3125–3130.

Goodwin, P. J., Leszcz, M., Koopmans, J., Arnold, A., Doll, R., Chochinov, H., Navarro, M., Butler, K., & Pritchard, K. I. (1996). Randomized trial of group psychosocial support in metastatic breast cancer: The BEST study. Breast-Expressive Supportive Therapy study. *Cancer Treatment Reviews* 22 (Suppl A), 91–96.

Greer, S., Morris, T., & Pettingale, K. W. (1979). Psychological response to breast cancer: Effect on outcome. *Lancet* 2(8146), 785–787.

Gruber, B., Hersh, S., Hall, N., Waletzky, L., Kunz, J., Carpenter, J., Kverno, K., & Weiss, S. (1993). Immunological responses of breast cancer patients to behavioral interventions. *Biofeedback and Self-Regulation* 18, 1–22.

Gruber, B. L., Hall, N. R., Hersh, S. P., & Dubois, P. (1988). Immune system and psychological changes in metastatic cancer patients using relaxation and guided imagery: A pilot study. *Scandinavian Journal of Behavior Therapy* 17, 25–46.

Halstead, M. T., & Fernsler, J. I. (1994). Coping strategies of long-term cancer survivors. *Cancer Nursing* 17, 94–100.

Herberman, R. (1985). Natural killer cells: Characteristics and possible role in resistance against tumor growth. In A. E. Reif & M. S. Mitchell (Eds.), *Immunity to cancer*. San Diego: Academic.

Hislop, T. G, Waxler, N. E., Coloman, A. I., Elwood, J. M., & Kan, L. (1987). The prognostic significance of psychosocial factors in women with breast cancer. *Journal of Chronic Diseases* 40, 729–735.

Holland, J. C., & Mastrovito, R. (1980) Psychologic adaptation to breast cancer. *Cancer* 46(4 Suppl), 1045–1052.

Ilnyckyj, A., Farber, J., Cheang, M., & Weinerman, B. (1994). A randomized controlled trial of psychotherapeutic intervention in cancer patients. *Annals of the Royal College of Physicians and Surgeons of Canada* 27, 93–96.

Jenkins, R. A., & Pargament, K. I. (1988). Cognitive appraisals and psychological adjustment in cancer patients. *Social Science and Medicine* 23, 286–196.

Jenkins, R. A., & Pargament, K. I. (1995). Religion and spirituality as resources for coping with cancer. Special Issue: Psychosocial resource variables in cancer studies: Conceptual and measurement issues. *Journal of Psychosocial Oncology* 13, 51–74.

Kaczorowski, J. M. (1989). Spiritual well-being and anxiety in adults diagnosed with cancer. *Hospital Journal* 5, 105–116.

Kissane, D. W., Clarke, D. M., Ikin, J., Bloch, S., Smith, G. C., Vitetta, L., & McKenzie, D. P. (1998). Psychological morbidity and quality of life in Australian women with early-stage breast cancer: A cross-sectional survey. *Medical Journal of Australia* 169, 192–196.

Linn, M. W., Linn, B. S., & Harris, R. (1982). Effects of counseling for late stage cancer. *Cancer* 49, 1048–1055.

Maunsell, E., Jacques, B., & Descrenes, L. (1995). Social support and survival among women with breast cancer. *Cancer* 76, 631–637.

McEwen, B.S. (1998). Protective and damaging effects of stress mediators. *New England Journal of Medicine* 338, 171–179.

Morgenstern, H., Gellert, C. A., Walter, S. D., Osteeld, A. M., & Siegel, B. S. (1984). The impact of a psychosocial support program on survival with breast cancer: The importance of selection bias in program evaluation. *Journal of Chronic Diseases* 37, 273–282.

Ramirez, A. J., Craig, T. K., Watson, J. P., Fentiman, I. S., North, W. R., Rubens, R. D. (1989). Stress and relapse of breast cancer. *British Medical Journal* 298, 291–293.

Reynolds, P., & Kaplan, G. A. (1990). Social connections and risk for cancer: Prospective evidence from the Alameda County Study. *Behavioral Medicine* 16, 101–110.

Richardson, I. L., Shelton, D. R., Krailo, M., & Levine, A. M. (1990). The effect of compliance with treatment on survival among patients with hematologic malignancies. *Journal of Clinical Oncology* 8, 356–364.

Rifkin, A., Doddi, S., Karagji, B., & Pollack, S. (1999). Religious and other predictors of psychosocial adjustment in cancer patients. *Psychosomatics* 40, 251–256.

Sapolsky, R. M., & Donnelly, T. M. (1985). Vulnerability to stress-induced tumor growth increases with age in rats: Role of glucocorticoids. *Endocrinology* 117, 662–666.

Sephton, S. E., Sapolsky, R. M., Kraemer, H. C., & Spiegel, D. (2000). Diurnal cortisol rhythm as a predictor of breast cancer survival. *Journal of the National Cancer Institute* 92, 994–1000.

Siegel, B. (1986). *Love, medicine and miracles.* New York: Harper & Row.

Somers, S., & Guillou, P. J. (1994). Tumour cell strategies for escaping immune control: Implications for psychoimmunotherapy. In C. E. Lewis, C. E. O'Sullivan, & J. Barraclough (Eds.), *The psychoimmunology of cancer: Mind and body in the fight for survival?* New York: Oxford University Press.

Souberbielle, B., & Dagleish, A. (1994). Anti-tumor immune mechanisms. In C.E. Lewis, C. O'Sullivan, & J. Barraclough (Eds.), *The psychoimmunology of cancer: Mind and body in the fight for survival?* New York: Oxford University Press.

Spiegel, D. (1998). Getting there is half the fun: Relating happiness to health. *Psychological Inquiry* 9, 66–68.

Spiegel, D., Bloom, J. R., Kraemer, H. C., & Gottheil, E. (1989). Effect of psychosocial treatment on survival of patients with metastatic breast cancer. *Lancet* 2(8668), 888–891.

Spiegel, D., Bloom, J. R., & Yalom, I. (1981). Group support for patients with metastatic cancer: A randomized outcome study. *Archives of General Psychiatry* 38, 527–533.

Spiegel, D., & Classen, C. (2000). *Group therapy for cancer patients: A research-based handbook of psychosocial care.* New York: Basic Books.

Spiegel, D., & Glafkides, M. C. (1983). Effects of group confrontation with death and dying. *International Journal of Group Psychotherapy* 33, 433–447.

Spiegel, D., & Kraemer, H. K. (1999). Cunning but careless: Analysis of a non-replication. *Psycho-Oncology* 8, 273–274.

Spiegel, D., Morrow, G. R., Classen, C., Raubertas, R., Stott, P. B., Mudaliar, N., Pierce, H. I., Flynn, P. J., Heard, L., & Riggs, G. (1999) Group psychotherapy for recently diagnosed breast cancer patients: A multicenter feasibility study. *Psycho-Oncology,* in press.

Spiegel, D., Sephton, S., Terr, A., & Stites, D. (1998). Effects of psychosocial treatment. In S. McCann, J. Lipton, E. Sternberg, G. Chrousos, P. Gold, & C. Smith (Eds.), *Prolonging cancer survival may be mediated by neuroimmune pathways in neuroimmunomodulation: Molecular aspects, integrative systems, and clinical advances.* New York: New York Academy of Sciences.

Spilka, B., Ladd, K., & David, J. (1993). *Religion and coping with breast cancer: Possible roles of prayer and forms of personal health.* Technical report. Atlanta: American Cancer Society.

Trinchieri, G. (1989). Biology of natural killer cells. *Advances in Immunology* 47, 187–376.

Wagner, M. K., Armstrong, D., & Laughlin, J. E. (1995). Cognitive determinants of quality of life after onset of cancer. *Psychological Reports* 77, 147–154.

Watson, M., Haviland, J. S., Greer, S., Davidson, J., & Bliss, J. M. (1999). Influence of psychological response on survival in breast cancer: A population-based cohort study. Lancet 354, 1331–1336.

Waxler-Morrison, N., Hislop, T. G., Mears, B., & Kan, L. (1991). Effects of social relationships on survival for women with breast cancer: A prospective study. *Social Science and Medicine* 33, 177–183.

Whiteside, T. L., & Herberman, R. 1995. The role of natural killer cells in immune surveillance of cancer. *Current Opinion in Immunology* 7, 704–710.

Yalom, I. D. (1980). *Existential psychotherapy.* New York: Basic Books.

Yates, J. W., Chalmer, B. J., St. James, P., Follansbee, M., & McKegney, F. P. (1981). Religion in patients with advanced cancer. *Medical and Pediatric Oncology* 9, 121–128.

Zhao, X.-Y., Malloy, P. J., Krishnan, A. V., Swami, S., Navone, N. M., Peehl, D. M., & Feldman, D. (2000). Glucocorticoids can promote androgen-independent growth of prostate cancer cells through a mutated androgen receptor. *Nature Medicine* 6, 703–706.

6

Psychosocial Stress, Social Networks, and Susceptibility to Infection

SHELDON COHEN

During the past several decades, support has grown for the premise that psychological and social factors can influence physical health. This includes evidence that enduring stressful life events and prolonged negative moods (e.g., depression, anxiety, anger) can increase risk for physical illness and early death (e.g., reviews by Booth-Kewley & Friedman, 1987; Cohen & Williamson, 1991; Schneiderman et al., 1989). It also includes evidence that those who participate in diverse social networks that include family, friends, workmates, neighbors, and fellow members of social and religious groups live longer and healthier lives than their less socially adept counterparts (e.g., Berkman & Syme, 1979; House et al., 1988; Vogt et al., 1992).

My own interests in this area have focused on the potential impact of psychological and social factors on the immune system, and consequently on our ability to fight off infectious disease. Here I begin by providing a selective overview of the evidence for the effects of psychosocial factors on the functional capabilities of the immune system. I then discuss similar data linking these same factors to the onset and progression of infectious disease. I provide only cursory reviews and refer the reader to Cohen and Herbert (1996), Cohen, Miller, et al. (2001), and Herbert and Cohen

(1993a, 1993b) for more detailed treatments. Finally, I suggest implications of this literature for understanding the role that religious participation might play in health.

Psychological Stress and Immunity

Over the last 15 years, dozens of studies have shown that stressful situations in people's lives are associated with alterations in immune function (see meta-analysis in Herbert & Cohen, 1993b). An example of this literature is a series of studies of the consequences of medical school examinations for cellular immune function reported by Glaser, Kiecolt-Glaser, and colleagues (e.g., Glaser, Pearson, Bonneau, et al., 1993; Glaser, Pearson, Jones, et al., 1991; Kiecolt-Glaser, Garner, et al., 1984). In these studies, medical students had their psychological stress responses and immune responses assessed during a low-stress baseline period (e.g., just following vacation) and again during a series of important exams. Students reported more stress during exams and showed a decrease in the function of cellular immune responses, including decreased NK activity, lymphocyte proliferation, and increased antibody to herpesviruses.

Chronic stressful events that last for a longer term (e.g., months or even years) have similar potential to influence the immune system. One example is the set of studies that assessed stress effects on residents of the area surrounding the Three Mile Island (TMI) nuclear power plant. TMI was the site of a serious accident in 1979 that released nuclear materials into the surrounding environment, and the level of distress among area residents remained quite high afterward (Baum et al., 1983). In fact, almost 10 years after the accident, McKinnon et al. (1989) found higher numbers of neutrophils and fewer B cells, suppressor/cytotoxic T cells, and NK cells in TMI residents than in demographically matched control subjects living in another area. They also found more antibody to herpesviruses in TMI residents, which suggests lower cellular immune competence.

Another chronic stressful event, providing care for Alzheimer's patients, has been associated with elevated levels of herpes antibodies (a marker of cellular immune suppression) (Kiecolt-Glaser & Glaser, 1987), and less production of antibody in response to an influenza immunization (Glaser, Kiecolt-Glaser, Malarkey, et al., 1998; Kiecolt-Glaser, Glaser, Gravenstein, et al., 1966).

Mood and Immunity

The effects of psychological stress on immunity are generally thought to be mediated by stress-elicited increases in negative mood. In turn, negative mood might trigger the release of immune-altering hormones, such as epinephrine, norepinephrine, and cortisol, or influence behaviors that might directly influence immune tissue, such as increased drinking and smoking and loss of sleep. Consequently, it is not surprising that the associations between negative moods and immunity generally parallel the psychological stress literature. For example, in nonclinical samples—that is, people who are not being treated for medical disorders—depressed mood is associated with decreased proliferative responses to mitogens (substances used to stimulate immune cell division) and decreased NK activity (see meta-analysis by Herbert & Cohen, 1993a). Moreover, similar (in quality) but more profound associations are found for clinically depressed patients.

Although it has received considerably less attention, anxiety appears to be associated with immune changes as well. For example, an anxious mood has been associated with decreased natural killer (NK) cell activity (Locke et al., 1984) and decreased proliferative response to both phytohemagglutinin (PHA) and concanavalin-A (Con-A), two commonly used laboratory mitogens (Linn, Linn, & Jensen, 1981).

Only a few studies have examined the association of positive mood states with immune outcomes. One daily diary study examined the relation between positive and negative mood states and antibody response to an orally ingested novel antigen over 8 weeks (Stone, Cox, et al., 1987). Antibody levels were higher on days when respondents reported high positive mood states and lower on days when they reported high negative mood states. These results were replicated in a subsequent study that monitored mood and antibody levels over a 12-week period (Stone, Neale, et al. 1994).

In two experimental studies, positive and negative affective states were induced in healthy subjects, and subsequent acute changes in immunity were documented. For example, Knapp et al. (1992) had subjects recall positive and negative experiences to induce "positive" and "negative" mood states. Both positive and negative moods were associated with decreased proliferative responses to PHA and increased numbers of neutrophils. Similar immune effects of positive and negative moods were attributed to the fact that all subjects reported increased levels of excitement (arousal) during the mood inductions, regardless of the direction, or valence, of the mood.

Futterman et al. (1994) used actors reading written scenarios that depicted four different emotional states—(1) high arousal with positive mood, (2) high arousal with negative mood, (3) low arousal with positive mood, and (4) low arousal with negative—to induce these mood states in experimental subjects. Although NK activity was not associated with mood condition, lymphocyte proliferation did increase following positive moods and decreased following negative moods.

Thus, different moods may be associated with different immune responses. Clear interpretation of this work is impeded by lack of consensus on the dimensions on which mood should be classified. However, existing work suggests that the dimensions of valence and arousal may be important ones in relating moods to immune function.

Psychological States and Susceptibility to Infection

Invasion of the body by a disease-causing agent is not sufficient cause for disease. Rather, disease occurs when the host's defenses are compromised or unable to recognize the foreign material as posing a threat. Therefore, psychological variables that influence immunity have the potential to influence the onset and progression of immune system–mediated diseases. What is less clear is whether psychologically induced changes in immunity are of the magnitude or type that would alter the ability of the body to fight disease (Cohen & Williamson, 1991; Laudenslager, 1987; O'Leary, 1990).

The following discussion is limited to studies that address the role of psychological factors in the onset and progression of upper respiratory viruses and herpesvirus. Chapter 8 contains a detailed discussion of the role of stress and related psychological barriers in human immunodeficiency virus (HIV) infection.

Upper Respiratory Infections

Early prospective work by Meyer and Haggerty (1962) indicated that both disruptive daily events and chronic family stress were associated with greater risk for upper respiratory infections. Similar results were reported by Graham et al. (1986), who collected measures of life stress from members of 94 families before and during a 6-month period in which diary data on subjects' respiratory symptoms also were collected daily. Illness episodes were validated by nose and throat cultures. Although high- and low-stress groups were almost identical with respect to demographics and health practices, the high-stress groups experienced more verified episodes of illness and more days with symptoms of respiratory illness.

In a study of susceptibility to influenza, Clover and colleagues (1989) assessed family relationships and individual stressful life events of 246 individuals in 58 families prior to the start of flu season. This study found that "stressed" families (i.e., those living in a rigid and chaotic environment) had a greater incidence of disease than nonstressed families (i.e., those living in a more "balanced," harmonious environment). Illness was not related to individual stressful life events in this study.

One might easily argue that the increased incidence of upper respiratory infections in individuals under stress in these studies may be attributable to stress-induced increases in exposure to infectious agents rather than to stress-induced immunosuppression. However, three recent viral-challenge trials suggest otherwise.

In a study of 394 volunteers, Cohen, Tyrrell, and Smith (1991, 1993) administered measures of stressful life events, perceived stress, and negative affect just before intentionally exposing subjects to one of five viruses that cause upper respiratory infections, better known as the common cold. We were interested in whether reports of stress could predict who would become ill. Only about 40% of exposed subjects develop colds, and all three stress measures predicted the probability of developing a cold, with greater stress linearly related to greater risk. Moreover, the relationships that we reported between increased stress and greater susceptibility to infection were found consistently across five different upper respiratory viruses. These results could not be explained by stress-elicited differences in health practices, such as smoking and alcohol consumption, or in the numbers of various white blood cell populations or total (nonspecific) antibody levels.

In another viral-challenge study, Stone, Bovbjerg, and colleagues (1992) replicated the relation between stressful life events and susceptibility to upper respiratory infections reported in Cohen, Tyrrell, and Smith (1991). Additionally, in a more recent study, Cohen, Frank, et al. (1998) demonstrated that although chronic stress predicted susceptibility to upper respiratory infections, acute stress did not. In this study, we administered a "life stressor" interview and psychological questionnaires to 276 volunteers and also collected blood and urine samples from this group. We then inoculated the volunteers with common cold viruses and monitored them for the onset of disease. Although severe acute stressful life events (less than 1 month long) were not associated with developing colds with exposure to a virus, severe chronic stressors (1 month or longer) were associated with a substantial increase in risk of disease. This relation was attributable primarily to underemployment or unemployment and to enduring interpersonal difficulties with family or friends. Interestingly, this study found that the association between chronic stressors and susceptibility to colds could not be fully explained by differences among stressed and nonstressed persons in social network characteristics, personality, health practices, or prechallenge endocrine or immune measures.

In another set of studies, we focused on psychological predictors of disease severity (rather than episode onset). We found that state (but not trait) negative affect measured just prior to viral exposure was associated with more severe colds and influenza, as measured by the amount of mucus produced over the course of the illness (Cohen, Doyle, Skoner, Fireman, et al., 1995). Another study focusing on the acute stress reported at the time of viral inoculation produced similar results. Indeed, those reporting greater stress had more severe illnesses after infection by an influenza virus (Cohen, Doyle, & Skoner, 1999). Moreover, the expression of illness symptoms was highly interrelated with the release of too much of a chemical messenger (IL-6, a pro-inflammatory cytokine). IL-6 is released as part of the immune system response to infection (see chapter 3). A stress-induced failure to "turn off" the release of this cytokine might be responsible for the increased severity of illness for those reporting more stress.

In sum, both stressful life events and psychological stress (perceptions and negative affect) are associated with increased susceptibility to upper respiratory infection. These effects are not generally explicable in terms of stress-elicited changes in health behaviors. Moreover, initial evidence suggests that these associations might occur because stress is associated with a dysregulation of immune response.

Herpes Simplex Virus Infection

Herpesviruses are thought to be responsible for cold sores, genital lesions, infectious mononucleosis and mononucleosis syndrome, and deafness in newborn infants (Kiecolt-Glaser & Glaser, 1987). Herpesviruses differ from most other known viruses in that after exposure, they are present in individuals all the time, although often in latent states. A robust cellular immune response plays a key role both in protection from initial herpes-virus infection and in keeping latent herpesviruses from becoming active (Glaser & Gotlieb-Stematsky, 1982).

Is stress associated with a recurrence of clinical disease (lesions) after a period of herpsvirus latency? A study of 125 college students provides an elegant test of the role of stress in herpes recurrence (Hoon et al., 1991). This work indicates that stress increases vulnerability to illness in general (nonherpes) and that it is this increase in nonspecific vulnerability that re-sults in herpes recurrence. Although Hoon and colleagues did not address the physiological basis (e.g., cellular immunity) for this nonspecific vul-nerability, they did find that the illness vulnerability measure was heavily influenced by highly prevalent infectious diseases (colds and influenza). Thus, an immune basis for this increased herpes recurrence is plausible.

The relationship between increased stress and increased susceptibility to herpes infection and recurrence is also supported by a series of studies of student nurses conducted in the 1970s. In these studies, negative moods at the beginning of the school year were generally associated with greater numbers of subsequent episodes of verified oral herpes (Friedmann et al., 1977, Katcher et al., 1973; Luborsky et al., 1976). Similar evidence for stress-induced recurrence is provided by both retrospective (e.g., Kemeny et al., 1989) and prospective studies of genital herpes (Goldmeier & John-son, 1982; McLarnon & Kaloupek, 1988; see critiques in Cohen & Williamson, 1991).

In sum, herpes studies generally support a relation between negative emotional states, including stress, and disease recurrence. However, the ev-idence is not entirely consistent, and methodological limitations warrant cautious interpretation of these results. Moreover, existing work does not establish the extent to which such effects are mediated through immune or behavioral pathways.

Social Relationships and Immunity

Substantial evidence implicates interpersonal relationships in the mainte-nance of health (Cohen, 1988; House et al., 1988). This is a heterogeneous literature with studies of a wide range of relationship concepts. These include whether or not one is involved in a relationship (e.g., marriage) or in multiple relationships (e.g., marriage, friendship, group member), whether they have a satisfactory marriage, whether they feel lonely, and whether they perceive that other people will provide them with social support when they need it. I provide only a short overview of social relationship research on immunity here, but refer the reader to Cohen, Underwood, and Gottlieb (2000) for detailed discussions of these concepts and the pathways through which they might influence health and to Cohen (1988), Cohen and Herbert (1996), Kiecolt-Glaser and Newton (in press), and Uchino et al. (1996) for reviews of this literature.

Probably the most provocative studies are a series of prospective community studies that show that people with diverse social networks—including spouse, friends, family members, neighbors, and fellow members of social and religious groups—suffer less illness and live longer than their more isolated counterparts (see reviews by Cohen, Gottlieb, & Underwood, 2000; House et al., 1988). The association between network diversity and mortality is extremely reliable among whites but is less clear among minority populations and more important for men than for women (House et al., 1988). There is no evidence at this time that the association between network diversity, morbidity, and mortality reported in the epidemiological literature can be explained in terms of the effects of social networks on the immune system.

One pathway through which the lack of social ties might influence health is through feelings of loneliness. In turn, the negative affective states triggered by loneliness, including depression and anxiety (Peplau & Perlman, 1982), might influence immunity. Several studies have examined the correlation between loneliness and immunity. For example, in their studies of first-year medical students, Kiecolt-Glaser and Glaser (Glaser, Kiecolt-Glaser, Speicher, et al., 1985; Kiecolt-Glaser, Garner, et al., 1984) found that persons higher in self-reported loneliness had lower NK activity and higher levels of herpesvirus antibody than those who described themselves as less lonely. In a related study, lonelier psychiatric inpatients had poorer NK cell function and lower proliferative responses to PHA than did patients who reported less loneliness (Kiecolt-Glaser, Ricker, et al., 1984b).

There is also substantial evidence that the loss of intimate social ties, especially marital disruptions (separation and divorce) are associated with poorer health (Verbrugge, 1979). In regard to marital discord and immunity, Kiecolt-Glaser, Fisher, and colleagues (1987) found that among 16 separated and divorced women there were higher levels of herpes anti-body, a lower percentage of NK cells, and lower lymphocyte proliferative response to PHA and Con-A than among a comparison group of 16 married women. In a similar study, Kiecolt-Glaser, Kennedy, and colleagues (1988) found that among 32 separated and divorced men there were more infectious illnesses and higher levels of herpes antibody than among their 32 married counterparts. Social conflicts with spouses have also been found to influence immune response. For example, a study that categorized newlywed couples on the basis of observed interactions (Kiecolt-Glaser, Malarkey, et al., 1993) found that those who exhibited more negative or hostile behaviors showed greater decreases over 24 hours in NK activity and proliferative response to PHA and Con-A.

Perceived availability of social support has also been associated with immune function. In a study of 256 elderly adults, Thomas and colleagues (1985) found that persons who reported they had "confiding" relationships had greater proliferative responses to PHA than those without confiding relationships. Moreover, this relationship was unchanged after controlling for psychological distress and health practices. Similar results were found in a study by Baron and colleagues (1990) among 23 spouses of patients with cancer. In this study, six different provisions of social support (including emotional and instrumental forms of support) were associated with higher NK activity and better proliferative response to PHA (but not to Con-A). Better immune response among "supported" persons could not be explained by greater depression or more numerous stressful life events among those with less social support.

In addition, Glaser, Kiecolt-Glaser, Bonneau, and colleagues (1992) found that medical students who reported more available social support produced more antibody in response to a hepatitis B vaccination than those reporting less support. However, two studies of HIV-positive men were less successful in establishing relations between social support and immunity (Goodkin et al., 1992; Perry et al., 1992). However, HIV infection compromises the immune system to a degree so severe that the relatively small effects of social support on immune function might be undetectable.

It is likely that many of the beneficial effects of social support on health can be attributed to the receipt of or perceived availability of emotional support—that is, someone to talk to about problems (Cohen & Wills, 1985). Indeed, studies examining the potential health benefits associated with a person's disclosure of traumatic events have found a positive relationship between the opportunity to disclose and better health indices. For example, Pennebaker and colleagues (1988) assigned 50 healthy under-graduates to write about either personal and traumatic events or trivial topics. They wrote for 20 minutes a day on 4 consecutive days. Immuno-logic data were collected before the study began (baseline), at the end of the intervention, and at 6-week and 4-month follow-ups.

This study found that blood drawn from subjects who wrote about traumatic events was more responsive to PHA (but not Con-A) than that from subjects who wrote about trivial events. There were no relations be-tween disclosure and alcohol intake, caffeine intake, or exercise over the course of the study. In addition, subjects revealing traumatic events made fewer visits to the health center in the 6 weeks following the intervention than did members of the control group. However, the data do not support an immune pathway because the lymphocyte proliferation data were *not* correlated with health center visits. This absence of correlation also sug-gests that increases in health center visits may be driven by psychological influences on decision processes rather than by influences on actual illness (Cohen & Williamson, 1991). Another effect of the disclosure interven-tion on immunity was found by Petrie and colleagues (1995). In this study, subjects who disclosed produced more antibody in response to sec-ondary immunization for hepatitis B than control subjects. Finally, a re-cent article has demonstrated associations between the disclosure manip-ulation and two diseases thought to be at least partly attributable to immune dysregulation (Smyth et al., 1999). Asthma patients who wrote about their problems had better lung function over the following 4 months than nontreatment controls. Rheumatoid arthritis patients who completed the intervention similarly demonstrated relative reduction in disease activity over the following 4 months in comparison with controls.

There have also been five studies of mortality in which cancer patients were randomly assigned either to social support groups in which they dis-cussed their feelings with other patients or to standard care control groups. Two of these studies found that group participation was associated with better disease outcomes (Fawzy et al., 1993; Spiegel et al., 1989), and three found no differences (Cunningham et al., 1998; Illnyckyj et al., 1994; Linn, Linn, & Harris, 1982). (See chapter 5 for more details on this literature.) Although we have only a tentative understanding of the condi-tions under which such groups might improve health or how they work (Cohen, Gottlieb, & Underwood, 2000; Helgeson & Gottlieb, 2000), this research illustrates that under certain circumstances—that are not yet en-

tirely clear—providing both psychological and social support can benefi-
cially affect the course of physical illness.

Social Relationships and Susceptibility to Infection

More direct evidence for the role of social relationships on immune functioning comes from studies of susceptibility to upper respiratory infections. Using the same paradigm as we used in our studies of psychological
stress and susceptibility to infection, Cohen, Doyle, Skoner, Rabin, et al.
(1997) recently assessed whether diverse ties to friends, family, work, and
community are associated with increased host resistance to infection. In
this study, a total of 276 healthy volunteers were assessed on the extent of
their participation in 12 types of social ties (spouse, parent, friend, work-
mate, member of social group, and others) and were then given nasal drops
containing one of two rhinoviruses and monitored for the development of
a common cold.

This study found that participants with more types of, or more diverse,
social ties were less susceptible to common colds (by either type of virus)
and when they did catch colds, they produced less mucus, were more effective in ciliary clearance of their nasal passages, and shed less virus than
those participants with fewer types of social ties. The participants' susceptibility to colds decreased in a dose-response manner with increased diversity of the social network. In fact, persons with the fewest social ties (1 to
3) had a 4.2 times greater adjusted relative risk of catching a cold than
those with the most (6 or more) types of social ties.

Interestingly, in a recent animal study, Cohen, Line, et al. (1997) found
that in Old World monkeys social status and not social stress was the factor most responsible for increasing susceptibility to viral infection. In this
study, we randomly assigned 60 male cynomolgus monkeys to either a
"stable" or "unstable" social (stress) condition for 15 months. Two markers of social status—social rank and percentage of behaviors that were
submissive—also were assessed at independent observation periods over
a 14-month period. Endocrine, immune, and behavioral responses were
each assessed (at 3-month intervals) during the ninth through fourteenth
months of the study. At the beginning of the fifteenth month, all animals
were exposed to a virus (adenovirus) that causes a common cold-like
illness.

Although the social instability manipulation was associated with increased agonistic behavior, as indicated by minor injuries and elevated norepinephrine responses to the unstable social condition, the manipulation did not influence the probability of being infected by the virus. However, low social status (as assessed by either marker) was associated with a substantially greater probability of being infected. It was also associated with less body weight, greater elevated cortisol responses to social reorganizations, and less aggressive behavior. None of these characteristics could account for the relation between social status and infection.

Religious Participation and Health

The most accepted association in the area of religion and health is that religious activities such as church attendance are associated with low morbidity and mortality (Ellison & Levin, 1998; McCullough et al., 2000; Oman & Reed, 1998). Specifically, prospective studies have found that greater frequency of attendance at religious services is associated with lower blood pressure, lower cause-specific mortality for coronary artery disease, lower incidence of physical disability, and lower all-cause mortality. An immune marker of ongoing inflammatory processes (the pro-inflammatory cytokine IL-6) has also been found to be lower among those who attend church more often (Koenig et al., 1997). Nevertheless, cautions have been raised in regard to methodological limitations of this literature and the fact that the effects often occur in some but not all subpopulations (Sloan et al., 1999).

The issue for this chapter is whether what we know about the role of stress and social relationships from research in health psychology, social epidemiology, and human psychoneuroimmunology can help us understand how and under what conditions religious participation might influence immune-related health. We suggest that there are two categories of pathways through which religious participation might influence health: (1) religious participation can contribute to the diversity of one's social network, enhancing beneficial cognitive and affective states, as well as promoting behaviors that benefit health, and (2) religious participation can provide the potential for reducing stress via the availability of coping resources.

We have discussed the provocative evidence that people with more diverse social networks live longer and healthier lives. In the realm of immune response, having a more diverse network (e.g., a spouse, children, friends, workmates, and fellow social and religious group members) is associated with greater resistance to infectious agents. Several possible reasons explain why those who participate in a diverse social network are healthier (Cohen, 1988; Cohen, Underwood, & Gottlieb, 2000; Uchino et al., 1996), and four of them are discussed here.

1. Being subject to social controls and peer pressures may influence normative health behaviors. For example, people's social networks might influence whether they exercise, consume alcohol, eat low-fat diets, or smoke.

2. Being integrated in a social network may provide a source of generalized positive affect, senses of predictability and stability, a sense of purpose, a sense of belonging and security, and a recognition of self-worth because of demonstrated ability to meet normative role expectations (Cassel, 1976; Hammer, 1981; Thoits, 1983; Wills, 1985). These positive psychological states are thought to be beneficial because they reduce psychological despair (Thoits, 1985) and result in greater motivation to care for oneself (e.g., Cohen & Syme, 1985).

3. Having a wide range of network ties provides multiple sources of information and thereby increases the probability of having access to an appropriate information source. Information could influence health-relevant behaviors or help one avoid or minimize stressful or other high-risk situations.

4. A social network may provide tangible and economic services that result in better health and better health care for network members. For example, network members could provide food, clothing, and housing that operate to prevent disease and limit exposure to risk factors.

In the case of stress buffering, social support can operate by preventing responses to stressful events that are inimical to health (Cohen, 1988; Cohen, Underwood, & Gottlieb, 2000; Cohen & Wills, 1985). Support may play a role at two different points in the causal chain that links stressors to illness (cf. Cohen & McKay, 1984; House, 1981). First, the belief that others will provide necessary resources may redefine the potential for harm posed by a situation and bolster one's perceived ability to cope with imposed demands, thereby preventing a particular situation from being appraised as highly stressful (Thoits, 1986). Second, support beliefs may reduce or eliminate the affective reaction to a stressful event, dampen physiological response to the event, or prevent or alter maladaptive behavior responses. The availability of persons to talk to about problems has also been found to reduce the intrusive thoughts that act to maintain chronic maladaptive responses to stressful events (Lepore et al., 1996).

The actual receipt of support in the face of stressful events could also play a role. Support may alleviate the impact of stress appraisal by providing a solution to the problem, by reducing the perceived importance of the problem, or by providing a distraction from the problem. It might also facilitate healthful behaviors such as exercise, personal hygiene, proper nutrition, rest, or adherence to medical regimens (cf. House, 1981; Cohen & Wills, 1985).

Participating in religious groups has the potential to influence all of these same mechanisms. In fact, in his summary of potential mechanisms that link religion to health, Pargament (1990) included reducing anxiety; enhancing the sense of meaning and purpose in life; and fostering personal growth, mastery, and control as possible explanations. He also included religious associations and beliefs as resources for coping with stress (e.g., Pargament, 1990, 1997; Pargament et al., 1990). Similarly, Ellison and Levin's (1998) list of mechanisms linking religion to health included regulation of health behaviors, promotion of positive self-perceptions, generation of positive emotions, and provision of social and coping resources.

One possibility is that religious participation is no different from other forms of social participation. In essence, being an active member of a church would be no different from being an active member of a bowling league or book club. In both cases, the other members of the group would be sources of recognition of self-worth, of information, of emotional and tangible resources, and so forth.

Alternatively, there could be something unique about religious participation. There are a number of possibilities here. One is that, for many, religious identification is a central social role with greater importance than others. It often involves greater commitment of time and a stronger identification with the beliefs and social norms of the group. For example, one would expect that, on the average, the health-relevant social norms of a religious group would have a greater impact on behavior than the consensual norms of fellow bowlers.

The breadth of social norms provided by religious identifications also may be major sources of structure, predictability, and purpose in life.

Moreover, religious groups often accept helping one another as a central assumption of their beliefs. In consequence, they might be more likely to provide support in time of need. Religious beliefs might play a role here as well. The stronger their beliefs, the greater their commitment would be to the group, and the greater the effects of the group on their behavior and affect. Finally, religious organizations may serve as an access point where individuals make contacts with other social domains, such as business, social, or recreational groups. Thus church attendance might have a synergistic effect on the size and diversity of a network and the resources it might provide (Ellison & George, 1994).

Evidence that religious participation enhances social resources is reported in data from large community samples. Bradley (1995) and Ellison and George (1994) report that frequent churchgoers have larger social networks, more contact with network members, more types of social support received, and more favorable perceptions of the quality of their social relationships than do nonmembers. These data are consistent with the hypothesis that churches may serve as an access point to other social domains but might also indicate self-selection of persons with interpersonal skills into church membership. In fact, Bradley (1995) found an overrepresentation of extroverted individuals and an underrepresentation of more neurotic persons among regular churchgoers.

In sum, belonging to a religious group should provide one with the same benefits of participating in any social domain. Moreover, certain characteristics of religious participation suggest that religious groups may be more effective at providing these benefits than other domains and that they may facilitate access to other social domains as well. However, the relative efficacy of religious participation in affecting health is not yet established, nor is it clear yet whether religious participation influences access to other social resources. Future research addressing these issues is imperative.

Moreover, this research should pay special attention to variables that might moderate the importance of church membership, such as individual commitment to the religious group and to its beliefs. The salience of norms for everyday living that contribute to feelings of self-esteem and self-control and of norms for a behavioral style that enhance health should be greatest among the more committed. Other potential important variables to consider include gender and physical well-being. Religious participation has been found to be more important for women than for men and for people who are ill than for those who are well (cf. Sloan et al., 1999). This is probably because women are more committed to their participation, and religion gains a new importance for those who are ill. Again, assessment of individual commitment might help clarify these data.

Finally, new work should also pay special attention to the geographic area under study—its overall rate of religious participation and of religious belief and commitment. Certainly, the extent to which the religious groups' norms are also the community norms should enhance their effectiveness.

Conclusions

There is growing evidence that psychological stress and social factors including network diversity and perceived availability of social support influence immunity and immune system–mediated disease. There also is substantial evidence that these factors can influence both cellular and humoral indicators of immune status and function, and, at least in the case of the less serious infectious diseases (colds, influenza, herpes), there is consistent and convincing evidence of links between stress and disease onset and progression.

A noteworthy aspect of this literature is the importance of participation in social networks for maintaining health and preventing and recovering from disease. These effects occur either through direct psychological and biological influences of our social contacts or through the buffering effects of these contacts when we face stressful life events. We argue in this chapter that the same mechanisms that link our relationships in other social domains to health are likely to link participation in religious organizations to health. Moreover, we suggest the possibility that religious participation may be an especially important social domain in relation to health.

ACKNOWLEDGMENTS

I would like to thank the Pittsburgh Mind-Body Center (HL65111 & HL65112) and the John D. and Catherine T. MacArthur Foundation Network on Socioeconomic Status and Health for their support. My participation was supported by a Senior Scientist Award from the NIMH (MH00721).

REFERENCES

Baron, R. S., Cutrona, C. E., Hicklin, D., Russell, D. W., & Lubaroff, D. M. (1990). Social support and immune function among spouses of cancer patients. *Journal of Personality and Social Psychology* 59, 344–352.

Baum, A., Gatchel, R. J., & Schaeffer, M. A. (1983). Emotional, behavioral, and physiological effects of chronic stress at Three Mile Island. *Journal of Consulting and Clinical Psychology* 51, 565–572.

Berkman, L. F., & Syme, S. L. (1979). Social networks, host resistance, and mortality. *American Journal of Epidemiology* 109, 186–204.

Booth-Kewley, S., & Friedman, H. S. (1987). Psychological predictors of heart disease: A quantitative review. *Psychological Bulletin* 101, 342–362.

Bradley, D. E. (1995). Religious involvement and social resources: Evidence from the data set, "Americans' Changing Lives." *Journal of the Scientific Study of Religion* 34, 259–267.

Cassel, J. (1976). The contribution of the social environment to host resistance: The Fourth Wade Hampton Frost Lecture. *American Journal of Epidemiology* 104, 107–123.

Clover, R. D., Abell, T., Becker, L. A., Crawford, S., & Ramsey, J. C. N. (1989). Family functioning and stress as predictors of influenza B infection. *Journal of Family Practice* 28, 535–539.

Cohen, S. (1988). Psychosocial models of the role of social support in the etiology of physical disease. *Health Psychology* 7, 269–297.

Cohen, S., Doyle, W. J., & Skoner, D. P. 1999. Psychological stress, cytokine production, and severity of upper respiratory symptoms. *Psychosomatic Medicine* 61, 175–180.

Cohen, S., Doyle, W. J., Skoner, D. P., Fireman, P., Gwaltney, J. M., Jr., & Newsom, J. T. (1995). State and trait negative affect as predictors of objective and subjective symptoms of respiratory viral infections. *Journal of Personality and Social Psychology* 68, 159–169.

Cohen, S., Doyle, W. J., Skoner, D. P., Rabin, B. S., & Gwaltney, J. M., Jr. (1997). Social ties and susceptibility to the common cold. *Journal of the American Medical Association* 277, 1940–1944.

Cohen, S., Frank, E., Doyle, W. J., Skoner, D. P., Rabin, B. S., & Gwaltney, J. M., Jr. (1998). Types of stressors that increase susceptibility to the common cold in healthy adults. *Health Psychology* 17, 214–223.

Cohen, S., & Herbert, T. B. (1996). Health psychology: Psychological factors and physical disease from the perspective of human psychoneuroimmunology. In J. T. Spence, J. M. Darley, & D. J. Foss (Eds.), *Annual review of psychology*, vol. 47. El Camino, CA: Annual Review, Inc.

Cohen, S., Line, S., Manuck, S. B., Rabin, B. S., Heise, E. R., & Kaplan, J. R. (1997). Chronic social stress, social status, and susceptibility to upper respiratory infections in nonhuman primates. *Psychosomatic Medicine* 59, 213–221.

Cohen, S., & McKay, G. (1984). Social support, stress, and the buffering hypothesis: A theoretical analysis. In A. Baum, J. E. Singer, & S. E. Taylor (Eds.), *Handbook of psychology and health*, vol. 4. Hillsdale, NJ: Erlbaum.

Cohen, S., Miller, G. E., & Rabin, B. S. (2001). Psychological stress and antibody response to antigenic challenge: A review. *Psychosomatic Medicine* 63, 7–18.

Cohen, S., & Syme, S. L. (1985). Issues in the study and application of social support. In S. Cohen & S. L. Syme (Eds.), *Social support and health*. New York: Academic.

Cohen, S., Tyrrell, D. A. J., & Smith, A. P. (1991). Psychological stress and susceptibility to the common cold. *New England Journal of Medicine* 325, 606–612.

Cohen, S., Tyrrell, D. A. J., & Smith, A. P. (1993). Negative life events, perceived stress, negative affect, and susceptibility to the common cold. *Journal of Personality and Social Psychology* 64, 131–40.

Cohen, S., Underwood, L. G., & Gottlieb, B. H. (Eds.). (2000). *Social support measurement and intervention*. New York: Oxford University Press.

Cohen, S., & Williamson, G. M. (1988). Perceived stress in a probability sample of the United States. In S. Spacapan & S. Oskamp (Eds.), *The social psychology of health*. Newbury CA: Sage.

Cohen, S., & Williamson, G. M. (1991). Stress and infectious disease in humans. *Psychological Bulletin* 109, 5–24.

Cohen, S., & Wills, T. A. (1985). Stress, social support, and the buffering hypothesis. *Psychological Bulletin* 109, 310–357.

Cunningham, A. J., Edmonds, C. V., Jenkins, G. P., Pollack, H., Lockwood, G. A., & Warr, D. (1998). A randomized controlled trial of the effects of group psychological therapy on survival in women with metastatic breast cancer. *Psycho-Oncology* 7, 508–517.

Ellison, C. G., & George, L. K. (1994). Religious involvement, social ties, and social support in a Southeastern community. *Journal of the Scientific Study of Religion* 33, 46–61.

Ellison, C. G., & Levin, J. S. (1998). The religion-health connection: Evidence, theory, and future directions. *Health Education and Behavior* 25, 700–720.

Fawzy, F. I., Fawzy, N. W., Hyun, C. S., Elashoff, R., Guthrie, D., Fahey, J. L., & Morton, D. L. (1993). Malignant melanoma: Effects of an early structured psychiatric intervention, coping, and affective state on recurrence and survival 6 years later. *Archives of General Psychiatry* 50, 681–689.

Friedmann, E., Katcher, A. H., & Brightman, V. J. (1977). Incidence of recurrent herpes labialis and upper respiratory infection: A prospective study of the influence of biologic, social and psychologic predictors. *Oral Surgery, Oral Medicine, and Oral Pathology* 43, 873–878.

Futterman, A. D., Kemeny, M. E., Shapiro, D., & Fahey, J. L. (1994). Immuno-logical and physiological changes associated with induced positive and nega-tive mood. *Psychosomatic Medicine* 56, 499–511.

Glaser, R., & Gottlieb-Stematsky, T. E. (1982). *Human herpesvirus infections: Clinical aspects.* New York: Marcel Dekker.

Glaser, R., Kiecolt-Glaser, J. K., Bonneau, R. H., Malarkey, W., Kennedy, S., & Hughes, J. (1992). Stress-induced modulation of immune response to re-combinant hepatitis B vaccine. *Psychsomatic Medicine* 54, 22–29.

Glaser, R., Kiecolt-Glaser, J. K., Malarkey, W. B., & Sheridan, J. F. (1998). The in-fluence of psychological stress on the immune response to vaccines. *Annals of the New York Academy of Science* 840, 649–655.

Glaser, R., Kiecolt-Glaser, J. K., Speicher, C. E., & Holliday, J. E. (1985). Stress, loneliness, and changes in herpesvirus latency. *Journal of Behavioral Medicine* 8, 249–260.

Glaser, R., Pearson, G. R., Bonneau, R. H., Esterling, B. A., Atkinson, C., & Kiecolt-Glaser, J. K. (1993). Stress and the memory T-cell response to the Epstein-Barr virus in healthy medical students. *Health Psychology* 12, 435–442.

Glaser, R., Pearson, G. R., Jones, J. F., Hillhouse, J., Kennedy, S., Mao, H. Y., Kiecolt-Glaser, J. K. (1991). Stress-related activation of Epstein-Barr virus. *Brain, Behavior, and Immunity* 5, 219–232.

Goldmeier, D., & Johnson, A. (1982). Does psychiatric illness affect the re-currence rate of genital herpes? *British Journal of Venereal Disease* 54, 40–43.

Goodkin, K., Blaney, N. T., Feaster, D., Fletcher, M. A., & Baum, A. (1992). Ac-tive coping style is associated with natural killer cell cytotoxicity in asympto-matic HIV-1 seropositive homosexual men. *Journal of Psychosomatic Re-search* 36, 635–650.

Graham, N. M. H, Douglas, R. B, & Ryan, P. 1986. Stress and acute respiratory infection. *American Journal of Epidemiology* 124, 389–401.

Hammer, M. (1981). Social supports, social networks, and schizophrenia. *Schiz-ophrenia Bulletin* 7, 45–57.

Helgeson, V. S., & Gottlieb, B. H. (2000). Support groups. In S. Cohen, L. G. Un-derwood, & B. H. Gottlieb (Eds.), *Social support measurement and interven-tion.* New York: Academic.

Herbert, T. B., & Cohen, S. (1993a). Depression and immunity: A meta-analytic review. *Psychological Bulletin* 113, 472–486.

Herbert, T. B, & Cohen, S. (1993b). Stress and immunity in humans: A meta-an-alytic review. *Psychosomatic Medicine* 55, 364–379.

Hoon, E. F., Hoon, P. W., Rand, K. H., Johnson, I., Hall, N. R., & Edwards, N. B. (1991). A psycho-behavioral model of genital herpes recurrence. *Journal of Psychosomatic Research* 35, 25–36.

House, J. S. (1981). *Work, stress, and social support*. Reading, MA: Addison-Wesley.

House, J. S., Landis, K. R., & Umberson, D. (1988). Social relationships and health. *Science* 241, 540–545.

Illnyckyj, A., Farber, J., Cheang, M., & Weinerman, B. (1994). A randomized controlled trial of psychotherapeutic intervention in cancer patients. *Annals of the Royal College of Physicians and Surgeons of Canada* 27, 93–96.

Katcher, A. H., Brightman, V. J., Luborsky, L., & Ship, I. (1973). Prediction of the incidence of recurrent herpes labialis and systemic illness from psychological measures. *Journal of Dental Research* 52, 49–58.

Kemeny, M. E., Cohen, F., & Zegens, L. (1989). Psychological and immunological predictors of genital herpes recurrence. *Psychosomatic Medicine* 51, 195–208.

Kiecolt-Glaser, J. K., Fisher, L. D., Ogrocki, P., Stout, J. C., Speicher, C. E, & Glaser, R. (1987). Marital quality, marital disruption, and immune function. *Psychosomatic Medicine* 49, 13–34.

Kiecolt-Glaser, J. K., Garner, W., Speicher, C. E., Penn, G. M., Holiday, J., & Glaser, R. 1984. Psychosocial modifiers of immunocompetence in medical students. *Psychosomatic Medicine* 46, 7–14.

Kiecolt-Glaser, J. K., & Glaser, R. (1987). Psychosocial influences on herpes virus latency. In E. Kurstak, Z. J. Lipowski, & P. V. Morozov (Eds.), *Viruses, immunity, and mental disorders*. New York: Plenum.

Kiecolt-Glaser, J. K., Glaser, R., Gravenstein, S., Malarkey, W. B., & Sheridan, J. F. (1966). Chronic stress alters the immune response to influenza virus vaccine in older adults. *Proceedings of the National Academy of Science* 93, 3043–3047.

Kiecolt-Glaser, J. K., Glaser, R., Shuttleworth, E. C., Dyer, C. S., Ogrocki, P., & Speicher, C. E. (1987). Chronic stress and immunity in family caregivers of Alzheimer's disease victims. *Psychosomatic Medicine* 49, 523–535.

Kiecolt-Glaser, J. K., Kennedy, S., Malkoff, S., Fisher, L., Speicher, C. E., & Glaser, R. 1988. Marital discord and immunity in males. *Psychosomatic Medicine* 50, 213–229.

Kiecolt-Glaser, J. K., Malarkey, W. B., Chee, M., Newton, T., & Cacioppo, J. T. (1993). Negative behavior during marital conflict is associated with immunological down-regulation. *Psychosomatic Medicine* 55, 395–409.

Kiecolt-Glaser, J. K., & Newton, T. (in press). Marriage and health: His and hers. *Psychological Bulletin*.

Kiecolt-Glaser, J. K., Ricker, D., George, J., Messick, G., Speicher, C. E., Garner, W., & Glaser, R. (1984). Urinary cortisol levels, cellular immunocompetency, and loneliness in psychiatric inpatients. *Psychosomatic Medicine* 46, 15–23.

Knapp, P. H., Levy, E. M., Giorgi, R. G., Black, P. H., Fox, B. H., & Heeren, T. C. (1992). Short-term immunological effects of induced emotion. *Psychosomatic Medicine* 54, 133–148.

Koenig, H. G., Cohen, H. J., George, L. K., Hays, J. C., Larson, D. B., & Blazer, D. G. (1997). Attendance at religious services, interleukin-6, and other biological parameters of immune function in older adults. *International Journal of Psychiatry in Medicine* 27, 233–250.

Laudenslager, M. L. (1987). Psychosocial stress and susceptibility to infectious disease. In E. Kurstak, Z. J. Lipowski, & P. Y. Morozov (Eds.), *Viruses, immunity and mental disorders*. New York: Plenum.

Lepore, S. J., Silver, R. C., Wortman, C. B., & Wayment, H. A. (1996). Social constraints, intrusive thoughts, and depressive symptoms among bereaved mothers. *Journal of Personality and Social Psychology* 70, 271–282.

Linn, B. S., Lin, M. W., & Jensen, J. (1981). Anxiety and immune responsiveness. *Psychology Reports* 49, 969–970.

Linn, M. W., Linn, B. S., & Harris, R (1982). Effects of counseling for late stage cancer patients. *Cancer* 49, 1048–1055.

Locke, S. E., Kraus, L., Leserman, J., Hurst, M. W., Heise,l J. S., & Williams, R. M. (1984). Life change stress, psychiatric symptoms, and natural killer cell activity. *Psychosomatic Medicine* 46, 441–453.

Luborsky, L., Mintz, J., Brightman, V. J., & Katcher, A. H. 1976. Herpes simplex virus and moods: A longitudinal study. *Journal of Psychosomatic Research* 20, 543–548.

McCullough, M. E., Hoyt, W. T., Larson, D. B., Koenig, H. G., & Thoresen, C. (2000). Religious involvement and mortality: A meta-analytic review. *Health Psychology* 19, 211–222.

McKinnon, W., Weisse, C. S., Reynolds, C. P., Bowles, C. A., & Baum, A. (1989). Chronic stress, leukocyte subpopulations, and humoral response to latent viruses. *Health Psychology* 8, 389–402.

McLarnon, L. D,, & Kaloupek, D. O. (1988). Psychological investigation of genital herpes recurrence: Prospective assessment and cognitive-behavioral intervention for a chronic physical disorder. *Health Psychology* 7, 231–249.

Meyer, R. J, & Haggerty, R. J. (1962). Streptococcal infections in families. *Pediatrics* 29, 539–549.

O'Leary, A. (1990). Stress, emotion, and human immune function. *Psychological Bulletin* 108, 363–382.

Oman, D., & Reed, D. (1998). Religion and mortality among the community-dwelling elderly. *American Journal of Public Health* 88, 1469–1475.

Pargament, K. I. (1990). God help me (II): Toward a theoretical framework of coping for the psychology of religion. *Research in the Social Scientific Study of Religion* 51, 195–224.

Pargament, K. I. (1997). *The psychology of religion and coping: Theory, research, practice*. New York: Guilford.

Pargament, K. I., Ensing, D. S., Falgout, K., Olsen, B., Van Haitsma, K., & Warren, R. (1990). God help me. I: Religious coping efforts as predictors of the outcomes to significant negative life events. *American Journal of Community Psychology* 18, 793–824.

Pennebaker, J. W., & Beau, S. K. (1986). Confronting a traumatic event: Toward an understanding of inhibition and disease. *Journal of Abnormal Psychology* 95, 274–281.

Pennebaker, J. W., Kiecolt-Glaser, J. K., & Glaser, R. (1988). Disclosures of traumas and immune function: Health implications for psychotherapy. *Journal of Consulting and Clinical Psychology* 56, 239–245.

Peplau, L. A., & Perlman, D. (Eds.). (1982). *Loneliness: A source book of current theory, research, and therapy.* New York: Wiley.

Perry, S., Fishman, B., Jacobsberg, L., & Frances, A. (1992). Relationships over 1 year between lymphocyte subsets and psychosocial variables among adults with infection by human immunodeficiency virus. *Archives of General Psychiatry* 49, 396–401.

Petrie, K. J., Booth, R. J., Pennebaker, J. W., Davison, K. P., & Thomas, M. G. 1995. Disclosure of trauma and immune response to a hepatitis B vaccination program. *Journal of Consulting and Clinical Psychology* 63, 787–792.

Schneiderman, N., Chesney, M. A, & Krantz, D. S. (1989). Biobehavioral aspects of cardiovascular disease: Progress and prospects. *Health Psychology* 8, 649–676.

Sloan, R. P., Bagiella, E., & Powell, T. (1999). Religion, spirituality, and medicine. *Lancet* 353, 664–667.

Smyth, J. M., Stone, A. A., Hurewitz, A., & Kaell, A. (1999) Effects of writing about stressful experiences on symptom reduction in patients with asthma or rheumatoid arthritis: A randomized trial. *Journal of the American Medical Association* 281, 1304–1309.

Spiegel, D., Bloom, J. R., Kraemer, H. C., & Gottheil, E. (1989). Effect of psychosocial treatment on survival of patients with metastatic breast cancer. *Lancet* 2, 888–891.

Stone, A. A., Bovbjerg, D. H., Neale, J. M., Napoli, A., Valdimarsdottir, H., Cox, D., Hayden, F. G., & Gwaltney, J. M. (1992). Development of common cold symptoms following experimental rhinovirus infection is related to prior stressful life events. *Behavioral Medicine* 8, 115–120.

Stone, A. A., Cox, D. S., Valdimarsdottir, H., Jandorf, L., & Neale, M. (1987). Evidence that secretory IgA antibody is associated with daily mood. *Journal of Personality and Social Psychology* 52, 988–993.

Stone, A. A., Neale, J. M., Cox, D. S., Napoli, A., Valdimarsdottir, H., & Kennedy-Moore, E. (1994). Daily events are associated with a secretory immune response to an oral antigen in men. *Health Psychology* 13, 440–446.

Thoits, P. A. (1983). Multiple identities and psychological well-being: A reformulation and test of the social isolation hypothesis. *American Sociological Review* 48, 174–187.

Thoits, P. A. (1985). Social support processes and psychological well-being: Theoretical possibilities. In I. G. Sarason & B. Sarason (Eds.), *Social support: Theory, research, and applications.* The Hague: Martinus Nijhoff.

Thoits, P. A. (1986). Social support as coping assistance. *Journal of Consulting and Clinical Psychology* 54, 416–423.

Thomas, P. D., Goodwin, J. M., & Goodwin, J. S. (1985). Effect of social support on stress-related changes in cholesterol level, uric acid level, and immune function in an elderly sample. *American Journal of Psychiatry* 142, 735–737.

Uchino, B. N., Cacioppo, J. T., & Kiecolt-Glaser, J. K. (1996). The relationship between social support and physiological processes. *Psychological Bulletin* 119, 488–531.

Verbrugge, L. M. (1979). Marital status and health. *Journal of Marriage and Family* 41, 267–285.

Vogt, T. M., Mullooly, J. P., Ernst, D., Pope, C. R., & Hollis, J. F. (1992). Social networks as predictors of ischemic heart disease, cancer, stroke, and hypertension. *Journal of Clinical Epidemiology* 45, 659–666.

Wills, T. A. (1985). Supportive functions and interpersonal relationships. In S. Cohen & S. L. Syme (Eds.), *Social support and health.* New York: Academic.

7

Psychosocial Factors, Immunity, and Wound Healing

HAROLD G. KOENIG & HARVEY JAY COHEN

In this chapter we review the work of Janice Kiecolt-Glaser, Ron Glaser, and others who have examined the effects of psychological stress and social support on immune functioning and wound healing. This area of research is of particular importance because of its potentially wide clinical application. If either individual or group support has an impact on immune function, the public health implications would be enormous. Likewise, if psychological stress affects wound healing in a clinically significant way, then stress-reducing interventions before and after surgical operations might significantly affect the speed of postsurgical recovery. We also explore in this chapter how such research advances may help inform future studies of the religion-health relationship and propose a number of research avenues to pursue. If religious involvement enhances social support and reduces stress, then investigations that explore the relationship between religion and immunity, wound healing, and postsurgical recovery may be worth pursuing.

Social Support and Immune Function

Social support has been shown to modify the psychological consequences of stress, thereby preventing or ameliorating adverse psychological outcomes such as depression (George, 1992; Uchino et al., 1996). Social isolation, in contrast, increases emotional distress that may lead to neuroendocrine and immune system changes that impair physical health. Studies in both nonhuman primates and humans bear this out. Sapolsky and colleagues (1997) examined the correlation between hypercorti-solism, social subordination, and isolation in 70 African yellow baboons. Baboons with the lowest ranking in the troop had postdexamethasone suppression test cortisols three times higher than levels found in dominant baboons. Socially isolated males also had elevated basal cortisol concentrations and tended to show dexamethasone resistance.

Studies in humans report similar findings. Early work with psychiatric patients and medical students discovered poorer immune function in those who were more isolated. Kiecolt-Glaser, Ricker, and George (1984) found in a sample of 33 psychiatric inpatients that those who scored above the median on the UCLA Loneliness Scale had significantly higher urinary cortisol levels, significantly lower levels of natural killer cell activity, and poorer T lymphocyte response to phytohemagglutinin. Similarly, in a hepatitis B vaccine study, medical students with greater social support during exam time mounted a stronger immune response to the vaccine than students with less support (Kiecolt-Glaser, Garner, & Spelcher, 1984). Likewise, Glaser et al. (1985), studying 49 first-year medical students, found that subjects scoring above the median in the UCLA Loneliness Scale had significantly higher Epstein-Barr virus antibody titers then low-loneliness subjects. The investigators concluded that the immunosuppression caused by loneliness and stress can significantly modulate herpesvirus latency.

Kiecolt-Glaser, Dura, and colleagues (1991) next examined stress levels, physical health, and immune function in 69 spousal caregivers of demented patients, comparing them with 69 sociodemographically matched controls. Caregivers reported significantly more days of infectious disease, primarily upper respiratory infections. Caregivers with lowest social support and highest stress at baseline showed the greatest and most uniform decrements in cellular immunity 13 months later. Likewise, Esterling et al. (1994) examined the effects of chronic stress and social support on alterations in natural killer (NK) cell response to cytokines in 14 active family caregivers of Alzheimer's patients, 17 former family caregivers of Alzheimer's patients, and 31 matched controls. Compared with controls, current and former caregivers demonstrated significantly poorer NK cell responses when exposed in vitro to recombinant interferon-gamma and interleukin-2. In a later study, comparing 28 current and former spousal caregivers of Alzheimer's patients and 29 controls, Esterling et al. (1996) found that NK cell activity was again positively related to emotional support and tangible social support. These findings were consistent with those of Baron et al. (1990), who had found that wives of cancer patients with higher levels of social support demonstrated greater natural killer cell cytotoxicity and phytohemagglutinin stimulation.

A series of marital studies that examined couples interacting in a laboratory paradigm demonstrated that lack of supportive relationships in the home may adversely affect immune functioning. Kiecolt-Glaser, Malarkey, Chee, et al. (1993) studied 90 newlywed couples to determine the relationship between negative behavior during marital conflict and immune function. The couples were brought into the hospital and catheters were placed in their arms soon after admission so that blood could be drawn as necessary. Subjects were asked to discuss an area of disagreement. The way in which couples disagreed was very much related to alterations in stress hormones and immune function. Spouses who displayed more negative or hostile behaviors during a 30-minute discussion of marital problems showed greater decreases in NK cell activity, less blastogenic response to two mitogens, weaker proliferative responses to monoclonal antibody, and larger increases in blood pressure that remained elevated longer. These effects were particularly strong in women.

Kiecolt-Glaser, Glaser, et al. (1997) next examined endocrine and immune correlates of marital conflict in 31 older couples who had been married an average of 42 years. Among wives, marital satisfaction and escalation of negative behavior during conflict correlated with substantial changes in cortisol, ACTH, and norepinephrine levels. Both men and women who displayed negative behaviors during conflict showed poorer immunological responses as measured by blastogenic response to T cell mitogens and antibody titers to latent Epstein-Barr virus. Investigators concluded from this series of studies that couples who engage in negative or hostile interactions—are sarcastic or demeaning when disagreeing about something—show much steeper increases in stress hormones and downturns in immune function.

Religious organizations could play an important role both in providing social support to members and in providing guidelines for marriage that help increase marital stability and decrease negative or hostile interactions. This may have value in terms of immune system functioning and ultimately the physical health of family members.

Social Support and Immune Function in Cancer

Associations between social support, immune function, and clinical outcomes are particularly notable in studies involving patients with cancer.

Levy et al. (1987) in a prospective study of 75 women with stage I or II breast cancer found cross-sectional correlations between lack of family support and lower NK cell activity both at baseline and at 3-month follow-up. Those who complained about lack of family support at baseline tended to show a decrease in NK activity at 3 months. Reduced activity of NK cells, in turn, was associated with shorter survival. In a later report on 66 women with early breast cancer, Levy and colleagues (1990) again found that women with higher social support had greater NK cell activity than those with low support.

If lack of support is associated with decreased immune functioning in cancer patients, perhaps interventions that increase social support might protect against these changes and improve health outcomes. To test this hypothesis, Spiegel and colleagues (1989) randomized 86 women with metastatic breast cancer to either psychosocial intervention or a control group with no intervention. The intervention was conducted over 12 months and consisted of weekly supportive group therapy. At 10-year follow-up, women receiving the support group intervention survived an average of 36.6 months compared with 18.9 months for those in the control group ($p < .0001$). Similarly, Fawzy and colleagues (1990, 1993) randomized patients with malignant melanoma to either a structured group intervention (which included stress management, relaxation, and social support) or a control group. Psychological, immunological, and disease characteristics were carefully measured at baseline and follow-up. Subjects receiving the intervention experienced significant increases in number of NK cells and in NK cytotoxic activity. At the 6-year follow-up, subjects receiving the intervention experienced fewer recurrences and lower mortality than those in the control group.

Given the relationship between social support and immune functioning, it is not surprising to find that greater social involvement is also associated with longer survival (Berkman & Syme, 1979; House et al., 1988; Vogt et al., 1992) and greater host resistance to infectious disease (Cohen et al., 1997; Glaser, Rabin, et al., 1999; Kiecolt-Glaser, Malarkey, Cacioppo, et al., 1994) in noncancer populations as well.

Religion and Social Support

As we learned in chapter 1, religious activity—whether personal and private, like prayer or scripture reading, or public and social, like attendance at religious services—is related to a greater amount of social support, quality of support, and satisfaction with support.

It is not quite clear how private religious activities enhance social support, although they may do so by affecting a person's attitude toward the value of both receiving support and giving support to others. Because of the relatively strong relationship between private and public religious activities, personal religious activity like prayer may also motivate persons to become more involved in the religious community—even if they don't feel like it (i.e., they are more introverted or physically less able). Private religious activity may reflect a deeper personal commitment to religion that motivates "other-oriented" activity as something that one ought to do, regardless of feelings. This, then, may result in more social contacts and greater support than would otherwise occur. Alternatively, persons engaged in private religious activities may simply perceive whatever social support they receive as being more adequate—either because it actually is of higher quality or because a more positive attitude makes them think it is. Finally, persons engaged in private religious activities may behave in a way that attracts others to them, thereby increasing actual support.

More obvious is the association between frequency of religious attendance and social support. Involvement in religious community activity increases a person's number of social contacts, particularly those likely to develop into personal relationships because of similar values and beliefs. Religious organizations typically provide numerous opportunities for engagement in social activities with other members of the congregation, which is often encouraged from the pulpit and also in religious scriptures. These social activities further link persons to a common vision and purpose, reinforcing interpersonal bonds. This is especially true for older adults, who because of relocation or health problems may have difficulty making new relationships or preserving old ones. One study conducted in the Midwestern United States found that more than half of older adults who were attending a geriatric medicine clinic stated that 80% or more of their closest friends came from their church congregation (Koenig et al., 1988). For some minority groups, particularly African Americans and Hispanic Americans, the church is often the organization that literally holds the community together (Delgado, 1981; Taylor, 1986; Taylor & Chatters, 1988).

The likelihood of having a supportive marital partner is also associated with religious involvement. In a review of research on religion and marital happiness or stability, we found 38 studies (Koenig et al., 2001). Almost all studies (35 of 38) found greater marital happiness or stability among the more religious or those from the same religious background. For example, Strawbridge et al. (1997) followed 5,286 participants in the Alameda County Study for 28 years, examining marital stability and other variables. Frequent church attenders (once per week or more) at baseline were only slightly more likely than less frequent attenders to be married (25% versus 23%). However, during the 28-year follow-up period, frequent attenders were 80% more likely to stay married than those who attended services less than once per week. Thus, religious involvement is associated with a more satisfying and stable marriage, which increases the likelihood of spousal support.

Religious Involvement, Social Support, and Immune Function

No research has yet examined the relationships between religious activity, social support, and immune function all in one study. Although religious involvement has been associated with greater social support, greater social support has been associated with better immune function, and greater religious involvement has been associated with better immune function, these associations have all been established in separate studies. The field is ripe for research that would examine the complex relationships between religious involvement, social support, and immune function as part of an observational study or clinical trial in which all these factors could be examined together in a single model.

For example, one might examine a population of stressed caregivers of demented relatives, study differences in social support and immune function in caregivers involved and not involved in religious activities, and assess changes in these parameters over time. Even more powerful would be an intervention study that randomized subjects to either religious involvement (or increased religious involvement) or a control group without such involvement, monitoring changes in social support and immune function over time. These are examples of studies that could utilize what we know about social support and immune functioning and apply it to better understand the relationship between religion and immunity.

Psychological Stress and Wound Healing

Studies suggest that meaning, acceptance, expectations of the surgery, and anxiety are all related to aspects of postsurgical wound healing (George,

1980; George & Scott, 1982). As noted in chapter 3, psychological stress (anticipatory stress of surgery or stress associated with trauma) activates the sympathetic nervous system, with consequent vasoconstriction and shunting of blood from skin to vital organs, such as the heart and brain. Although this response in the acute setting has adaptive value, its persistence over time results in peripheral tissue hypoxia. Likewise, cortisol, the primary adrenal glucocorticoid released in response to hypothalamic-pituitary-adrenal activation, alters the inflammatory response after injury. Although the exact mechanism is unknown, cortisol probably affects wound healing by alterations in collagen synthesis, blood flow, and substrate metabolism (Durant et al., 1986). Studies have shown that stress-induced elevations of epinephrine, norepinephrine, and cortisol inhibit fibroblast growth in postoperative patients, interfering with wound healing (Saito et al., 1997). Reduction of psychological stress should both reduce serum cortisol levels and limit catecholamine-induced vasoconstriction and wound hypoxia, thereby increasing fibroblast growth and wound closure. Furthermore, wound healing involves a cascade of immunological events, with later stages heavily dependent on the success of earlier stages (Barbul, 1990; Hubner et al., 1996; Lowry, 1993). Both cytokines and T cells, influenced by hormonal factors, play important roles in this process (Schaffer & Barbul, 1998).

Studies on Stress and Wound Healing

Interested in the health consequences of changes in immune function, Kiecolt-Glaser and colleagues have conducted a series of studies on stress and wound healing. Because most surgical wounds are sutured wounds, it is difficult to measure the closure of a wound that has already been closed artificially. For that reason, these investigators created a small, uniform punch biopsy about the size of a pencil eraser (3.5 mm) on the skin (full-thickness wound). Speed of healing was then measured by photography of the wound and response to hydrogen peroxide.

In the first of these studies, Kiecolt-Glaser, Marucha, et al. (1996) wounded 13 stressed family caregivers of patients with Alzheimer's disease and 13 very well matched noncaregiver controls. Wound healing took 24% longer for caregivers than for noncaregivers (or approximately 9 days longer). Analyses of the production of interleukin (IL)-1β in response to lipopolysaccharide stimulation showed that caregivers' peripheral blood leukocytes produced less of this substance than did the leukocytes of controls. The IL-1β data provide evidence for an immunological mechanism that may have been responsible for caregivers' deficits in wound repair.

This finding has now been replicated with a mouse model. Padgett et al. (1998) wounded mice with a 3.5-mm punch biopsy, applying restraint stress to the test group but not to controls. Female, hairless mice, 6 to 8 weeks of age, were subjected to restraint stress 3 days before and for 5 days following dorsal application of a 3.5-mm sterile punch wound. Control mice received the dorsal application of the 3.5-mm wound but were not restrained. By means of photography and image analysis, the rate of wound healing for the two groups was compared. Wounds on control mice healed an average of 3.1 days sooner than did those on restraint-treated mice. In other words, wounds on stressed mice took a significant 27% longer to heal than those on mice who were not stressed. Analysis of skin layers revealed reduced inflammation surrounding the wounds of restraint-treated mice. Investigators also found that serum cortisol levels were significantly higher in the stressed mice than in controls (162.5 ng/ml vs. 35.7 ng/ml). More-over, when mice were treated with a glucocorticoid receptor antagonist, healing rates in stressed mice increased to those of control animals, sug-gesting that delayed healing resulted from stress-induced elevations of serum cortisol.

Next, to determine whether more usual everyday stress could have sim-ilar effects on wound healing, Marucha et al. (1998) studied 11 dental stu-dents, wounding them on their buccal mucosa and then looking at the same individuals at two different points in time. Two 3.5-mm punch biop-sies were performed. The first one took place at the end of summer vaca-tion. The second biopsy was performed on the other side of the mouth, 3 days before the first major exam of the term. Each individual, then, had two identical wounds. Investigators discovered that 8 days were required at the end of summer vacation to fully heal the wounds, whereas 11 days were required during the exam period (40% difference to heal identical wounds). The same methods were used to assess healing as in the Kiecolt-Glaser, Marucha, et al. (1996) study cited previously. Again, production of IL-1 declined by 68% during examinations, similar to the finding in their earlier study.

Mechanism of Effect

What was interesting in this study was the timing of the healing. After the students survived the exam, stress stopped abruptly, but wounds did not close abruptly. The wound healing continued but didn't suddenly catch up to that of nonstressed students. This can be understood in terms of the immunological cascade already noted that takes place early in wound healing. If early events in this cascade are impaired by stress, then later events will likewise be affected, and wound healing down the road could be delayed.

Recall that previous studies suggested that levels of proinflammatory cytokines in the local wound environment may play a role. Cytokines such as IL-1 and tumor necrosis factor help protect against infection, prepare injured tissue for repair by enhancing the function of white blood cells, and regulate the ability of fibroblasts and epithelial cells to remodel the wound (Lowry, 1993). In particular, IL-1 stimulates the production of other cytokines necessary for wound healing, including IL-2, IL-6, and IL-8. Consequently, anything that reduces IL-1 levels early during the process of wound repair (particularly in the first 24 hours) could adversely affect later events in the immunological cascade involved in wound healing.

How might proinflammatory cytokines in the local wound environment be affected? Investigators believe that serum cortisol may play a key role. Recall that glucocorticoids were shown to play a critical role in the delayed healing of restraint-stressed mice (Padgett et al., 1998), a finding also reported by others (Hubner et al., 1996). In this way, stress may reduce levels of proinflammatory cytokines like IL-1 that play a crucial role in the early immunological events required for complete wound healing.

Glaser, Kiecolt-Glaser, et al. (1999) recently discovered evidence that psychological stress significantly affects levels of proinflammatory cytokines in the local wound environment, acting through serum cortisol. Using a suction device, these investigators placed skin blisters (wounds) on the forearms of 36 female subjects (average age 57 years). Investigators placed a plastic template over the blister wounds, filling up the wells thus formed with 70% autologous serum in buffer. At 5 and 24 hours after the suction blisters were placed, specimens were aspirated from these chamber wells. Subjects with higher levels of perceived stress (assessed using the 10-item Perceived Stress Scale) had significantly lower levels of IL-1 and IL-8 at the wound sites. Likewise, subjects who reported more stress and negative affect (assessed using the 20-item Positive and Negative Affect Schedule) had low levels of both cytokines and higher levels of salivary cortisol at 24 hours. Glaser et al. concluded that psychological stress delays wound healing by adversely affecting levels of proinflammatory cytokines (such as IL-1 and IL-8) in the local wound. This study is important because it provides further evidence for a subcellular mechanism explaining the effects of psychological stress on wound healing.

From a clinical standpoint, there is a relatively large surgical literature on psychosocial stress and surgical recovery. Nearly 200 intervention studies, starting around 1965 and continuing to the present, have examined the benefits for psychosocial interventions prior to surgery, demonstrating that such interventions decrease anxiety and stress, reduce hospital stays, and result in fewer postoperative complications, better treatment compliance, and less need for pain medication (Contrada et al., 1994; Johnston & Vogele, 1993). Most recently, Scheier et al. (1999) found that depressive symptoms were a significant predictor of infection-related hospital readmission following coronary artery bypass graft surgery. Considering the information learned from recent studies on immunological aspects of wound healing, things begin to make sense. The process of wound healing involves an immunological cascade in which early events in that cascade are crucial. If stress delays those important early events, this will delay the cascade and ultimately impair wound closure.

Religion and Wound Healing

If religious beliefs and practices improve coping, reduce stress, and increase hope and optimism, then there is reason to think that religion might also affect the speed of wound healing and ultimately influence surgical outcomes. No studies, however, have examined this relationship directly. Several naturalistic studies have reported that religious activity predicts improved surgical outcomes, such as longer walking distances after hip surgery (Pressman et al., 1990), greater survival after open-heart surgery (Oxman et al., 1995), and improved health after heart transplantation (Harris et al., 1995). A few studies report less need for pain medication and shorter hospital stays after surgery for patients who receive religious interventions, particularly chaplain visits (Bliss et al., 1995; Florell, 1973).

A variety of studies could be done with surgical patients—in terms of naturalistic and intervention studies—to determine whether religiosity or religious practices influence wound healing and recovery from surgery. For example, religious beliefs and practices of patients prior to surgery could be measured and related to the speed of wound healing and likelihood of infection or other complications. Effects on surgical outcomes of personal religiousness or private religious activity could be compared with those of public or social religious activity. Alternatively, subjects prior to surgery might be randomized to either a religious intervention (such as chaplain visits, personal or group prayer, or other religious ritual) or to a control group, and postsurgical outcomes could be assessed. To avoid problems of uniformity of wound size and surgical technique, an investigator might apply an experimental wound to the skin or soft palate in the same way that Kiecolt-Glaser's group did in their studies, using photography and hydrogen peroxide fizzing to measure the speed of wound healing. Neuroendocrine (cortisol) and immune measures (IL-1, IL-8) should also be assessed so that the mechanism of the effect can be identified. If funding is limited for such work, then simply adding a religious measure (chapter 15) to ongoing PNI studies of wound healing and/or surgical outcome would help provide clues about this relationship.

If a simple religious or spiritual intervention—such as prayer, visits from a pastor or chaplain, or support from a religious community—could be shown to reduce the stress of surgery, improve immune functioning, and thereby speed wound healing, this would provide important information to health care providers. Such a religious intervention or practice would be inexpensive and widely accepted by religious patients, and it would empower them to positively affect the course of their recovery. Many of these religious practices are and will continue to be performed by patients and families regardless of whether they are encouraged or not by health professionals. Nevertheless, it would be useful for clinicians to know if such activities have any objective impact on wound closure or surgical outcome so that they could more effectively utilize the religious resources of patients to speed the healing process.

References

Barbul, A. (1990). Immune aspects of wound repair. *Clinics in Plastic Surgery* 17, 433–442.
Baron, R. S., Cutrona, C. E., Hicklin, D., Russel, D. W., & Lubaroff, D. M. (1990). Social support and immune function among spouses of cancer patients. *Journal of Personality and Social Psychology* 59, 344–352.
Berkman, L. F., & Syme, S. L. (1979). Social networks, colds resistance, and mortality. *American Journal of Epidemiology* 109, 186–204.
Bliss, J. R., McSherry, E., & Fassett, J. (1995). Chaplain intervention reduces costs in major DRGs: An experimental study. In H. Heffernan, E. McSherry, & R. Fitzgerald (Eds.), *Proceedings NIH clinical center conference on spirituality*

and health care outcomes, March 21. Bethesda, MD: Department of Spiritual Ministry, NIH Clinical Center.

Cohen, S., Doyle, W. J., Skoner, D. P., Rabin, B. S., & Gwaltney, J. M. (1997). Social ties and susceptibility to the common cold. *Journal of the American Medical Association* 277, 1940–1944.

Contrada, R. J., Leventhal, E. A., & Anderson, J. R. (1994). Psychological preparation for surgery: Marshalling individual and social resources to optimize self-regulation. In S. Maes, H. Leventhal, & M. Johnston (Eds.), *International review of health psychology* (pp. 219–266). Chichester, England: Wiley.

Delgado, M. (1981). Ethnic and cultural variations in the care of the aged Hispanic elderly and natural support systems: A special focus on Puerto Ricans. *Journal of Geriatric Psychiatry* 15(2), 239–251.

Durant, S., Duval, D., & Homo-Delarche, F. (1986). Factors involved in the control of fibroblast proliferation by glucocorticoids: A review. *Endocrinology Review* 7, 254–269.

Esterling, B. A., Kiecolt-Glaser, J. K., Bodnar, J. C., & Glaser, R. (1994). Chronic stress, social support, and persistent alterations in the natural killer cell response to cytokines in older adults. *Health Psychology* 13, 291–298.

Esterling, B. A., Kiecolt-Glaser, J. K., & Glaser, R. (1996). Psychosocial modulation of cytokine-induced natural killer cell activity in older adults. *Psychosomatic Medicine* 58, 264–272.

Fawzy, F. I., Kemeny, M. E., Fawzy, N. W., Elashoff, R., Morton, D., Cousins, N., & Fahey, J. L. (1990). A structured psychiatric intervention for cancer patients: II. Changes over time in immunological measures. *Archives of General Psychiatry* 47, 729–735.

Fawzy, F. I., Fawzy, N. W., Hyun, C., Elashoff, R., Guthrie, D., Fahey, J. L., & Morton, D. L. (1993). Malignant melanoma: Effects of an earlier structured psychiatric intervention, coping, and affective state on recurrence and survival six years later. *Archives of General Psychiatry* 50, 681–689.

Florell, J. L. (1973). Crisis-intervention in orthopedic surgery: Empirical evidence of the effectiveness of a chaplain working with surgery patients. *Bulletin of the American Protestant Hospital Association* 37(2), 29–36.

George, J. M. (1980). The effects of psychological factors and physical trauma on recovery from oral surgery. *Journal of Behavioral Medicine* 3, 291–310.

George, J. M., & Scott, D. S. (1982). The effects of psychological factors on recovery from surgery. *Journal of the American Dental Association* 105, 251–258.

George, L. K. (1992). Social factors and the onset and outcome of depression. In K. W. Schaie, D. Blazer, & J. S. House (Eds.), *Aging, health behaviors, and health outcomes* (pp. 137–159). Hillsdale, NJ: Erlbaum.

Glaser, R., Kiecolt-Glaser, J. K., Marucha, P. T., MacCallum, R. C., Laskowski, B. F., & Malarkey, W. B. (1999). Stress-related changes in proinflammatory cytokine production in wounds. *Archives of General Psychiatry* 56, 450–456.

Glaser, R., Kiecolt-Glaser, J. K., Speicher, C. E., & Holliday, J. E. (1985). Stress, loneliness, and changes in herpes virus latency. *Journal of Behavioral Medicine* 8, 249–260.

Glaser, R., Rabin, B., Chesney, M., Cohen, S., & Natelson, B. (1999). Stress-induced immunomodulation: Implications for infectious diseases? *Journal of the American Medical Association* 281, 2268–2270.

Harris, R. C., Dew, M. A., Lee, A., Amaya, M., Buches, L., Reetz, D., & Coleman, G. (1995). The role of religion in heart transplant recipients' health and well-being. *Journal of Religion and Health* 34(1), 17–32.

House, J. S., Landis, K. R., & Umberson, D. (1988). Social relationships and health. *Science* 241, 540–545.

Hubner, G., Brauchle, M., Smola, H., Madlener, M., Fassler, R., & Werner, S. (1996). Differential regulation of pro-inflammatory cytokines during wound healing in normal and glucocorticoid-treated mice. *Cytokine* 8, 548–556.

Johnston, M., & Vogele, C. (1993). Benefits of psychological preparation for surgery: A meta-analysis. *Annals of Behavioral Medicine* 15, 245–256.

Kiecolt-Glaser, J. K., Dura, J. R., Speicher, C. E., Trask, O. J., & Glaser, R. (1991). Spousal caregivers of dementia victims: Longitudinal changes in immunity and health. *Psychosomatic Medicine* 53, 345–362.

Kiecolt-Glaser, J. K., Garner, W., & Spelcher, C. (1984). Psychosocial modifiers of immunocompetence in medical students. *Psychosomatic Medicine* 46, 7–14.

Kiecolt-Glaser, J. K., Glaser, R., Cacioppo, J. T., MacCallum, R. C., Snydersmith, M., Kim. C., & Malarkey, W. B. (1997). Marital conflict in older adults: Endocrinological and immunological correlates. *Psychosomatic Medicine* 49, 339–349.

Kiecolt-Glaser, J. K., Malarkey, W. B., Cacioppo, J. T., & Glaser, R. (1994). Stressful personal relationships: Immune and into credit function. In R. Glaser & J. Kiecolt-Glaser (Eds.), *Handbook of human stress and immunity* (pp. 321–339). San Diego, CA: Academic Press.

Kiecolt-Glaser, J. K., Malarkey, W. B., Chee, M., Newton, T., Cacioppo, J. T., Mao, H. Y., & Glaser, R. (1993). Negative behavior during marital conflict is associated with immunological down-regulation. *Psychosomatic Medicine* 55, 395–409.

Kiecolt-Glaser, J. K., Marucha, P. T., Malarkey, W. B., Mercado, A. M., & Glaser, R. (1996). Slowing of wound healing by psychological stress. *Lancet* 346(8984), 1194–1196.

Kiecolt-Glaser, J. K., Ricker, D., & George, J. (1984). Urinary cortisol levels, cellular immunocompetence, and loneliness in psychiatric inpatients. *Psychosomatic Medicine* 46, 15–23.

Koenig, H. G., McCullough, M., & Larson, D. B. (2001). *Handbook of religion and health*. New York: Oxford University Press.

Koenig, H. G., Moberg, D. O., & Kvale, J. N. (1988). Religious activities and attitudes of older adults in a geriatric assessment clinic. *Journal of the American Geriatrics Society* 36, 362–374.

Levy, S., Herberman, R. B., Lee, J., Whiteside, I., Kirkwood, J., & McFeeley, S. (1990). Estrogen receptor concentration and social factors as predictors of natural killer cell activity in early-stage breast cancer patients. *Natural Immunity and Cell Growth Regulation* 9, 313–324.

Levy, S., Lippman, M., & d'Angelo, T. (1987). Correlation of stress factors with sustained suppression of natural killer cell activity and predictive prognosis in patients with breast cancer. *Journal of Clinical Oncology* 5, 348–353.

Lowry, S. F. (1993). Cytokine mediators of immunity and inflammation. *Archives of Surgery* 28, 1235–1241.

Marucha, P. T., Kiecolt-Glaser, J. K., & Favagehi, M. (1998). Mucosal wound healing is impaired by examinations stress. *Psychosomatic Medicine* 60, 362–365.

Oxman, T. E., Freeman, D. H., & Manheimer, E. D. (1995). Lack of social participation or religious strength and comfort as risk factors for death after cardiac surgery in the elderly. *Psychosomatic Medicine* 57, 5–15.

Padgett, D. A., Marucha, P. T., & Sheridan, J. F. (1998). Restraint stress slows cutaneous wound healing in mice. *Brain, Behavior, and Immunity* 12, 64–73.

Pressman, P., Lyons, J. S., Larson, D. B., & Strain, J. J. (1990). Religious belief, depression, and ambulation status in elderly women with broken hips. *American Journal of Psychiatry* 147, 758–759.

Saito, T., Tazawa, K., Yokoyama, Y., & Saito, M. (1997). Surgical stress inhibits the growth of fibroblasts through the elevation of plasma catecholamine and cortisol concentrations. *Surgery Today* 27(7), 627–631.

Sapolsky, R. M., Alberts, S. C., & Altman, J. (1997). Hypercortisolism associated with social subordinance or social isolation among wild baboons. *Archives of General Psychiatry* 54, 1137–1143.

Schaffer, M., & Barbul, A. (1998). Lymphocyte function and wound healing following injury. *British Journal of Surgery* 85, 444–460.

Scheier, M. F., Matthews, K. A., Owens, J. F., Schultz, R., Bridges, M. W., Magovern, G. J., & Carver, C. S. (1999). Optimism and re-hospitalization following coronary artery bypass graft surgery. *Archives of Internal Medicine* 159, 829–835.

Spiegel, D., Bloom, J. R., Kraemer, H. C., & Gottheil, E. (1989). Effect of psychosocial treatment on survival of patients with metastatic breast cancer. *Lancet* 2(8668), 888–891.

Strawbridge, W. J., Cohen, R. D., Shema, S. J., & Kaplan, G. A. (1997). Frequent attendance at religious services and mortality over 28 years. *American Journal of Public Health* 87, 957–961.

Taylor, R. J. (1986). Religious participation among elderly blacks. *Gerontologist* 26, 630–635.

Taylor, R. J., & Chatters, L. M. (1988). Church members as a source of informal social support. *Review of Religious Research* 30, 193–203.

Uchino, B. N., Cacioppo, J. R., & Kiecolt-Glaser, J. K. (1996). The relationship between social support and physiological processes: A review with emphasis on underlying mechanisms and implications for health. *Psychological Bulletin* 119, 488–531.

Vogt, T. M., Lullooly, J. P., Ernst, D., Pope, C. R., & Hollis, J. F. (1992). Social networks as predictors of ischemic heart disease, cancer, stroke and hypertension. *Journal of Clinical Epidemiology* 45, 659–666.

8

Psychosocial Factors, Spirituality/ Religiousness, and Immune Function in HIV/AIDS Patients

GAIL IRONSON & NEIL SCHNEIDERMAN

In 2000, it was estimated that 36 million people worldwide had been infected with the human immunodeficiency virus (HIV) and that 15,000 people were being newly infected with the virus each day (CDC, 2000). In 1999 alone, 3 million people worldwide died of acquired immunodeficiency syndrome (AIDS) (CDC, 2000). Although the HIV epidemic has created an unprecedented challenge for medical researchers throughout the world attempting to understand how the virus infects and overwhelms its host, it has become increasingly clear over the years that, in many ways, HIV is no different from all the other infectious diseases, both viral and bacterial, that have threatened humankind throughout the millennia.

In fact, just as diseases such as tuberculosis and herpes have been found to be prone to influence by psychological and social factors that affect immunological resistance to them, so, too, has HIV. Because HIV is a disease characterized by immune system dysfunction and is also resisted by the immune system, it would seem that PNI effects on immune functions might have an even greater impact on the course of HIV infection than on the course of other infectious diseases. In particular, it appears people's psychological health, how they cope with stressors, their social connections, and their beliefs and attitudes can play a significant role in the course of HIV infection. It also appears that individuals' religious and spiritual beliefs can affect these factors, thereby indirectly playing a role in the course of HIV infection as well.

In this chapter, we briefly explore the pathogenesis of HIV and its treatment and the various psychosocial factors known to play a role in the progression of HIV to AIDS. We also examine the impact of religious and spiritual beliefs and practices on these psychosocial factors and the implications of this relationship for the treatment of HIV/AIDS.

The Pathogenesis of HIV

HIV is a highly infective retrovirus that has the ability to incorporate itself into the DNA of its host's immune cells, which it enters via specific cell surface receptors (e.g., CD4 and others). Shortly after exposure, HIV enters and spreads throughout the lymphoid tissues (such as the lymph nodes, spleen, and tonsils) and various organs that contain lymphatic tissues (e.g., intestines) or resident macrophage cells (e.g., brain microglia).

During this early "acute" phase,[1] no measurable anti-HIV antibodies are found in the blood, even though persistent viral replication, or viremia, begins. Viremia is partially controlled by the immune response to the virus during the acute phase, particularly by CD8 cells, until eventually immune depletion occurs. After the acute phase is over, individuals enter into what may be a prolonged phase, during which their immune systems begin making antibodies, or seroconvert, to HIV (i.e., become HIV-positive) (CDC group 2). During this second phase, the infected individual has antibodies to HIV (i.e., has seroconverted) and is symptom-free, or asymptomatic, yet 90% of those infected experience some form of CD4 (helper T cell) cell decline within 5 years (Fauci, 1988). Because of this prolonged asymptomatic phase, infected individuals often are unaware of their HIV status and may unknowingly spread the disease.

The next phase (CDC group 3) occurs as CD4 cells drop below $500/mm^3$ (normal CD4 lymphocyte values range from 800 to $1200/mm^3$). This stage is characterized by persistent generalized lymphadenopathy, or inflammation and swelling of the lymph nodes, although this condition does not occur in all HIV-infected individuals. Many HIV-infected individuals in this stage experience a variety of other symptoms, such as diarrhea, fatigue, oral candidiasis (a fungal infection), fever, night sweats, and weight loss, that precede AIDS.

The final stage of HIV infection (CDC group 4) is characterized by an AIDS diagnosis, which is made when an individual's CD4 count drops below $200/mm^3$. At this stage, HIV-infected individuals typically begin displaying a range of clinical symptoms of severe immune dysfunction, including hairy leukoplakia (irregular white spots or patches on the mucous membranes of the tongue or cheek), *Pneumocystis carinii* pneumonia, Kaposi's sarcoma, non-Hodgkin's lymphoma, or AIDS-related dementia. Not surprisingly, during this last phase, viral load increases, and so does the rate of infectivity.

Strategies for Treating HIV Infection

Until recently, it was estimated that 30% of HIV-infected individuals would progress from initial exposure to full-blown AIDS within 5 years. Within 15 years, 90% of those infected would be diagnosed with AIDS (Stine, 1996). The average length of time for most individuals from initial infection to the development of symptomatic AIDS was about 10 years.

However, because of the wealth of knowledge regarding the mode of transmission and the pathogenesis of the disease gained through basic and clinical research, the clinical course of HIV infection has improved dramatically, particularly during the last decade. In fact, new pharmacological and other approaches to treating HIV infection have radically changed the course of this disease from a virtual death sentence on account of the progressive deterioration of the immune system to a chronic but manageable condition in which many immune markers remain suppressed but stable. Therefore, today, most individuals with HIV can live relatively normal lives.

Pharmacological Approaches. The reasons for this dramatic change in prognosis of HIV infection include the introduction of a class of potent antiviral agents, beginning with zidovudine (AZT) in 1987 (Blaxhult & Lidman, 1998), leading to the newer reverse transcriptase inhibitors and HIV-specific "protease" inhibitors in the mid-1990s. With the advent of these drugs, particularly the use of combination therapies, in which the virus is attacked on a number of fronts, there has been a significant improvement both in delaying the onset of AIDS and in delaying mortality (Sendi et al., 1999). Indeed, between 1994 and 1998 mortality declined from 20.2 deaths per 100 person years to 8.4 deaths per 100 person years. Approximately 60% of patients who received protease-inhibitor therapy achieved undetectable viral load (Moore and Chaisson, 1999).

Although these drugs are very successful, viral resistance may develop, especially when doses of these complex regimens are missed. Genotyping of the specific drug-resistant strain is often used to guide the choice of a "salvage" regimen, which has led to improved selection of medications successful in reducing viral load (Durant et al., 1999).

Other Approaches. Research conducted over the past decade has found a variety of other factors associated with differences in the rate of progression of HIV infection among individuals, including genetic, constitutional, viral (different strains of HIV), immune, and psychological and social factors (see Balbin et al., 1999, for a discussion of this research). The application of that knowledge to clinical practice has added to the improved prognosis of individuals with HIV.

Because much of this research is beyond the scope of this chapter, the present discussion focuses on research on the relationship between HIV and psychosocial factors, including religion and spirituality. It also discusses the implications of this research for the treatment of HIV and AIDS.

Psychosocial Predictors of Disease Progression in HIV/AIDS

Several psychosocial factors have been explored as possible predictors of disease progression in HIV infection, including life stressors, depression and distress, coping, social support and loss, disclosure and emotional expression, and adherence.

Life Stressors and Bereavement. Major negative life events, such as loss of a partner or spouse, have been implicated as factors in HIV disease progression, although the association between stress and HIV progression is not completely clear. In the primate model of AIDS, simian immunodeficiency virus (SIV) infection, for example, the stress of changes in housing and separations from the social group in a 90-day period before SIV inoculation and in a 30-day period after inoculation has been found to correlate with decreased survival (Capitano & Lerche, 1998). Similarly, in humans, Evans and colleagues (1997) followed 93 initially asymptomatic HIV-positive gay men for up to 42 months and assessed their status every 6 months. These investigators found that higher severe life stress increased the odds of HIV progression fourfold in those followed for at least 2 years.

Bereavement, defined as prolonged grief over the loss of a loved one or close friend, has been shown to affect the progression of HIV infection. Cole and Kemeny (1991), for example, found that death of friends and lovers from AIDS predicted the development of symptoms of AIDS in previously asymptomatic HIV-infected individuals. Furthermore, Kemeny and Dean (1995) investigated the relationship between early AIDS-related bereavement and subsequent changes in CD4 T cell levels and health over a 3- to 4-year follow-up period in 85 HIV-positive gay men. These investigators found that individuals who had experienced an AIDS-related bereavement event prior to study entry lost CD4 T cells more rapidly over time than those individuals who had not suffered an AIDS-related bereavement event. This relationship persisted even after the investigators controlled for other factors known to affect HIV progression, including age, initial health status, and use of antiretroviral drugs, sedatives, recreational drugs, cigarettes, and alcohol. The investigators also assessed two psychological responses to loss—grief and depression—and found that grief was unrelated to CD4 decline and symptom onset. By contrast, depression, specifically the self-reproach aspect of depression, was predictive of CD4 loss.

Bereavement has also been shown to negatively affect a number of other immune markers longitudinally, including numbers of natural killer cells and CD8 lymphocytes (Leserman et al., 1997), NK cytotoxicity, and T cell proliferation to phytohemagglutinin (an immune-stimulating mitogen) (Goodkin et al., 1996).

However, not all studies have found that life stress and bereavement affect HIV disease progression. For example, Kessler et al. (1991) found that there was no relationship between 24 separate stressor events and either CD4 declines or the development of AIDS symptoms. Rabkin, Williams, et al. (1991) also found no relationship between stress and subsequent CD4 or CD8 change over 6 months. However, they did find a "suggestive" relationship between depression and symptom development.

Depression. Like stress and bereavement, there have been conflicting findings regarding the effects of depression on HIV infection and its progression to AIDS. For example, in 1993, two major large longitudinal studies published simultaneously in the *Journal of the American Medical Association* (Burack et al., 1993; Lyketsos et al., 1993) came to opposite conclusions regarding the predictive power of depression for HIV progression. The first study by Burack et al. (1993) found depression was related to subsequent CD4 decline over 5.5 years in a cohort of 277 HIV-positive men. In contrast, Lyketsos and colleagues (1993) found that depression did not predict a faster CD4 decline in a sample of 1,809 gay men followed for 8 years.

Although neither of these studies found a statistically significant relationship between depression and mortality, three subsequent studies did: a longitudinal study of 402 HIV-positive gay men followed for up to 7.5 years (Mayne et al., 1996); a longitudinal study of 765 HIV-positive women followed for up to 7 years (Ickovics et al., 2001); and a longitudinal study of 414 HIV-positive men followed for up to 5 years (Patterson et al., 1996). As noted previously, Rabkin, Williams, and colleagues (1991) found a suggestive relationship between depression and symptoms, and Leserman et al. (2000) found a relationship between depression and progression to AIDS in a longitudinal sample followed for up to 7 years.

Vassend et al. (1997) found that negative affect (anxiety, distress, tension) was related to subjective symptoms but not immune markers. Emotional distress predicted disease progression in another cohort over 12 months (Vedhara et al., 1997).

Based on several studies, it is possible that these conflicting results are due to the fact that the impact of depression (and distress) may be different at different levels of CD4 lymphocytes. For example, Solano et al. (1993) found that psychological distress predicted development of symptoms, but only in a group of HIV-positive individuals with low initial CD4 numbers. In contrast, Burack et al. (1993) found a faster decline in CD4 counts for depression only in those with high CD4 counts.

A study by Kemeny and colleagues (1990) suggests that chronic, rather than acute, depression may be important in affecting HIV disease progression. This study found that when depression was sustained (over a 2-year period) there was a faster decline in CD4 counts than in not chronically depressed counterparts over a 5-year period. In other studies, Kemeny et al. (1994) tried to disentangle depression from bereavement and found that depression was related to HIV progression only in the nonbereaved group. In this study, the investigators assessed immunological parameters in 45 HIV-positive and HIV-negative gay men who had recently experienced the deaths of close friends and 45 matched nonbereaved men. No immune differences were found between bereaved and nonbereaved men. However, among the HIV-positive nonbereaved men, higher depressed mood was significantly associated with fewer CD4 (helper/inducer) T lymphocytes, more activated CD8 (suppressor/cytotoxic) T cells, and lower proliferative responses to the mitogen phytohemagglutinin. In other words, the HIV-positive men who reported higher levels of depressed mood not associated with bereavement demonstrated immunological patterns consistent with HIV activity and progression.

A study by Perry and colleagues (1992) found no relationship between 22 psychosocial variables and CD4 cell numbers. However, there was a significant association for hopelessness (an aspect of depression) and CD4 counts. Similarly, Rabkin, Goetz, et al. (1997), in a study of 112 HIV-positive and 52 HIV-negative homosexual men followed over a 4-year period, found that there was no increase in rates of clinical depression and anxiety over the 4 years despite substantial HIV illness progression. Indeed, on all occasions, the mean "psychopathology" symptom ratings were within the normal or "not depressed" range. Not surprisingly, compared with the HIV-negative men, the HIV-positive men had slightly more anxiety and somatic depressive symptoms throughout. The only measure that showed an increase in distress over time was orientation to the future; among the HIV-positive men, hopes for the future waned across assessments.

In summary, while the evidence is not entirely consistent, there does appear to be a relationship between depression and HIV disease progression. This relationship may be strong in certain circumstances, such as more severe chronic depression, depression unrelated to bereavement, and in hopelessness. Furthermore, depression during bereavement may represent a normal working through of loss, whereas depression not related to bereavement may be indicative of something more chronic and severe.

Interestingly, depressive disorders are the exception and not the rule in HIV patients (Perry, 1994), occurring in about 1 of 10 individuals. In fact, rather than being depressed, many patients with HIV have a surprisingly strong will to live, and many feel that life with HIV is better than it was before they became infected (Tsevat et al., 1999).

Coping with Stress. A number of studies have investigated the relationship between styles of coping and subsequent health in HIV-infected individuals. For the most part, these studies have found that active coping (i.e., taking constructive steps to deal with one's problems) can slow the progression of HIV infection, whereas denial or disengagement contributes to HIV infectivity. Ironson, Friedman, and colleagues (1994), for example, found that those individuals who at the beginning of the study reacted to the news that they were seropositive for HIV with denial and behavioral disengagement had a greater CD4 decline and lower T cell proliferative response at 1-year follow-up and a greater likelihood of AIDS symptoms or death at 2-year follow-up than individuals who used more active coping styles. Similarly, Solano et al. (1993) found that individuals with high levels of denial and repression were likely to develop symptoms of AIDS at 6-month and 12-month follow-up.

In contrast, Blomkvist et al. (1994) demonstrated in a study of HIV-positive hemophiliac patients that "active optimistic coping behavior" was negatively related to mortality over 1 to 7 years. Similarly, Mulder, Antoni, et al. (1995) found that "active confrontational" coping was related to decreased clinical progression at 1-year follow-up in a cohort of gay men. Finally, Vassend et al. (1997) found that HIV-positive individuals who had lower scores on measures of active problem-focused coping (such as positive reappraisal and seeking social support) were more likely to have developed AIDS at subsequent follow-up.

Unfortunately, based on these studies alone, one cannot make the assumption that denial of one's HIV status is bad and that active coping is good. Indeed, Reed, Kemeny, Taylor, Wang, et al. (1994) showed that "realistic" acceptance was a significant predictor of decreased survival time. In addition, Mulder, de Vroome, et al. (1999) recently found that "avoidance" coping was associated with a lower rate of CD4 decline over 7 years and less appearance of syncytium-inducing HIV variants.

Although these findings seem to contradict one another, on closer examination, it is possible to find some reconciliation. In fact, earlier presentations of avoidance coping referred to this construct as "distraction" rather than denial (Mulder, Antoni, et al., 1995). Additionally, a closer look at the previous "realistic acceptance" findings (Reed, Kemeny, Taylor, Wang, et al., 1994) shows that one of the items ("prepare myself for the worst") in fact may be measuring a sense of fatalism or pessimism, which has been found to negatively affect HIV-positive health status (see next section). Thus, in coping with HIV infection, it may be most effective to avoid obsessive rumination with a healthy dose of distraction.

Cognitive Mindset. Other studies have explored how a constellation of variables, referred to as "cognitive mindset" (i.e., negative expectancies, optimism, and finding meaning), may affect the course of HIV disease. Several studies suggest that a negative mindset leads to faster progression of HIV infectivity. As noted before, the study by Reed, Kemeny, Taylor, Wang, et al. (1994) found that a variable relating to fatalism was a significant predictor of decreased survival time. In a more recent study, the same researchers found that negative expectancies in combination with bereavement predicted faster time to AIDS-related symptoms in the next 2.5 to 3.5 years among initially asymptomatic HIV-positive gay men

(Reed, Kemeny, Taylor, & Visscher, 1999). Negative attributions (in particular, attributing negative events to aspects of the self) also significantly predicted faster CD4 decline (Segerstrom et al., 1996).

Additionally, Byrnes and colleagues (1998) studied whether stressful negative life events and pessimism were associated with lower NK cell cytotoxicity and T cytotoxic/suppressor cell (CD8+, CD3+) percentage in black women co-infected with human immunodeficiency virus type 1 (HIV-1) and human papillomavirus (HPV), a viral initiator of cervical cancer. This study found that a higher level of pessimism was related to lower levels of NK cell cytotoxicity and fewer cytotoxic/suppressor cells after controlling for presence or absence of two types of HPV, behavioral-lifestyle factors, and the subjective impact of negative life events. Thus the researchers concluded that a pessimistic attitude may be associated with immune decrements and possibly poorer control over HPV infection, as well as an increased risk for future progression of cervical dysplasia to invasive cervical cancer in HIV-positive minority women co-infected with HPV.

Conversely, research suggests that a positive mindset may be protective against the progression of HIV infection. For example, Blomkvist and colleagues (1994) found that an optimistic outlook, including looking forward to future activities, was related to lower mortality during follow-up in a group of HIV-infected hemophiliacs. Additionally, an intriguing study by Bower et al. (1998) found that those who found "meaning" in response to an HIV-related stressor had a slower CD4 decline and lower mortality over a 2- to 3-year period than those who did not find meaning in the stressor.

In summary, a negative mindset, characterized by a fatalistic or pessimistic outlook on both past and future events, appears to be related to faster HIV infection progression. In contrast, a positive, optimistic mindset, in which an individual finds meaning in the illness rather than disillusionment with life, appears to be protective of health, at least in the short term.

Social Support. The relationship between social support and HIV-related health status, in general, is not yet clear. Theorell and colleagues (1995), for example, found that high social support was associated with a slower drop in CD4 count over subsequent years in a cohort of hemophiliacs. Similarly, Patterson et al. (1996) found that large network sizes predicted longevity among those with AIDS, but not among other subjects. Solano and colleagues (1993) also found that low social support was related to the development of symptoms only in those with low CD4 numbers.

Conversely, in their recent review of the literature on social support and HIV, Miller and Cole (1998) noted accelerated disease progression for gay men in the early stages of infection who had extensive networks of personal relationships. Miller and colleagues (1997) also found that, contrary to their expectation, lower levels of loneliness predicted more rapid levels of CD4 declines, and loneliness was not related to mortality or development of symptoms. Furthermore, Eich-Höchli et al. (1997) found that social resources were not related to disease progression after 2 years.

Leserman and colleagues (1999) recently evaluated the effects of three psychosocial variables—stress, depressive symptoms, and social support—in a prospective longitudinal study with repeated (6-month) assessments of immune status in a sample of HIV-infected individuals. This study found that more cumulative stressful life events, more cumulative depressive symptoms, and less cumulative social support were associated with faster progression to AIDS. When all three variables were analyzed together, stress and social support remained significant in the model. Indeed, at 5.5 years, the probability of getting AIDS was two to three times as high among those above the median for stress or below the median for social support. Even two moderate stressors increased AIDS risk twofold compared with no stressors. This study is important for utilizing cumulative measures and a clinical outcome (AIDS) rather than "surrogate" markers of progression.

These studies suggest that social support can often be helpful for HIV infections, particularly as one becomes sicker. However, social networks can also be deleterious, especially for gay men during early stages of infection.

Other Psychosocial Variables. A number of other psychosocial variables have been shown to affect the progression of HIV. Cole, Kemeny, Taylor, and Visscher (1996), for example, investigated the role of disclosure and found that gay men who concealed their sexual orientation had a faster course of HIV infection by 1.5 to 2 years than those who had disclosed their sexual orientation. In subsequent research, however, Cole, Kemeny, and Taylor (1997) found that a subset of gay men who were sensitive to "rejection" did better if they kept their homosexual orientation concealed. Perhaps related, our group (O'Cleirigh et al., 1999) demonstrated that long-term survivors of AIDS had higher levels of emotional expression than an HIV-positive comparison group. Furthermore, in studies of long-term survivors (Balbin et al., 1999; Ironson et al., 1998), we also found that individuals in this "unusual" group had higher scores than an HIV comparison group on a number of other psychological variables, including collaborative relationships with their doctors, life involvement, being part-nered, and hopefulness.

In another study examining the effects of stress management on HIV progression, we found that the practice of relaxation techniques, doing homework, and attending stress management sessions were significantly related to disease progression to AIDS at a 2-year follow-up period (Iron-son, Friedman, et al., 1994). Thus, individual differences in the amount of effort people put into an intervention rather than merely being part of an intervention may be important in affecting disease progression.

Last, studies have shown a connection between HIV survival and hardi-ness—that is, a sense of commitment and control and an ability to see ad-versity as a challenge. For example, Solomon et al. (1987) demonstrated that HIV-infected individuals who were emotionally hardy were more likely to be alive at follow-up than less-hardy individuals were.

Thus, disclosure, emotional expression, and hardiness appear to influ-ence the progression of HIV infection. Specifically, those HIV-infected in-dividuals who are able to disclose their sexual orientation (if they are gay), who are able to express their emotions, and who are emotionally hardy ap-pear to have an immunological advantage.

Religion, Spirituality, and HIV

Health and Long Survival

A number of recent findings suggest that religion and spirituality may be an essential component to health and well-being in individuals with HIV. For example, Ironson et al. (2000) and Ironson et al. (in press) recently con-ducted a study of the role of religion in the lives of long-term HIV survivors (it had been at least 4 years since they had an AIDS-defining symptom be-fore starting on protease inhibitors) versus an HIV-positive comparison group (most of whom would not become long-term survivors). These two groups were compared on two measures relevant to religion: (1) a 25-item scale (a short form of the IWORSHIP scale; Ironson et al., in press) that has 4 subscales measuring aspects of spirituality/religiousness: a sense of peace, faith in God, religious behavior, and compassion for others, and (2) use of religion as a coping strategy. This study found that long-term survivors scored significantly higher than the comparison group on all 4 subscales of the IWORSHIP (Ironson et al., in press). More specifically, long-term survivors were more likely than the HIV-positive comparison group (Ironson et al., in press) to report a more compassionate, respectful view of others; to participate more frequently in religious behaviors, such as attending services, praying, or meditating; to have faith in God; to have a sense of peace; and to use religion as a coping strategy (Ironson et al., 2000).

Similarly, Barroso (1999) recently interviewed 25 men and women who were long-term nonprogressors (HIV positive for 7 or more years, CD4 counts of at least $500/mm^3$, and free from opportunistic infections and/or AIDS-defining illnesses) to determine psychological and social factors that might help account for their resistance to the disease. A content analysis used to elicit "themes" found that viewing HIV as a manageable illness, taking care of one's physical health, valuing human connectedness, taking care of one's emotional and mental health, and spirituality were all deemed as important to these nonprogressors.

Coping, Psychological Well-Being, and Risk Behaviors

Research indicates that many people with HIV view religion and spirituality as a bridge between hopelessness and meaningfulness in life. For example, Woods and Ironson (1999) found that HIV/AIDS patients appear to use spirituality more than religion in coping with their illness. The investigators made this finding by using a semistructured interview with 60 patients suffering from cancer, heart attacks, or HIV/AIDS. Specifically, these patients were asked to identify themselves as religious, spiritual, or both, as well as to report on how their illness was affected by their religious and spiritual beliefs. This study found that the HIV/AIDS patients were more likely to identify themselves as spiritual (70%), whereas heart attack patients were more likely to identify themselves as primarily religious (65%). Cancer patients were evenly divided, with 35% identifying themselves as spiritual, 35% as religious, and 30% as both. In fact, the HIV patients in this study appeared to be alienated from their religion (only 10% identified themselves as being solely religious).

Additionally, although both religious and spiritual people felt that their beliefs influenced their recoveries, there were marked differences in their explanations for how this was accomplished. The spiritually oriented individuals noted that their beliefs influenced their recovery through self-empowerment (e.g., giving them courage or knowledge of how to heal, giving them optimism, helping them cope and relax). In contrast, those identifying themselves as primarily religious stated that their beliefs helped them through something done to them directly (e.g., their prayers would be answered), through others (e.g., asking guidance from doctors, asking others to pray for them), or through religious rules governing specific health-affecting behaviors (e.g., alcohol, tobacco use, etc.). Moreover, there were significant differences between these two groups in their overall views of God, self, world, and others.

Several studies have found a relationship between spirituality/religiousness and lower reported levels of distress. In a diverse sample of 279 HIV-positive people Ironson et al. (in press) found significant correlations between high spirituality/religiousness and lower anxiety, less perceived distress, less hopelessness, and more optimism. In addition, spirituality/religiousness was also related to lower levels of the stress hormone cortisol.

Woods et al. (1999a) recently examined the relationship between religiosity and the affective and immune status of 106 HIV-positive, mildly symptomatic gay men. This study found that religious coping (e.g., placing trust in God, seeking comfort in religion) was significantly associated with lower scores on the Beck Depression Inventory, but not with specific immune markers. In contrast, religious behavior (e.g., service attendance, prayer, spiritual discussion, reading religious literature) was significantly associated with higher T-helper-inducer cell (CD4+) counts and higher CD4+ percentages, but not with depression. Regression analyses indicated that religiosity's associations with affect and immune status was not mediated by the subjects' sense of self-efficacy or ability to actively cope with their health situation. The associations between religiosity, affect, and immune status also appeared to be independent of symptom status. Self-efficacy, however, did appear to contribute uniquely and significantly to lower depression scores.

In another study, Woods et al. (1999b) examined the relationship between religiosity, emotional affect, and immune status in 33 HIV-positive African American women (stage 2, CDC HIV status). Investigators found that religious coping was significantly associated with lower levels of depression and anxiety. Statistical analysis revealed that the effect of religious coping on depressive symptoms appeared to be mediated by an "active" coping style. Then again, the association between religious coping and lower levels of anxiety did not appear to be mediated by either active coping or a sense of self-efficacy (personal empowerment). In addition, contrary to the result of their other study in HIV-positive gay men (Woods et al., 1999a), this study did not find a statistically significant association between religious behavior and immune status.

There is some evidence that spirituality has a beneficial effect on psychological well-being in HIV-infected individuals. Fryback and Reinert (1999), for example, found in a small study of patients with HIV and cancer that those who had found "meaning" in their disease through spirituality believed that they had a better quality of life at the time of the interview than they had had before their diagnosis. Similarly, in a large cross-sectional study, Coleman and Holzemer (1999) measured depression, hope, and state-trait anxiety in a sample of 117 African American men and women living with HIV disease to explore the relationship of spiritual well-being and HIV symptoms to these factors. Investigators found that existential well-being—a spiritual indicator of meaning and purpose—was significantly related to the participants' psychological well-being. In addition, HIV symptoms were found to be significant predictors of psychological well-being.

Finally, there is evidence that higher spirituality/religiousness is related to a variety of risk-related behaviors such as safe sex, decreased use of alcohol, and positive behaviors such as helping others (Ironson et al., in press).

Therefore, more research is needed to further delineate the effects of religious-spiritual beliefs and behaviors on the course of HIV illness. However, the research to date suggests that certain spiritual behaviors and beliefs can indeed help HIV-infected people cope with their illness and give them a better quality of life by improving their psychological well-being.

Conclusions and Implications for the Treatment of HIV/AIDS

HIV infection is a complex condition with many manifestations. Although just a few years ago most of those infected would go on to develop full-blown AIDS and die, recent advances in pharmacological treatments for this condition have significantly prolonged survival. Nevertheless, there is still no cure for this disease, and the course of infection with HIV varies widely among individuals. It has been hypothesized that some of the variation is due to psychosocial factors, including stressful life events, psychological distress, ways of coping with HIV infection, and the quality of the social network. The data discussed in this chapter support the hypothesis that coping with HIV infection is a complex phenomenon that involves multiple interacting variables.

Religion and spirituality represent one mechanism by which individuals with HIV/AIDS may cope with their illness. Although only a few studies on the relationship between religion/spirituality and physical and psychological health have been done to date in HIV populations, there is certainly enough data to suggest that this area warrants significantly more attention by the medical community.

Indeed, in this chapter we have shown that religion and spirituality do seem to help long-term HIV survivors, particularly once they start developing symptoms. What is not known yet, however, is whether religion and spirituality play a role in increasing survival in individuals infected with HIV, although preliminary data from the Ironson et al. (in press) study of long-term survivors suggest it may have a role. Nevertheless, there appears to be sufficient evidence demonstrating the ability of religion and spirituality to affect coping and distress, cortisol, and risky behaviors in HIV-positive individuals, factors that can potentially play a significant role in affecting the progression of HIV infection to full-blown AIDS. It is possible, therefore, that religious and spiritual beliefs are analogous to cognitive-behavioral interventions, which have been shown to enhance coping and social support in HIV-infected individuals and to contribute to improved quality of life factors, such as emotional functioning, social functioning, and sense of well-being (Lutgendorf et al., 1994).

Before attempting to incorporate this research into clinical practice, however, it is important to keep in mind that we still know relatively little about what the constructs "religion" and "spirituality" truly represent. Indeed, the studies we have highlighted demonstrate that while HIV-infected individuals may embrace spirituality, they may have a more fearful view of what they perceive religion to be. This is because the two major routes of acquiring HIV are through homosexual contact and intravenous drug abuse, two behaviors that are frowned upon and even denounced by mainstream religious traditions. Therefore, before attempting to use religious or spiritual interventions in this population, we need to better understand what the individual's spiritual or religious views are and whether these views are helpful and comforting or cause fear and anxiety. Those spiritual and religious beliefs and practices that promote a sense of comfort in God, a feeling of connection to others, and a willingness to forgive oneself and others for transgressions can all be extremely helpful psychologically, whereas spiritual and religious beliefs that provoke a sense of fear of God, alienation from others, and rumination about one's own or others' flaws are likely to have negative cognitive and emotional consequences.

We also need a better understanding of whether it is helpful or harmful to encourage new religious or spiritual beliefs in individuals who have few or none. Although it may not be damaging to make the nonreligious patient aware of information on the relationship between spirituality and health in a nonjudgmental way, there are many ethical reasons why openly encouraging a patient to engage in specific religious or spiritual practice may be detrimental (see chapter 14 in this volume).

There is currently an urgent need for longitudinal studies to determine if people become more religious as a result of illness or if the people who are more religious are somehow protected from disease progression. If the latter turns out to be the case, then we may have an opportunity to begin intervening at the moment an HIV diagnosis is made, when many people start reexamining and rethinking their relationship with their religious beliefs. By quickly identifying which beliefs may help them and which may harm them, we will have another important tool to use against this devastating illness.

NOTE

1. The Centers for Disease Control and Prevention has categorized HIV infection into four different groups based on the presence or absence of disease and clinical or laboratory findings. The four groups are (1) an acute infection, (2) an asymptomatic infection, (3) persistent generalized lymphadenopathy, and (4) acquired immunodeficiency syndrome (AIDS).

REFERENCES

Balbin, E. G., Ironson, G. H., & Solomon, G. F. (1999). Stress and coping: The psychoneuroimmunology of HIV/AIDS. *Baillieres Clinical Endocrinology and Metabolism* 13, 125–143.

Barroso, J. (1999). Long-term nonprogressors with HIV disease. *Nursing Research* 48, 242–249.

Blaxhult, A., & Lidman, K. (1998). Current treatment of HIV infection. *Nordisk Medicin* 113, 290–292, 296.

Blomkvist, V., Theorell, T., Jonsson, H., Schulman, S., Berntorp, E., & Stiegendal, L. (1994). Psychosocial self-prognosis in relation to mortality and morbidity in hemophiliacs with HIV infection. *Psychotherapy and Psychosomatics* 62, 185–192.

Bower, J. E., Kemeny, M. E., Taylor, S. E., & Fahey, J. L. (1998). Cognitive processing, discovery of meaning: CD4 decline, and AIDS-related mortality among bereaved HIV-seropositive men. *Journal of Consulting and Clinical Psychology* 66, 979–986.

Burack, J. H., Barrett, D. C., Stall, R. D., Chesney, M. A., Ekstrand, M. L., & Coates, T. J. (1993). Depressive symptoms and CD4 lymphocyte decline among HIV-infected men. *Journal of the American Medical Association* 270, 2568–2573.

Byrnes, D. M., Antoni, M. H., Goodkin, K., Efantis-Potter, J., Asthana, D., Simon, T., Munajj, J., Ironson, G., & Fletcher, M. A. (1998). Stressful events, pessimism, natural killer cell cytotoxicity, and cytotoxic/suppressor T cells in HIV+ black women at risk for cervical cancer. *Psychosomatic Medicine* 60, 714–722.

Capitano, J. P., & Lerche, N. W. (1998). Social separation, housing relocation, and survival in simian AIDS: A retrospective analysis. *Psychosomatic Medicine* 60, 235–244.

Centers for Disease Control and Prevention (2000). *HIV/AIDS Surveillance Report* 12(1).

Cole, S. W., & Kemeny, M. E. (1991). Psychosocial influences in the progression of HIV infection. In R. A. Ader, D. L. Felten, & N. Cohen (Eds.), *Psychoneuroimmunology*, 3rd ed. San Diego: Academic Press.

Cole, S. W., Kemeny, M. E., & Taylor, S. E. (1997). Social identify and physical health: Accelerated HIV progression in rejection-sensitive gay men. *Journal of Personality and Social Psychology* 72, 320–335.

Cole, S. W., Kemeny, M. E., Taylor, S. E., & Visscher, B. R. (1996). Elevated physical health risk among gay men who conceal their homosexual identity. *Health Psychology* 15, 243–251.

Coleman, C. L., & Holzemer, W. L. (1999). Spirituality, psychological well-being, and HIV symptoms for African Americans living with HIV disease. *Journal of the Association of Nurses in AIDS Care* 10, 42–50.

Durant, J., Clevenbergh, P., Halfon, P., Delgiudice, P., Porsin, S., Simonet, P., Montagne, N., Boucher, C. A., Schapiro, J. M., & Dellamonica, P. (1999). Drug-resistance genotyping in HIV-l therapy: The VIRADAPT randomized controlled trial. *Lancet* 353, 2195–2199.

Eich-Höchli, D., Niklowitz, M. W., Lüthy, R., & Opravil, M. (1997). Are immunological markers, social and personal resources, or a complaint-free state predictors of progression among HIV-infected patients? *Acta Psychiatrica Scandinavica* 95, 476–484.

Evans, D. L., Leserman, J., Perkins, D. O., Stern, R. A., Murphy, C., Zheng, B., Gettes, D., Longmate, J. A., Silva, S. G., van der Horst, C. M., Hall, C. D., Folds, J. D., Golden, R. N., & Petitto, J. M. (1997). Severe life stress as a predictor of early disease progression in HIV infection. *American Journal of Psychiatry* 154, 630–634.

Fauci, A. S. (1988). The scientific agenda for AIDS. *Issues in Science and Technology* 4, 33–42.

Fryback, P. B., & Reinert, B. R. (1999). Spirituality and people with potentially fatal diagnoses. *Nursing Forum* 34, 13–22.

Goodkin, K., Feaster, D. J., Tuttle, R., Blaney, N. T., Kumar, M., Baum, M. K., Slapshak, P., & Fletcher, M. A. (1996). Bereavement is associated with time-dependent decrements in cellular immune function in asymptomatic human immunodeficiency virus type 1-seropositive homosexual men. *Clinical and Diagnostic Laboratory Immunolo*gy 3, 109–118.

Ickovics, J. R., Hamburger, M. E., Vlahov, D., Schoenbaum, E. E., Schuman, P., Boland, R. J., Moore, J., for the HIV Epidemiology Research Study Group (2001). Mortality, CD4 cell count decline, and depressive symptoms among HIV-seropositive women: Longitudinal analysis from the HIV epidemiology research study. *Journal of the American Medical Association* 285(11), 1–22.

Ironson, G., Friedman, A., Klimas, N., Antoni, M. H., Fletcher, M. A., LaPerriere, A., Simoneau, J., & Schneiderman, N. (1994). Distress, denial, and low adherence to behavioral interventions predict faster disease progression in gay men infected with human immunodeficiency virus. *International Journal of Behavioral Medicine* 1, 90–105.

Ironson, G., Solomon, G., Balbin, E. B., O'Cleirigh, C., George, A., Kumar, M., Larson, D., and Woods, T. (in press). Spirituality, cortisol and long survival with HIV/AIDS: Examining associations with a measure of both spirituality and religiousness. *Annals of Behavioral Medicine* (special issue on religion and health).

Ironson, G., Solomon, G. F., Balbin, E., O'Cleirigh, C., George, A., Schneiderman, N., & Woods, T. (March 1998). Characteristics of long-term survivors of AIDS. Paper presented at the annual meeting of the American Psychosomatic Society, Clearwater, FL.

Ironson, G., Solomon, G. F., Balbin, E., O'Cleirigh, C., George, A., Schneiderman, N., & Woods, T. (March 2000). Religious behavior, religious coping, and compassionate view of others associated with long-term survival with AIDS. Abstract presented at the fifty-eighth annual American Psychosomatic Society meeting, Savannah, GA. Abstract # 1415 (published in *Pyschosomatic Medicine* 62, 113).

Kemeny, M. E., & Dean, L. (1995). Effects of AIDS-related bereavement on HIV progression among New York City gay men. *AIDS Education and Prevention* 7 (supplement), 36–47.

Kemeny, M., Duran, R., Taylor, S., Weiner, H., Visscher, B., & Fahey, J. (1990). Chronic depression predicts CD4 decline over a five-year period in HIV-seropositive men. Paper presented at the Sixth International Conference on AIDS, San Francisco, CA.

Kemeny, M. E., Weiner, H., Taylor, S. E., Schneider, S., Visscher, B., & Fahey, J. L. (1994). Repeated bereavement, depressed mood, and immune parameters in HIV seropositive and seronegative gay men. *Health Psychology* 13, 14–24.

Kessler, R. C., Foster, C., Joseph, J., Ostrow, D., Wortman, C., Phair, J., & Chmiel, J. (1991). Stressful life events and symptom onset in HIV infection. *American Journal of Psychiatry* 148, 733–738.

Leserman, J., Jackson, E. D., Petitto, J. M., Golden, R. N., Silva, S. G., Perkins, D. O., Cai, J., Folds, J. D., & Evans, D. L. (1999). Progression to AIDS: The effects of stress, depressive symptoms, and social support. *Psychosomatic Medicine* 61, 397–406.

Leserman, J., Petitto, J. M., Golden, R. N., Gaynes, B. N., Gu, H., Perkins, D. O., Silva, S. G., Folds, J. D., and Evans, D. L. (2000). Impact of stressful life events, depression, social support, coping, and cortisol on progression to AIDS. *American Journal of Psychiatry* 157, 1221–1228.

Leserman, J., Petitto, J. M., Perkins, D. O., Folds, J. D., Golden, R. N., & Evans, D. L. (1997). Severe stress, depressive symptoms, and changes in lymphocyte subsets in human immunodeficiency virus-infected men. *Archives of General Psychiatry* 54, 279–285.

Lutgendorf, S., Antoni, M. H., Schneiderman, N., & Fletcher M. A. (1994). Psychosocial counseling to improve quality of life in HIV infection. *Patient Education and Counseling* 24, 217–235.

Lyketsos, C. G., Hoover, D. R., Guccione, M., Senterfitt, W., Dew, M. A., Wesch, J., VanRanen, M. J., Treisman, G. J., & Morgenstern, H. (1993). Depressive symptoms as predictors of medical outcomes in HIV infection. Multicenter AIDS Cohort Study. *Journal of the American Medical Association* 270, 2563–2567.

Mayne, T. J., Vittinghoff, E., Chesney, M. A., Barrett, D. C., & Coates, T. J. (1996). Depressive affect and survival among gay and bisexual men infected with HIV. *Archives of Internal Medicine* 156, 2233–2238.

Miller, G. E., and Cole, S. W. (1998). Social relationships and the progression of human immunodeficiency virus infection: A review of evidence and possible underlying mechanisms. *Annals of Behavioral Medicine* 20, 181–189.

Miller, G. E., Kemeny, M. E., Taylor, S. E., Cole, S. W., and Visscher, B. R. (1997). Social relationships and immune processes in HIV seropositive gay and bisexual men. *Annals of Behavioral Medicine* 19, 139–151.

Moore, R. D., and Chaisson, R. E. (1999). Natural history of HIV infection in the era of combination therapy. *AIDS* 1, 1933–1942.

Mulder, C. L., Antoni, M. H., Dulvenvoorden, H. J., Kauffmann, R. H., & Goodkin, K. (1995). Active confrontational coping predicts decreased clinical progression over a one-year period in HIV-infected homosexual men. *Journal of Psychosomatic Research* 39, 957–965.

Mulder, C. L., de Vroome, E. M., van Griensven, G., & Antoni, M. (1995). Distraction as a predictor of the biological course of HIV-1 infection over a 7-year period in gay men. *Psychosomatic Medicine* 57:67 (abstract).

Mulder, C. L., de Vroome, E. M. M., van Griensven, G. J., Antoni, M. H., & Sandfort, T. G. (1999). Avoidance as a predictor of the biological course of HIV infection over a 7-year period in gay men. *Health Psychology* 10, 107–113.

O'Cleirigh, C., Ironson, G. H, Balbin, E. G., Ohata, J., Scheiderman, N., Fletcher, M. A., & Solomon, G. (April 1999). Emotional expression is associated with long-term survival of patients with AIDS. Poster presented at the annual meeting of the Society of Behavioral Medicine, San Diego.

Patterson, T. L., Shaw, W. S., Semple, S. J., Cherner, M., McCutchan, J. A., Atkinson, J. H., Grant, I., & Nannis, E. (1996). Relationship of psychosocial factors to HIV disease progression. *Annals of Behavioral Medicine* 18, 30–39.

Perry, S., Fishman, B., Jacobsberg, L., & Frances, A. (1992). Relationships over 1 year between lymphocyte subsets and psychosocial variables among adults with infection by human immunodeficiency virus. *Archives of General Psychiatry* 49, 396–401.

Perry, S. W., III (1994). HIV-related depression. *Research Publications—Association for Research in Nervous and Mental Disease* 72, 223–238.

Rabkin, J. G., Goetz, R. R., Remien, R. H., Williams, J. B., Todak, G., & Gorman, J. M. (1997). Stability of mood despite HIV illness progression in a group of homosexual men. *American Journal of Psychiatry* 154, 231–238.

Rabkin, J. G., Williams, J. B. W., Remien, R. H., Goetz, R., Kertzner, R., & Gorman, J. M. (1991). Depression, distress, lymphocyte subsets, and human immunodeficiency virus symptoms on two occasions in HIV-positive homosexual men. *Archives of General Psychiatry* 40, 111–119.

Reed, G. M., Kemeny, M. E., Taylor, S. E., Visscher, B. R. (1999). Negative HIV-specific expectancies and AIDS-related bereavement as predictors of symptom onset in asymptomatic HIV-positive gay men. *Health Psychology* 10, 354–363.

Reed, G. M., Kemeny, M. E., Taylor, S. E., Wang, H. Y., & Visscher, B. R. (1994). Realistic acceptance as a predictor of decreased survival time in gay men with AIDS. *Health Psychology* 13, 299–307.

Segerstrom, S. C., Taylor, S. E., Kemeny, M. E., Reed, G. M., & Visscher, B. R. (1996). Casual attributions predict rate of immune decline in HIV-seropositive gay men. *Health Psychology* 15, 485–493.

Sendi, P. P., Bucher, H. C., Craig, B. A., Pfluger, D., & Battegay, M. (1999). Estimating AIDS-free survival in a severely immunosuppressed asymptomatic HIV-infected population in the era of antiretroviral triple combination therapy. *Journal of Acquired Immune Deficiency Syndromes and Human Retrovirology* 20, 376–381.

Solano, L., Costa, M., Salvati, S., Coda, R., Aiuti, F., Mezzaroma, I., & Bertini, M. (1993). Psychosocial factors and clinical evolution in HIV-1 infection: A longitudinal study. *Journal of Psychosomatic Research* 37, 39–51.

Solomon, G., Temoshok, L., O'Leary, A., & Zich, J. (1987). An intensive psy-choimmunologic study of long-surviving persons with AIDS. Pilot work, background studies, hypotheses, and methods. *Annals of the New York Academy of Sciences* 496, 647–655.

Stine, G. J. (1996). *AIDS update*. Upper Saddle River, NJ: Prentice Hall.

Theorell, T., Blomkvist, V., Jonsson, H., Schulman, S., Berntorp, E., & Stigendal, L. (1995). Social support and the development of immune function in human immunodeficiency virus infection. *Psychosomatic Medicine* 57, 32–36.

Tsevat, J., Sherman, S. N., McElwee, J. A., Mandell, K. L., Simbartl, L. A., Son-nenberg, F. A., & Fowler, F. J. Jr. (1999). The will to live among HIV-infected patients. *Annals of Internal Medicine* 131, 194–198.

Vassend, O., Eskild, A., & Halvorsen, R. (1997). Negative effectivity, coping, immune status, and disease progression in HIV-infected individuals. *Psychological Health* 12, 375–388.

Vedhara, K., Nott, K. H., Bradbeer, C. S., Davidson, E. A. F., Ong, E. L. C., Snow, M. H., Palmer, D., & Nayagam, A. T. (1997). Greater emotional distress is associated with accelerated CD4+ cell decline in HIV infection. *Journal of Psychosomatic Research* 42, 379–390.

Woods, T. E., Antoni, M. H., Ironson, G. H., & Kling, D. W. (1999a). Religiosity is associated with affective and immune status in symptomatic HIV-infected gay men. *Journal of Psychosomatic Research* 46, 165–176.

Woods, T. E., Antoni, M. H., Ironson, G. H., & Kling, D. W. (1999b). Religiosity is associated with affective status in symptomatic HIV-infected African-American women. *Journal of Health Psychology* 4, 317–326.

Woods, T. E., & Ironson, G. H. (1999). Religion and spirituality in the face of illness. *Journal of Health Psychology* 4, 393–412.

9

Hostility, Neuroendocrine Changes, and Health Outcomes

REDFORD B. WILLIAMS

Research conducted over the past several decades has demonstrated a moderately strong association between chronic negative emotional states, such as hostility and anger, and negative health outcomes. The interdisciplinary field of psychoneuroimmunology (PNI) provides a good environment for studying the effects of hostility on health because of the complex sequelae of events in the central nervous system, endocrine system, immune system, blood, and heart, all of which are set in motion as a consequence of chronic negative emotions. The emphasis of many religious and spiritual traditions on mastering or controlling anger and other negative emotions may offer opportunities not only for studying the hostility phenomenon but also for understanding ways that the health-damaging effects of hostility may be thwarted.

Hostility and Health

Research on the health consequences of hostility and anger essentially began with Friedman and Rosenman's pioneering work to identify persons at high risk of developing coronary disease. Friedman and Rosenman (1974) identified a "type A" behavior pattern, which they characterized as a competitive, impatient, hurrying behavioral and emotional style. Furthermore, hostility was considered a key component of the type A behavior pattern.

Beginning in the early 1980s, Williams, Haney, and colleagues (1980) demonstrated that scores on a 50-item hostility scale (Ho) correlated positively with coronary artery disease (CAD) severity. In fact, Ho scores cor-related with CAD independently of type A and just as strongly as type A, and in women as well as in men. Because the Ho scale is part of the Min-nesota Multiphasic Personality Inventory (MMPI), a psychological assess-ment scale that was originally developed in the 1950s, in the 1980s several groups began rescoring old MMPIs for the Ho scale to determine if, in-deed, Ho scores predicted increased coronary heart disease (CHD) risk. For example, Shekelle and coworkers (1983) in the Western Electric Study found those with high Ho scores were also more likely to die of all causes, including cancer. In another study of this type, Barefoot et al. (1983) followed up 255 doctors who had taken the MMPI in medical school 25 years earlier. They found that those with higher Ho scores in medical school were nearly *seven* times more likely than their less hostile counterparts to be dead by age 50.

Although some of these follow-up studies failed to demonstrate the Ho scale's ability to predict health outcomes (Hearn et al., 1989; Leon et al., 1988; McCranie et al., 1986), a number of other studies, using other corrob-orating self-report measures of hostility and related constructs, especially behavioral assessments of interview data (Brummett et al., 1998; Williams, Barefoot, et al., 1988), strongly suggest that hostility does predict increased risk of coronary disease, as well as all-cause morbidity and mortality. Indeed, Williams, Barefoot, and colleagues (1988) analyzed risk-factor, behavioral, and angiographic data collected on 2,289 patients who were undergoing diagnostic coronary angiography at Duke University Medical Center be-tween 1974 and 1980 to determine the relationship between type A behav-ior pattern and angiographically documented CAD. This study showed that type A behavior as assessed by the Structured Interview was significantly as-sociated with CAD severity, even after controlling for known risk factors for CAD, including age, sex, hyperlipidemia (elevated blood lipid levels), smok-ing, hypertension, and their various significant interactions.

This relationship, however, *was* age-dependent; among patients age 45 or younger, type As had more severe CAD than did type Bs; among pa-tients age 46 to 54, CAD severity was similar between type As and type Bs; and among patients 55 and older, there was a trend toward more severe CAD among type Bs than among type As. Williams, Barefoot, and col-leagues concluded that "inadequate sample sizes, use of assessment tools other than the SI [Structured Interview], and failure to consider the Type A by age interaction could account for failures to find a Type A-CAD rela-tionship in other studies."

Recently, Haney et al. (1996) used the Interpersonal Hostility Assessment Technique (IHAT) to measure hostility from verbal behavior. In the IHAT, four types of behaviors are scored as hostility: (1) evading the question, (2) irritation, and (3) indirect and (4) direct challenges to the interviewer. The sum of the frequencies of these acts is a Hostile Behavior Index, which is divided into two components: (1) verbal, scored with speech content in mind, and (2) paraverbal, based on vocal stylistics. This study examined characteristics of IHAT assessments in 129 male coronary patients and found that the Hostile Behavior Index score correlated highly with CAD severity after controlling for traditional risk factors.

Results from laboratory studies provide further support that chronic hostility is damaging to health. Suarez and Williams (1989) demonstrated that laboratory-induced "harassment" produced significantly greater cardiovascular overreaction, or hyperreactivity, in the high hostility (high Ho) scoring subjects. Another important finding of this study was that high anger and irritation ratings were significantly associated with enhanced cardiovascular reactivity only in subjects who scored high for hostility. Indeed, for low Ho subjects, becoming irritated when harassed was uncorrelated with cardiovascular reactivity.

Suarez and colleagues have since demonstrated that men who score high for hostility show "excessive" behaviorally induced cardiovascular and neuroendocrine responsivity, as well as anger to interpersonally challenging situations (Suarez, Kuhn, et al. 1998). In fact, "harassed" subjects with high Ho scores exhibited enhanced and prolonged blood pressures, heart rate, forearm blood flow, forearm vascular resistance, norepinephrine, testosterone, and cortisol responses relative to low Ho subjects in the harassed condition and both high and low Ho subjects in the nonharassed condition. Heightened physiological reactivity in high Ho subjects was correlated with arousal of negative affects (e.g., anger). Additionally, Suarez, Shiller, and collaborators (1997) found that compared with low-hostility men, high-hostility men report a greater frequency of anger, longer duration of anger, more frequent brooding, and a more hostile outlook.

Potential Mechanisms

What potential mechanisms explain the increased morbidity and mortality among high Ho individuals? One may be that hostility influences health through lifestyle. For example, Siegler's Alumni Heart Study (Siegler et al., 1992) found that those students who had higher Ho scores when they were in college in the 1960s had an increased incidence of health-damaging behaviors 21 to 23 years later. Indeed, they consumed more caffeine, were more likely to be current smokers, were heavier, and had higher lipid ratios than those with lower hostility scores during college. Siegler and colleagues concluded that "these associations are large enough to have possible public health significance." These findings, along with complementary findings from the CARDIA study (Scherwitz et al., 1992), show that hostile persons are placing themselves at higher risk for health problems indirectly by eating more, drinking more alcohol, and smoking more cigarettes.

Hostility and Impaired Autonomic Balance

However, growing evidence indicates that chronic hostility may also have direct negative effects on health through physiological processes. In a study in the late 1980s, for example, Muranaka and colleagues (1988) found that type A men have a shorter and less pronounced vagally mediated decrease in heart rate during elicitation of the "dive" reflex, which suggests that a weaker parasympathetic function exists in coronary-prone persons. This finding was confirmed by Fukudo and colleagues (1992) in a subsequent study, which showed that the extent to which cardiac stimulation with isoproterenol is enhanced by atropine pretreatment—a measure of the amount of vagal antagonism of sympathetic nervous system effects on the myocardium in the normal state—is strongly correlated with lower scores on several different hostility and anger scales. In other words, high Ho subjects show weaker vagal antagonism of sympathetic nervous system effects on the heart. Sloan et al. (1993) further confirmed this result by showing a negative correlation between Ho scores and a measure of vagal tone (heart period variability) in ambulatory Holter ECG records.

Hostility and Impaired Clotting Response

High Ho individuals also appear to have altered platelet reactivity to psychological stress. Markovitz et al. (1996), for example, recently found that β-thromboglobulin (BTG) levels were increased (a sign of increased clotting that could lead to a myocardial infarction) in a group of men after they had been subjected to a laboratory stressor (i.e., a "type A" Structured Interview and speech task). The group of men included 14 who had suffered and recovered from a heart attack and 15 healthy men of similar age.

This study found that increases in BTG with stress were related to both higher Structured Interview ratings of Potential for Hostility and type A behavior. Even after statistical adjustment for the fact that men taking aspirin and other platelet inhibitors before the study had less change in BTG with stress, Structured Interview ratings of Potential for Hostility were still "strongly" related to increases in BTG with stress. Increases in BTG, however, were not related to Cook-Medley hostility scores. In addition, contrary to expectations, healthy men tended to have greater change in BTG with stress than the post– myocardial infarction men.

Hostility and Impaired Immune Response

Persons with high levels of hostility show differential changes in expression of cytokines, which are low-molecular-weight proteins that are released by immune cells (as well as other cells in the body) in response to infectious agents, such as bacteria, viruses, fungi, and parasites (Rabin, 1999, p. 64). For example, Suarez et al. (2000) recently examined the relationship between levels of tryptophan (a precursor of the neurotransmitter serotonin, which, when depleted, has been linked to aggressive behavior) in cerebrospinal fluid (CSF) and stress-induced changes in the expression of cytokines and adhesion molecules on blood monocytes from 56 healthy adults, age 18 to 49. The stress protocol involved reading aloud an anger and sad recall. Blood samples for monocyte markers were taken before and immediately after the completion of the protocol. This study found that CSF-tryptophan was positively associated with stress-induced changes in the cytokine tumor necrosis factor-α (TNF-α) for women, and negatively for men. CSF-tryptophan also was significantly associated with changes in the cytokine interleukin 1-α (IL-1α), indicating that lower CSF tryptophan was associated with greater stress-induced changes in IL-1α in both men and women. Results of this study suggest that stress-related enhancement of pro-inflammatory cytokines (i.e., TNF-α and IL-1α) on blood monocytes, which are known to promote the formation of plaques on the walls of arteries, is associated with low levels of tryptophan, a characteristic associated with behavioral risk factors for atherosclerosis (hardening of the arteries).

Hostility and Altered Serotonergic Activity

Recent research suggests that hostility is associated with low brain serotonergic function. Indeed, low levels of central nervous system serotonergic activity have been found to correlate inversely with human aggressive behavior, as well as depression in some individuals. For example, Ravindran and colleagues (1999) recently showed that lowering tryptophan levels in male subjects (with no personal or family history of depression) by feeding them a tryptophan-deficient diet reduced plasma tryptophan and serotonin and increased negative moods (particularly depression and anger). This mood change was directly related to the extent of the tryptophan or serotonin reductions. Furthermore, studies have shown that fluoxetine, a selective serotonin reuptake inhibitor that increases extracellular concentrations of serotonin in brain regions, reduces aggressive behavior in animals and decreases aggressive behavior and feelings of anger or hostility in humans as well (see Fuller, 1996, for a review of this data).

Low serotonergic central nervous system activity can also result from inherited factors. Indeed, variations, or polymorphisms, of the genes involved in the processing of serotonin have been implicated in the hostile personality type. Heils et al. (1997), for example, found a functional polymorphism in the transcriptional control region upstream of the serotonin transporter gene at the *SLC6A4* locus. The transcriptional promoter activity of the short (*s*) form was less than that of the long (*l*) form of the serotonin transporter promoter gene. In addition, they found individuals with the *s* form were more likely to have neurotic characteristics (e.g., anxiety, anger, hostility, and depression).

Although a later study by Ohara and colleagues (1998) failed to find an association between the *l/s* polymorphism of the serotonin transporter gene and mood disorders, a more recent study by Manuck and collaborators (1999) found a strong association between hostile behavior and polymorphisms of the gene coding for tryptophan hydroxylase (TPH), the rate-limiting enzyme in serotonin biosynthesis. In this study, men and women ($n = 251$) were genotyped for the A218C polymorphism located on intron 7 of the TPH gene. All subjects were administered a standard interview to measure aggression and anger-related traits of personality; in a portion of subjects, central nervous system serotonergic activity was assessed by neuropsychopharmacological challenge (prolactin response to fenfluramine hydrochloride). As expected, individuals who had a specific TPH gene type, or *U* allele, scored significantly higher on measures of aggression, had a tendency to experience unprovoked anger and were more likely to report expressing their anger outwardly than individuals homozygous for the alternate L allele. In men, but not women, peak prolactin response to fenfluramine was also attenuated among subjects having any U allele, relative to LL homozygotes. Manuck et al. thus concluded that "individual differences in aggressive disposition are associated with an intronic polymorphism of the TPH gene."

Emotional trauma, especially at an early age, also has been implicated in the development of low central nervous system serotonergic levels in hostile individuals. Indeed, animal research shows that harsh environmental conditions early in life can cause long-lasting biobehavioral changes through effects on serotonergic systems. Higley, Thompson, and colleagues (1993) have found that rhesus monkeys deprived of normal maternal care during the first 6 months of life grow up to have reduced brain serotonin function. Further, monkeys with low central nervous system serotonin levels early in life also have increased mortality from aggressive behavior later in life (Higley, Mehlman, et al., 1996), increased biological reactivity to stress and increased alcohol preference (Higley & Bennett, 1999), and impaired social behaviors (Higley & Linnoila, 1997). In contrast, Meaney and colleagues (1993) have shown that rats receiving *increased* maternal attention during the first 7 days of life show fewer biological response to stress later in life and are less fearful.

Potential Explanatory Models

Whatever the mechanisms mediating the effects of hostility on health, it is likely that reduced brain serotonergic function in high Ho individuals accounts, in part, for the clustering of health-damaging behavior characteristics in hostile persons. Deficient central nervous system serotonergic function also has been implicated in depression (Risch & Nemeroff, 1992). Additional support for the hypothesis that serotonin deficiency can adversely affect health comes from a consideration of recent research that links low cholesterol with certain types of mortality. Muldoon et al. (1990), in their review of the cholesterol-lowering trials, found an increase in nonillness mortality, chiefly due to accidents, suicide, and violence, in the cholesterol-lowering groups. Cohort studies have found a similar increase in violent deaths among persons with low cholesterol levels (Multiple Risk Factor Intervention Trial Research Group, 1992).

In a fascinating series of studies, the groups at Bowman Gray School of Medicine and Pittsburgh (Kaplan, Manuck, & Shively, 1991; Kaplan, Mann, et al., 1992) found that monkeys with low cholesterol levels exhibit more aggressive and fewer affiliative behaviors than their high-cholesterol counterparts. Moreover, these investigators propose that the "antisocial" behavioral effects of low cholesterol are mediated by reduced central nervous system serotonin function, as indexed by both smaller prolactin responses to fenfluramine and lower CSF 5-HIAA (tryptophan) levels in animals with lower cholesterol levels.

More direct support for this explanation comes from Engelberg (1992), who cites evidence showing decreased brain serotonin receptor numbers in the setting of low cholesterol as providing a specific mechanism whereby low cholesterol could bring about a brain serotonin deficiency state leading to the behavioral changes that predispose to violent forms of death.

In contrast to the preceding scenario, where decreased central nervous system serotonergic function and the consequent behavioral changes are secondary to decreased cholesterol concentrations, in the hostility syndrome it seems more likely that low central nervous system serotonergic function is the primary state, whether due to early environmental influences on development or to genetic factors, that leads to behavioral and physiological changes.

If additional research confirms that a serotonin deficiency is the cause of the hostility syndrome, it would have far-reaching implications for prevention and treatment of the medical disorders to which hostile persons are prone. A growing proliferation of drugs enhance central nervous system serotonin function, including selective serotonin reuptake inhibitors (e.g., fluoxetine, sertraline, paroxetine, and fluvoxamine) and specific serotonin receptor agonists (e.g., buspirone). Although developed with treatment of psychiatric disorders in mind, it may soon become evident to all that these agents could have an equally, if not more, important application in preventing the health-damaging consequences of the hostility syndrome.

Goodkin and Appels (1997) have proposed an overarching theoretical model to explain the proposed feedback relationship between behavior (e.g., hostility), associated neuroendocrine changes (e.g., serotonin), immunological responses, and the pathogenesis of coronary artery disease. They have proposed a two-stage model with the first stage consisting of a long-term chronic hostility, prolonged occupational overexertion (e.g., the "driven" type A personality), and exposure to other life stressors, such as marital discord. This stage eventually terminates in a much shorter second stage, which Goodkin and Appels have dubbed "vital exhaustion."

According to Goodkin and Appels (1997), vital exhaustion is characterized by stressor-associated neuroendocrine changes, which result in immunosuppression leading to reactivation of latent, systemic infections (such as cytomegalovirus) and potentially to autoimmune reactions as well. The consequent release of pro-inflammatory cytokines exacerbates fatigue and induces a stimulus for cytokine production in the brain. This cytokine production, in turn, stimulates a chronically activated, overcompensated limbic-hypothalamic-pituitary-adrenal axis (limbic-HPA). A chronically activated limbic-HPA system results in a dampened response, continued exhaustion, and a potential "reverberating circuit" between behavior, neuroendocrine change, cytokine release, and coronary artery occlusion. According to this model, the end of this second phase culminates in a heart attack.

Spirituality/Religion and Hostility

How might spirituality/religion have an impact on hostility? For starters, a core principle taught in both Judaism and Christianity is that people should love their neighbors as themselves; a similar precept can also be found in Eastern traditions (Haskins, 1991). The ultimate goal of Buddhism, for example, is Nirvana, which Buddha defined as the end of desire. It also means freedom, inward peace and joy, and a state in which birth, age, sickness, pain, and death cease. Nirvana, as taught by Buddhists, means a state of no flame or selfish desire—that is, no passion (Haskins, 1991). Furthermore, in Hinduism, the major religion of India, a person can achieve freedom from the sense of individuality and separateness from the universe only by completely changing one's way of thinking and of seeing the world. Thus, one must acquire certain virtues, the five most important of which are purity, self-control, detachment, truth, and nonviolence. At the same time, one must suppress the six deadly sins or passions: desire or lust, anger, greed, infatuation, pride, and envy (Parrinder, 1984).

It is striking to note, therefore, that items on the Ho (Cook-Medley) scale are in direct contrast to these precepts and teachings. For example, people who score high on the Ho scale endorse statements to the effect that (1) most people are selfish, mean, and not to be trusted; (2) I harbor a lot of anger toward others; and (3) I don't bother to hide my poor opinion of another to spare their feelings, and when I'm angry, you're going to know it (Cook & Medley, 1954).

Thus, most of the world's major religions promote a less hostile pattern of thinking, feeling, and acting. According to Kaplan (1992), although the evolution of the type A hypothesis is well documented, the "protective" corresponding type B construct has not evolved similarly. Kaplan proposes the study of four neglected protective processes that are commonly found in religious and spiritual traditions: (1) uniqueness/self-esteem/autonomy, (2) forgiveness, (3) sociability, and (4) "causal" wisdom attributions. Among these four, the forgiveness construct has received the most scientific scrutiny to date, albeit few empirical studies exist on this construct (Worthington, 1999). It would also be interesting to see if these processes have any effect on tryptophan and serotonin levels in people who practice them on a regular basis.

Summary and Conclusions

It is remarkable that recent behavioral medicine research has been uncovering psychosocial factors—hostility, depression, social isolation—that increase risk of major illness and mortality and, at the same time, appear *opposite* in many respects to characteristics the world's religions have been promoting as desirable for over 2,000 years. In addition, this research has identified risky health behaviors, biological characteristics, and neurobiological underpinnings that could account for the increased disease risk associated with psychosocial risk factors.

This confluence of scientific and religious findings and thought seems to me a most interesting example of "ancient truths find modern proofs." To those who might ask whether this means that the religious teachings are now more "believable," or that the scientific findings are more "satisfying," I would simply quote a Zen proverb: If a finger points to the moon in the night sky, which is more worthy of our attention, the finger, or the moon to which it points?

REFERENCES

Barefoot, J. C., Dahlstrom, W. G., & Williams, R. B. (1983). Hostility, CHD incidence, and total mortality: A 25-year follow-up study of 255 physicians. *Psychosomatic Medicine* 45, 59–63.

Brummett, B. H., Babyak, M. A., Barefoot, J. C., Bosworth, H. B., Clapp-Channing, N. E., Siegler, I. C., Williams, R. B., Jr., & Mark, D. B. (1998). Social support and hostility as predictors of depressive symptoms in cardiac patients one month after hospitalization: a prospective study. *Psychosomatic Medicine* 60, 707–713.

Cook, W., & Medley, D. (1954). Proposed hostility and pharasaic-virtue scales of the MMPI. *Journal of Applied Psychology* 38, 414–418.

Engelberg, H. (1992). Low serum cholesterol and suicide. *Lancet* 339, 727–729.

Friedman, M., & Rosenman, R. H. (1974). *Type A behavior and your heart.* Greenwich, CT: Fawcett.

Fukudo, S., Lane, J. D., Anderson, N. B., Kuhn, C. M., Schanberg, S. M., McCown, N., Muranaka, M., Suzuki, J., Williams, R. B., Jr. (1992). Accentuated vagal antagonism of beta-adrenergic effects on ventricular repolarization: Evidence of weaker antagonism in hostile type A men. *Circulation* 85, 2045–2053.

Fuller, R. W. (1996). Fluoxetine effects on serotonin function and aggressive behavior. *Annals of the New York Academy of Sciences* 794, 90–97.

Goodkin, K., & Appels, A. (1997). Behavioral-neuroendocrine-immunologic interactions in myocardial infarction. *Medical Hypotheses* 48, 209–214.

Haney, T. L., Maynard, K. E., Houseworth, S. J., Scherwitz, L. W., Williams, R. B., & Barefoot, J. C. (1996). The Interpersonal Hostility Assessment Technique: Description and validation against the criterion of coronary artery disease. *Journal of Personality Assessment* 66, 386–401.

Haskins, J. (1991). *Religions of the world,* rev. ed. New York: Hippocrene.

Hearn, M. D., Murray, D. M., & Luepker, R. B. (1989). Hostility, coronary heart disease, and total mortality: A 33-year follow-up study of university students. *Journal of Behavioral Medicine* 12, 105–121.

Heils, A., Mossner, R., & Lesch, K. P. T. I. (1997). The human serotonin transporter gene polymorphism: Basic research and clinical implications. *Journal of Neural Transmission* 104, 1005–1014.

Higley, J. D., & Bennett, A. J. (1999). Central nervous system serotonin and personality as variables contributing to excessive alcohol consumption in nonhuman primates. *Alcohol and Alcoholism* 34, 402–418.

Higley, J. D., & Linnoila, M. (1997). A nonhuman primate model of excessive alcohol intake. Personality and neurobiological parallels of type I- and type II-like alcoholism. *Recent Developments in Alcoholism* 13, 191–219.

Higley, J. D., Mehlman, P. T., Higley, S. B., Fernald, B., Vickers, J., Lindell, S. G., Taub, D. M., Suomi, S. J., & Linnoila, M. (1996). Excessive mortality in young free-ranging male nonhuman primates with low cerebrospinal fluid 5-hydroxyindoleacetic acid concentrations. *Archives of General Psychiatry* 53, 537–543.

Higley, J. D., Thompson, W. W., Champoux, M., Goldman, D., Hasert, M. F., Kraemer, G. W., Scanlan, J. M., Suomi, S. J., & Linnoila, M. (1993). Paternal and maternal genetic and enviromental contributions to cerebrospinal fluid monamine metabolites in Rhesus monkeys (*Macaca mulatta*). *Archives of General Psychiatry* 50, 615–623.

Kaplan, B. H. (1992). Social health and the forgiving heart: The type B story. *Journal of Behavioral Medicine* 15, 3–14.

Kaplan, J. R., Manuck, S. B., & Shively, C. A. (1991). The effects of fat and cholesterol on aggressive behavior in monkeys. *Psychosomatic Medicine* 53, 634–642.

Kaplan, J. R., Shively, C. A., Fontenot, M. B., Morgan, T. M., Howell, S. M., Manuck, S. B., Muldoon, M. F., & Mann, J. J. (1994). Demonstration of an association among dietary cholesterol, central serotonergic activity, and social behavior in monkeys. *Psychosomatic Medicine* 56, 479–484.

Leon, G. R., Finn, S. E., Murray, D., & Bailey, J. M. (1988). Inability to predict cardiovascular disease from hostility scores or MMPI items related to Type A behavior. *Journal of Consulting and Clinical Psychology* 56, 597–600.

Manuck, S. B., Flory, J. D., Ferrell, R. E., Dent, K. M., Mann, J. J., & Muldoon, M. F. (1999). Aggression and anger-related traits associated with a polymorphism of the tryptophan hydroxylase gene. *Biological Psychiatry* 45, 603–614.

Markovitz, J. H., Matthews, K. A., Kiss, J., & Smitherman, T. C. (1996). Effects of hostility on platelet reactivity to psychological stress in coronary heart disease patients and in healthy controls. *Psychosomatic Medicine* 58, 143–149.

McCranie, E. W., Watkins, L. A., Brandsma, J. M., & Sisson, B. D. (1986). Hostility, coronary heart disease (CHD), incidence, and total mortality: Lack of association in a 25-year follow-up study of 478 physicians. *Journal of Behavioral Medicine* 9, 119–125.

Meaney, M. J., Bhatnagan, S., Dioria, J., Larocque, S., Francis, D., O'Donnell, D., Shanks, N., Sharma, S., Smythe, J., and Viau, V. (1993). Molecular basis for the development of individual differences in the hypothalamic-pituitary-adrenal stress response. *Cellular and Molecular Neurobiology* 13, 321–347.

Muldoon, M. F., Manuck, S. B., & Mathews, K. M. (1990). Lowering cholesterol concentrations and mortality: A quantitative review of primary prevention trials. *British Medical Journal* 301, 309–314.

Multiple Risk Factor Intervention Trial Research Group. (1992). Serum cholesterol level and mortality. *Archives of Internal Medicine* 152, 1490–1500.

Muranaka, M., Lane, J. D., Suarez, E. C., Anderson, N. B., Suzuki, J., & Williams, R. B., Jr. (1988). Stimulus-specific patterns of cardiovascular reactivity in type A and B subjects: Evidence for enhanced vagal reactivity in type B. *Psychophysiology* 25, 330–338.

Ohara, K., Nagai, M., Tsukamoto, T., Tani, K., Suzuki, Y., & Ohara, K. (1998). Functional polymorphism in the serotonin transporter promoter at the SLC6A4 locus and mood disorders. *Biological Psychiatry* 44, 550–554.

Parrinder, G. (Ed.) (1984). *World religions: From ancient history to present*, rev. ed. New York: Facts on File.

Rabin, B. S. (1999). *Stress, Immune Function, and Health: The Connection*. New York: Wiley-Liss & Sons.

Ravindran, A. V., Griffiths, J., Merali, Z., Knott, V. J., & Anisman, H. (1999). Influence of acute tryptophan depletion on mood and immune measures in healthy males. *Psychoneuroendocrinology* 24, 99–113.

Risch, S. C., & Nemeroff, C. B. (1992). Neurochemical alterations of serotonergic neuronal systems in depression. *Journal of Clinical Psychiatry* 53(supplement), 3–7.

Scherwitz, L. W., Perkins, L. L., Chesney, M. A., Hughes, G. H., Sidney, S., & Manolio, T. A. (1992). Hostility and health behaviors in young adults: The CARDIA study. *American Journal of Epidemiology* 136, 136–145.

Shekelle, R. B., Gale, M., Ostfeld, A. M., & Paul, O. (1983). Hostility, risk of coronary disease, and mortality. *Psychosomatic Medicine* 45, 219–228.

Siegler, I. C., Peterson, B. L., Barefoot, J. C., & Williams, R. B. (1992). Hostility during late adolescence predicts coronary risk factors at mid-life. *American Journal of Epidemiology* 136, 146–154.

Sloan, R. P., Shapiro, P. A., Bagiella, E., et al. (1993). Cardiovascular autonomic control and hostility. *Psychosomatic Medicine* 55, 102.

Suarez, E. C., et al. (2000). Paper presented at the annual meeting of the Society of Behavioral Medicine, Seattle, WA.

Suarez, E. C., Kuhn, C. M., Schanberg, S. M., Williams, R. B., Jr., & Zimmermann, E. A. (1998). Neuroendocrine, cardiovascular, and emotional responses of hostile men: The role of interpersonal challenge. *Psychosomatic Medicine* 60, 78–88.

Suarez, E. C., Shiller, A. D., Kuhn, C. M., Schanberg, S., Williams, R. B., Jr., & Zimmermann, E. A. T. (1997). The relationship between hostility and beta-adrenergic receptor physiology in health young males. *Psychosomatic Medicine* 59, 481–487.

Suarez, E. C., & Williams, R. B. (1989). Situational determinants of cardiovascular and emotional reactivity in high and low hostile men. *Psychosomatic Medicine* 51: 404–418.

Williams, R. B., Haney, T. B., Lee, K. L., Kong, Y. H., Blumenthal, J. A., & Whalen, R. E. (1980). Type A behavior, hostility, and coronary atherosclerosis. *Psychosomatic Medicine* 42, 539–549.

Williams, R. B. Jr., Barefoot, J. C., Haney, T. L., Harrell, F. E., Jr., Blumenthal, J. A., Pryor. D. B., & Peterson, B. (1988). Type A behavior and angiographically documented coronary atherosclerosis in a sample of 2,289 patients. *Psychosomatic Medicine* 50, 139–152.

Worthington, E. L. (Ed.). (1999). *Dimensions of forgiveness: Psychological research and theological perspectives*. Radnor, PA: John Templeton Press.

10

Psychological Stress and Autoimmune Disease

HAROLD G. KOENIG & HARVEY JAY COHEN

Because chemicals produced by immune cells signal the brain, and the brain in turn sends chemical signals to regulate the immune system, the two systems are able to signal each other continuously and rapidly in response to external or internal threats to homeostasis. Just as the brain can send hormonal and nervous system signals that suppress immune functioning in response to stress, disruption of the regulatory influence of the brain on the immune system can lead to increased immune activity and, if directed against the body's own tissues and organs, greater susceptibility to inflammatory and autoimmune disease (Sternberg & Gold, 1997). For instance, animals whose brain-immune communications have been disrupted experimentally are at much greater risk for adverse outcomes from inflammatory disease. Reestablishment of those communications can reduce inflammation and moderate immune activity.

This chapter examines autoimmune disorders that are associated with excessive immune activity and inflammation and discusses research that links the onset and course of autoimmune conditions with psychosocial stress. The use of religion by patients to cope with autoimmune disorders such as psoriasis, rheumatoid arthritis, and systemic lupus erythematosus also is explored, as are the effects of religious-spiritual interventions on the disease course. Throughout most of this book thus far, the effects of psychological stress and emotional distress have been discussed in terms of their ability to weaken or suppress immune function. There is another effect, however, that stress can have on the immune system that appears to be the exact opposite. Psychosocial stress may interfere with the ability of the body to regulate immune functioning, resulting in the excessive or exaggerated responses seen in autoimmune diseases. How it does this is discussed here.

Autoimmune Diseases

Before reviewing the mechanisms by which stress may lead to exaggerated immune function, it is important to describe what happens during the course of autoimmune disorders. Autoimmune diseases occur when the immune system reacts to the body's own healthy tissue, such as the skin, kidneys, adrenals, central nervous system, tendons, cartilage, joint spaces, thyroid, muscles, intestines, or insulin-producing cells of the pancreas, as if this "self" tissue were a foreign invader that needs eradication. In some autoimmune diseases, such as insulin-dependent diabetes, in which the pancreatic cells that produce insulin are completely destroyed by the person's own lymphocytes, the immune assault ends in the same way that elimination of an infectious agent ends the immune response. However, in most autoimmune disorders, the immune system fails to eliminate the healthy tissue; rather, it continues to produce ongoing damage to the tissue over time (such as rheumatoid arthritis). This can result in chronic pain, inflammation, and physical disability.

Not only does the immune process associated with autoimmune diseases produce tissue damage but also it affects one's mood and sense of vigor. It does so because activated immune cells produce blood proteins called cytokines that may induce feelings of tiredness, fatigue, and depression (Sternberg & Gold, 1997). This especially is seen in diseases such as chronic fatigue syndrome and fibromyalgia, as well as in rheumatoid and other types of inflammatory arthritis.

There also is evidence from studies in animals and humans that autoimmune disorders may shorten life span. For example, certain strains of mice that spontaneously develop autoimmune diseases have a shorter duration of life than mice that do not develop autoimmune disease (Kubo et al., 1992; Mihara et al., 1987; Wofsy & Seaman, 1985). Autoimmune processes also may increase the risk of early death in humans (Aho, 1980), and studies of centenarians suggest that autoimmune responses may be less common in these persons than in those persons who die at younger ages (Mariotti et al., 1992). Autoimmune processes may directly damage tissue necessary for survival or may indirectly affect survival by interfering with normal immune responses—thereby increasing susceptibility to infection, delaying wound-healing, or affecting the development or course of a malignancy.

Autoimmune disorders probably arise through a number of different mechanisms. The immune system has a way of eliminating lymphocytes that recognize "self" through a process known as the development of immune tolerance (Rabin, 1999). For B lymphocytes, this usually occurs in the bone marrow or in the germinal centers of lymph nodes before they are sufficiently mature to become functionally active. For T lymphocytes, the thymus gland eliminates those that are reactive to self or normal tissues during maturation; if they escape removal in the thymus, autoreactive T lymphocytes also can be destroyed once they reach the peripheral circulation through a peripheral tolerance mechanism (see Rabin, 1999, p. 234). If either of these mechanisms is disrupted by invading viruses or tissue inflammation, lymphocytes sensitized to self may survive and initiate an autoimmune process.

Stress, the Stress Response, and Autoimmune Disease

Psychosocial stress can affect the development and course of autoimmune disease in a number of ways. First, severe stress during early development (stress affecting the child directly after birth or indirectly via the mother during the intrauterine period) may impair the body's later ability to respond to stress, such as the capacity to secrete corticotropin-releasing factor (CRF). An impaired stress response has been causally associated with susceptibility to autoimmune inflammatory disease by pharmacological and surgical experiments in animals and humans (Cutolo et al., 1999). Treatment of certain strains of mice with drugs that block cortisol receptors increases the severity of autoimmune disease, whereas injecting cortisol into rats with autoimmune disorders reduces their inflammatory responses (Sternberg et al., 1989). Furthermore, removing the pituitary gland (which secretes CRF) or the adrenal glands (which secrete cortisol) from animals normally resistant to inflammatory disease increases their susceptibility to these conditions (Sternberg, 1997). Implanting normal hypothalamic tissue into rats with autoimmune diseases has been shown to decrease their sensitivity to inflammation (Misiewicz et al., 1997). Thus, any disruption of the neuroendocrine stress response system can increase susceptibility to autoimmune inflammatory disease.

A second and more likely way that psychosocial stress can either increase the risk of autoimmune disease or adversely affect its course is by impairing the regulatory component of the immune system that is responsible for controlling exaggerated immune responses (Rabin, 1999). As noted earlier in this chapter, neuroendocrine and immune mechanisms exist to prevent the immune system from reacting to and attempting to destroy the body's healthy tissue; these mechanisms also turn off the immune system responses after foreign invaders have been removed. Psychological stress may impair this regulatory component of the immune system sufficiently so that when infection leads to tissue damage, exposure of previously "hidden" tissue to the immune system results in the formation of autoantibodies that subsequently cross-react with normal healthy tissues. Alternatively, the immune system may develop antibodies to the invading virus or other pathogen that subsequently cross-react with normal tissue located in joints, skin, or other body organs. In either case, the immune system forms antibodies to normal healthy tissue and attempts to destroy it, resulting in autoimmune disease.

A number of other theories seek to explain the relationship between stress and increased immune activity. Elenkov and Chrousos (1999) suggest that stress may have both systemic and local effects that affect the immune system in different ways. Systemically, stress may induce a shift of T helper I (Th1) to T helper II (Th2) cells, impairing immunity against viruses, bacteria, and neoplastic degeneration; locally, stress may induce pro-inflammatory activities through neural activation of the peripheral CRF–mast cell–histamine axis. Studying inflammation in rat and human tissues, these investigators found that CRF-activated mast cells (via a CRF receptor type 1–dependent mechanism) led to a release of histamine, vasodilation, and increased vascular permeability (Elenkov et al., 1999).

Van Eden (2000) discusses how the discovery of highly immunological heat shock proteins (HSPs) in humans may help explain the relationship between stress and autoimmune disorders. Increased immune reactivity may result from stress-induced upregulation of self-HSPs during inflammation and tissue destruction. Especially exciting is the possibility that immunization with sequences of microbial-HSPs may increase resistance to autoimmune diseases. Thus, immune reactivity directed toward self-HSPs may be part of a regulatory immune mechanism that contributes both to the maintenance of self-tolerance and to the boosting of the body's anti-inflammatory activity.

Let us now examine specific autoimmune conditions thought to be influenced by stress, including such common conditions as psoriasis, rheumatoid arthritis, Graves's disease, and multiple sclerosis. Because of space limitations, we do not discuss other autoimmune disorders that may be stress related, including insulin-dependent diabetes mellitus, systemic lupus erythematosus, inflammatory bowel disease, ulcerative colitis, and Crohn's disease, although the mechanism by which stress induces or exacerbates these diseases may be similar to that in psoriasis and the other conditions discussed here. Autoimmune disorders that involve red blood cells, platelets, or white blood cells, such as autoimmune hemolytic anemia, autoimmune thrombocytopenia, or autoimmune agranulocytosis, are not thought to be influenced by psychosocial stressors.

Psoriasis

Psoriasis is a disease of the skin associated with the development of pinkish or reddish plaques covered by white or silvery scales. Lesions are typically located around the elbows, forearms, knees, cleft of the buttocks, and scalp. The plaques tend to worsen and then remit over time, sometimes in response to psychological and environmental factors. Microscopic examination of these plaques shows dilated blood vessels surrounded by white blood cells. T lymphocytes and their products are believed to mediate this autoimmune disorder, and treatments that block cytokines produced by T lymphocytes (cyclosporine) improve the disease (Valdimarsson et al., 1997). Streptococcal bacterial infections of the skin have sometimes been associated with psoriatic lesions and therefore may have something to do with the development of lymphocytes that attack both these bacteria and normal components of the skin (Rassmusen, 2000).

Numerous studies report that psychological factors and stress are associated with the onset or exacerbation of skin symptoms in patients with psoriasis (Al'Abadie et al., 1994; Gaston et al, 1991; Gupta et al., 1996; Harvima et al., 1996; Polenghi et al., 1989). Behavioral interventions such as hypnosis and meditation have resulted in significant improvements in disease activity, particularly when combined with photochemotherapy (Istvan et al., 1998; Kabat-Zinn et al., 1998; Tausk & Whitmore, 1999).

For example, Kabat-Zinn and colleagues (1998) randomized 37 subjects with psoriasis to either a mindfulness meditation stress-reduction intervention (guided by audiotaped instructions during light treatments) or to a control condition of phototherapy treatments alone. Mindfulness meditation has its roots in Theravada Buddhism (insight meditation), Mahayana Buddhism (Zen practices), and Yogic traditions that follow the teachings of Krishnamurti and others. In this study, psoriasis status was assessed by direct inspection and by evaluation of photographs of psoriasis lesions by physicians who were unaware of the subjects' study group. Investigators concluded that meditation-induced stress reduction increases the rate of resolution of psoriatic lesions, particularly when performed at the same time as ultraviolet light therapy.

Other studies have found that a variety of relaxation therapies can reduce the severity of disease activity in psoriasis, possibly because of their effect of reducing sympathetic nervous system activity (Winchell & Watts, 1988; Zachariae et al., 1996). Another mechanism involves skin mast cells. Animal studies indicate that acute psychological stress can cause skin mast cell degranulation, which worsens disease activity in psoriasis; mast cell degranulation is dependent on several neuropeptides, including corticotropin-releasing hormone, neurotensin, and substance P (Singh et al., 1999).

Rheumatoid Arthritis

Rheumatoid arthritis is an autoimmune disorder associated with pain and inflammation of tissue surrounding the small joints of the hands, wrists, and feet, and as the disease progresses, it involves larger joints such as elbows, shoulders, and knees. Rheumatoid arthritis affects nearly 5 million Americans, about 2% of adults. On pathological examination, a large accumulation of lymphocytes and plasma cells is typically found in the synovial membranes that surround the affected joints, suggesting an autoimmune etiology. These immune cells contribute to the destruction of articular and periarticular structures, which results in severe pain, limitation of movement, and crippling deformities. There is almost certainly a genetic predisposition to this disease, and an HLA-DRB1 genotype may be a prognostic marker for the disease. The course of rheumatoid and other types of inflammatory arthritis tends to fluctuate over time, with relapses and remissions, and may be influenced by stress (Harbuz, 1999).

There is evidence in humans that physiological responses to psychological stress, measured either by sympathetic nervous system or hypothalamic-pituitary axis (HPA) activation, are blunted in subjects with rheumatoid arthritis. Geenen and colleagues (1996) compared sympathetic nervous system responses to a mental challenge stress task in a sample of rheumatoid arthritis patients with those of control subjects without rheumatoid arthritis. Subjects with this arthritis—especially those with the worst pain—had the lowest sympathetic activation, suggesting an impaired stress response. Whether blunting of sympathetic nervous system responses occurs prior to or after the development of rheumatoid arthritis is unknown. Other investigators have documented abnormal HPA responses to immune and inflammatory stimuli in patients with rheumatoid arthritis (Chikanza et al., 1992). These findings are consistent with reports from animal models showing greater autoimmune activity in mice with impaired CRF and cortisol responses (Calogero et al., 1992; Sternberg, 1995).

Studies in both animals and humans suggest that stress may influence the course of the disease, either one way or the other. For example, Rogers and colleagues (1980) were able to experimentally induce arthritis in rats by immunizing them with collagen. To stress them, some of the rats were exposed to cats. Not only did cat-exposed rats experience an improvement in their disease but also simply handling and transporting the control rats ameliorated disease symptoms. This finding suggests that psychological stress may result in an *improvement* in disease symptoms in autoimmune arthritis, presumably by increasing production of CRF and cortisol, which subsequently decrease immune system activity and reduce inflammation.

Studies in humans report conflicting results. Some investigators find that interpersonal stressors predict increases in disease activity in patients with rheumatoid arthritis (Arango & Cano, 1998; Zautra et al., 1997, 1999). For example, Zautra et al. (1997) examined the effects of changes in interpersonal stress on disease activity in 41 women. Measures of everyday stressful events were collected weekly for 12 weeks and related to disease activity. Subjects who experienced increased interpersonal stress showed elevations in DR+CD3 cells, sIL-2R, clinicians' rating of disease, and self-reported joint tenderness.

The findings of Potter and Zautra (1997) may help explain why certain stressful events are associated with a decrease in disease activity in rheumatoid arthritis, whereas other stressful events are associated with increased inflammation and symptoms. These investigators followed a 53-year-old woman with rheumatoid arthritis for a 12-week period, during which she experienced two unexpected family deaths and also encountered a number of small events associated with negative affect. Investigators found a large decrease in disease symptoms and signs immediately following the two major losses (family members); however, negative affect and small events were related to a worsening of disease status. These observations were confirmed in an analysis of 25 other subjects with this arthritis, which suggests that major life events and small life events have opposite effects on disease activity. Other studies report that the presence or absence of rheumatoid factor may determine whether the onset or course of rheumatoid arthritis is stress related (Stewart et al., 1994).

Of particular importance are studies showing that stress-reducing psychological or behavioral interventions help to ameliorate disease symptoms and objective measures of disease activity in patients with rheumatoid arthritis. Smyth et al. (1999) examined whether writing about stressful experiences might affect disease symptoms in patients with rheumatoid arthritis: controls were asked to write about an emotionally neutral topic; subjects wrote for 20 minutes on 3 consecutive days a week, and outcomes were assessed at 2 weeks, 2 months, and 4 months after writing. Symptom improvement among rheumatoid arthritis patients did occur, but not until the 4-month assessment. This study confirmed the positive effects that emotional disclosure (even when disclosure occurs only in the form of writing) may have on disease activity (Kelly et al., 1997).

Other investigators also have found that psychological interventions designed to reduce stress produce a small but significant improvement in clinical activity among patients with this disease (Bradley et al., 1987; Parker et al., 1991). Even if they do not reduce disease activity, such interventions can decrease the pain perceived by these patients (Young, 1993). Pain reduction may result from increased opioid production (within the central nervous system and/or peripherally) or may be due to a reduction in immune system activity that actually diminishes inflammation itself.

Psychological factors also may influence the effect that the disease has on physical functioning. There is evidence that a "sense of coherence" (Antonovsky, 1979) may be a mediator between actual disability level and degree of handicap perceived by rheumatoid arthritis patients. Sense of coherence involves holding a worldview that provides meaning and purpose; life events fit together into a coherent whole that is understandable and predictable. Among other factors, religion is said to provide believers with a sense of coherence (Kark et al., 1996). Schnyder and colleagues (1999) examined the association between disability, handicap, and sense of coherence in a sample of 89 subjects with rheumatoid arthritis. Objective measures of illness severity were used to measure disability, whereas subjects' judgment concerning their condition was used as a measure of handicap. Significant correlations were found between sense of coherence and all handicap variables, whereas there was no association between sense of coherence and disability variables. These findings suggest that sense of coherence may mediate between disability and handicap in rheumatoid arthritis patients.

Graves's Disease

Graves's disease is an autoimmune disorder that affects the thyroid gland. Antibodies are directed at thyroid-stimulating hormone (TSH) receptors located on the gland. These antibodies act like TSH itself, stimulating the thyroid cells to enlarge and produce large quantities of thyroid hormone, making the person hyperthyroid. This is one of the most common causes of hyperthyroidism. People with Graves's disease experience symptoms of increased perspiration, heat intolerance, increased appetite, irritability, thyroid enlargement, and sometimes protrusion of the eyes. In Graves's disease, the antibody stimulating the release of thyroid hormones is not TSH, and so there is no negative feedback loop shutting off hormone production, as there is with TSH. Thyroid hormone production increases are uncontrolled, speeding up the body's metabolism and resulting in the symptoms just noted.

There is some evidence that psychological stress may affect the disorder. Studies in humans have found that subjects with Graves's disease (particularly women) are more likely than control subjects to have encountered high levels of stress prior to the diagnosis. Lidz (1955) and then Bennett and Cambor (1961) were among the first to report that emotional factors were important in the etiology of hyperthyroidism. Subsequently, other investigators have confirmed that an increase in negative life events precedes the disorder (Harris et al., 1992; Kung, 1995; Sonono et al., 1993; Winsa et al., 1991; Yoshiuchi et al., 1998). It is unclear, however, whether excess reports of life events prior to diagnosis are due to an actual increased number of events or to increased *reporting* of events because of the psychological alterations caused by high levels of circulating thyroid hormone.

Rabin (1999) provides two possible explanations for the role that stress plays in Graves's disease. First, the altered immune system regulation seen

in this disorder may result from a genetic defect that alters immune surveillance. This defect might cause the loss of a *suppressor* T lymphocyte
that then allows autoreactive lymphocytes to produce the TSH-like antibodies that stimulate the gland (Volpe 1977, 1993).

Second, stress may alter the functioning of the thyroid gland by decreasing TSH production through its effects on the pituitary or the hypothalamus. Studies in animals have shown that chronic stress is associated
with increased weight of the thyroid gland, despite decreased concentrations of TSH and decreased production of thyroid hormone (Servatius et
al., 1994). If chronic stress decreases TSH production, it may be accompanied by an increased production of the TSH receptor in the thyroid gland.
If the excess TSH receptors are shed into the general circulation, this may
allow lymphocytes to become sensitized and produce antibodies to the receptor. Because TSH receptors usually are attached to the thyroid cell
membrane, immunological tolerance may not develop.

Multiple Sclerosis

Multiple sclerosis (MS) is a chronic autoimmune disease of the central
nervous system characterized by intermittent inflammation of the myelin
sheath that covers nerve cell axons in the brain and spinal cord. The damaged areas that result are called plaques. MS produces visual changes and
muscle weakness or paralysis in an inconsistent pattern. As the disease
worsens, different nerves are affected at different times, producing an exacerbation of current symptoms, as well as new symptoms. Microscopic examination of affected axons shows infiltration by T lymphocytes, macrophages, and plasma cells. Lymphocytes and macrophages release cytokines,
proteolytic enzymes, and immunoglobulins that cause the inflammatory
damage seen in plaques. Although the initiating event for MS is unknown,
both genetic and environmental factors are believed to play a role.

Stress has been reported to exacerbate symptoms in MS, and there are
immunological mechanisms present that may help explain this association. Oro and colleagues (1996) found that MS patients had a low likelihood of having IgE-mediated diseases, suggesting an increase in the activity of Th1 lymphocytes (known to be stimulated by psychological stress).
Indeed, approximately 80% of MS patients report stressful life events in
the year prior to onset of the disorder, compared with 35 to 50% of neurological and healthy controls (Grant et al., 1989; Warren et al., 1982).

Stressful life events often involve interpersonal or financial difficulties. MS patients also report significantly more stressful life events in the months prior to the disease's exacerbations than in symptom-free intervals (Franklin et al., 1988; Stip & Truelle, 1994).

For example, Schwartz and colleagues (1999) followed 96 healthy controls and 101 MS patients for 6 years, comparing self-reported stressful events and changes in health status between groups. They found a bidirectional relationship between stress and illness, with increased risk of disease progression when reported stressful events were higher and an increased risk of reported stressful events when rate of disease progression was higher. Investigators concluded that MS patients demonstrate a vicious cycle between stress and disease exacerbations.

Nevertheless, severe acute psychological stress may in some cases improve symptoms. During the Persian Gulf War, Nisipeanu and Korczyn (1993) reported fewer exacerbations of MS among those with this condition, and this suggests that intense psychological stress may suppress immune activity responsible for the disease. Thus, immune alterations that affect disease activity may depend on the severity and chronicity of the stressor. Ackerman et al. (1996, 1998) found that immune alterations remain intact in patients who have MS and are exposed to mild psychosocial stressors. In response to giving a 5-minute videotape speech under stressful conditions, both patients with MS and controls without the disease demonstrated similar transient increases in number and activity of neutrophils, monocytes, macrophages (and cytokine production), T lymphocytes, and NK cells. As with other autoimmune disorders, severe stress appears to mobilize anti-inflammatory stress hormones that improve disease symptoms, whereas milder stress often precedes either the onset of the disease or exacerbation of symptoms.

There is also an association between viral infections and the onset of the disease. For many years, epidemiologists have reported that multiple sclerosis tends to be more common in northern climates. Panitch and colleagues (1987) found that infection with a respiratory viral infection often preceded disease exacerbations. According to Rabin (1999), this apparent association can be explained in three ways. First, stress may suppress immune functioning, increasing susceptibility to viral infection with respiratory viruses and viruses capable of infecting nerve cells in the central nervous system. Once the acute stressor passes and immune function is restored, immune activity may be directed at the virus in infected nerve cells, causing damage to those cells and their axons. Second, stress may suppress immune system function, resulting in an increased risk of respiratory infection. A latent virus (unrelated to the respiratory infection) becomes activated in nerve cells because of stress-induced immune system suppression. Consequently, immune activation directed at removing the latent virus produces damage to nerve cells. Third, psychological stress reduces immune system functioning, allowing for viral respiratory infection. Stress-induced changes in immune system function (again unrelated to the respiratory infection) produce increases in CD8 cells, NK cells, and Th1 lymphocytes, which result in destruction of nerve tissue by reacting to autologous antigens present in myelin. Recall that Ackerman and colleagues (1996, 1998) demonstrated that the immune systems of MS patients react normally to acute stress by increases in these cell types.

Van Noort and colleagues (2000) sum up the current thinking about the relationship between viral infection, immune functioning, and multiple sclerosis, and produce their own theory to explain this association. They note several possible mechanisms for the relationship between viral infection and myelin-directed autoimmunity, including molecular mimicry and bystander activation. To help explain why this disease occurs only in humans, however, the investigators propose that peripheral microbial infections of lymphoid cells prime human T cells not only to microbial antigens but also to the stress protein α B-crystallin that is expressed in infected lymphoid cells. As a result, stress-induced accumulation of this "self-antigen" in oligodendrocytes and/or myelin provokes inflammation as the recruited T cells then mistake the self-antigen for the microbial antigen.

Whatever the mechanism, it is clear that stress-induced immune system alterations may predispose people to the development or exacerbation of multiple sclerosis. As with the other stress-related autoimmune disorders, psychosocial or behavioral interventions that reduce stress and facilitate coping may help to either prevent the disease or moderate its course.

Psychological and Behavioral Interventions in Autoimmune Diseases

To date, the majority of studies of psychological and behavioral interventions for autoimmune disorders have focused on two conditions, diabetes and arthritis. The following briefly provides an overview of the types of studies conducted in these two conditions.

Diabetes

Stress has long been suspected as having major effects on both elevated blood glucose levels and decreased insulin action. Thus, stress is a potential contributor to chronic hyperglycemia in diabetes, although its exact role is unclear (Surwit & Schneider, 1993). Although human studies on the role of stress on the course of diabetes are few, studies suggest that psychological and behavioral interventions to manage stress may contribute significantly to diabetes treatment.

Mendez and Belendez (1997), for example, have demonstrated that a behavioral intervention in young diabetics can bring significant changes in compliance and social interactions. Improvements were shown in acquiring diabetes information (patients and their parents), adherence, handling daily hassles, quality of social interactions, frequency of blood glucose checks, blood glucose estimate errors, and negative family support (parents).

Grey and colleagues have demonstrated in a series of elegant studies that behavioral interventions can significantly improve the prognosis for diabetes patients. In one study, Grey, Boland, Davidson, Yu, Sullivan-Bolyai, et al. (1998) randomly assigned a total of 65 youths between the ages of 13 and 20 years to one of two groups: (1) intensive insulin management combined with coping skills training and (2) intensive management without such training. The training consisted of a series of small-group efforts designed to teach adolescents the coping skills of social problem solving, social skills training, cognitive behavior modification, and conflict resolution. This study found that adolescents who received coping skills training had lower hemoglobin A1c (HbA1c), a marker for diabetic control, as well as better diabetes "self-efficacy" (i.e., a sense of control). Individuals in the behavioral intervention group also were less "upset" about coping with diabetes than adolescents receiving intensive insulin management alone. Further, adolescents who received the training found it easier to cope with diabetes and experienced less of a negative impact of diabetes on quality of life than those who did not receive it.

In a follow-up study, Grey, Boland, Davidson, Yu, and Tamborlane (1999) randomly assigned 77 youths (age 12 to 20 years) who were beginning intensive insulin therapy to one of two groups: intensive management with or without coping skills training. After 6 months, again, subjects who received the training had better metabolic control and better general self-efficacy; they reported less negative impact of diabetes on quality of life and had fewer worries about diabetes. More recently, Grey, Boland, Davidson, Li, et al. (2000) demonstrated that behavioral training intervention can be used to improve metabolic control and quality of life in adolescents who have had diabetes for more than 1 year.

Rheumatoid Arthritis

As previously noted, the role of stress in the etiology of rheumatoid arthritis has sometimes been questioned. Nevertheless, several intervention studies support the notion that stress plays a role in the clinical manifestations of this illness. For example, Young et al. (1995) reported that a multicomponent cognitive-behavioral intervention including biofeedback was associated with reductions in disease-related clinic visits and days hospitalized, as well as reductions in the overall costs of medical services. More recently, Sinclair and colleagues (1998) evaluated the effectiveness of a cognitive-behavioral intervention for women with this arthritis. In that study, 90 adult women participated in 1 of 14 nurse-led groups over an 18-month period. Personal coping resources, pain-coping behaviors, psychological well-being, and disease symptomatology were measured at four time periods. There were significant changes on all measures of personal coping resources and psychological well-being, half of the pain-coping behaviors, and one indicator of disease symptoms from the start to the end of the intervention. Furthermore, the positive changes brought about by the program were maintained over a 3-month follow-up period.

Similarly, Barlow and colleagues (1999) administered the Arthritis Self-Management Programme (ASMP) to 89 people with rheumatoid arthritis or osteoarthritis and found that after 4 months participants demonstrated significant increases in arthritis self-efficacy, cognitive symptom management, communication with doctors, exercise, and relaxation. In addition, there was a significant decrease in pain and visits to other health professionals.

In summary, the available evidence indicates that psychological and behavioral stress-control interventions produce significant and positive changes in quality of life, pain, and functional disabilities in patients with diabetes, rheumatoid arthritis, and, as shown previously, psoriasis.

Religion and Autoimmune Diseases

If we can make the case that religion and/or spirituality buffers the psychological stress caused by negative life events, decreases the likelihood of stressful events, or promotes better immune functioning by other mechanisms, then a plausible link between religion and autoimmune disorders may exist. As noted in chapter 1, religious beliefs and practices are associated with improved coping, less anxiety, lower rates of depression, and quicker recovery from depression, especially during periods of high stress (medical illness, financial stress, or relationship loss). Similarly, religion is associated with greater social support (that itself may buffer against stress) and fewer negative health behaviors (cigarette smoking, alcohol use) that may impair immune functioning just as psychological stress does.

Research on the relationship between religiousness or spirituality and either the onset or the course of autoimmune inflammatory diseases, however, is scant. We review what research exists next, including studies that examine whether patients with these conditions cope better with stress if they are religious.

Miller (1985) examined the relationship between loneliness and spiritual well-being in 54 patients with rheumatoid arthritis who attended a rheumatology clinic in Milwaukee, Wisconsin, and 64 healthy adults. The investigator found an inverse relationship between spiritual well-being and loneliness in both arthritis patients ($-.27$, $p < .01$) and healthy adults ($-.39$, $p < .001$). Arthritis patients had higher spiritual well-being (94.3 vs. 83.7, $p < .01$) and religious well-being (48.0 vs. 38.2, $p < .0001$) scores than healthy subjects. Miller concluded that "chronic illness may be a factor in stimulating the person's valuing religion, having faith in God, and having a relationship with God" (p. 83).

In a qualitative study of 109 Hispanic women with arthritis who attended a rheumatology clinic in New York City, Abraido-Lanza et al. (1996) asked a series of open-ended questions to determine how patients coped with arthritis. Women in the sample were of lower socioeconomic status and had a mean age of 51 years; approximately half of them had a diagnosis of rheumatoid arthritis, 16% of systemic lupus erythematosus, and 16% of osteoarthritis. The most common coping strategy reported by respondents was engaging in activities; the second most important spontaneously reported strategy was use of religion (38.1% of the sample).

At least two studies have examined the effects of religious interventions on symptom course in patients with autoimmune disorders. As noted, Kabat-Zinn et al. (1998) randomized 37 psoriasis patients to either the Buddhist practice of mindfulness meditation or to a control group; both groups received phototherapy treatments. Patients assigned to the meditation group experienced more resolution of psoriatic lesions than the controls did. This study suggests that reducing stress by religious meditation or prayer may help to ameliorate the inflammatory lesions of psoriasis.

Similarly, Matthews and colleagues (1999) conducted a randomized clinical trial to examine the effects of intercessory Christian prayer as an adjunct to standard medical care for patients with rheumatoid arthritis. Forty patients (82% female, all white, mean age 62) who had moderately active arthritis were given a 3-day intercessory prayer intervention that included 6 hours of instruction and 6 hours of direct-contact prayer ("laying on of hands"). Half of the group was also randomized in double-blind conditions to receive intercessory prayer at a distance for 6 months. Subjects were assessed at 3 and 12 months after intervention. Prayed-for subjects demonstrated significant overall improvement ($p < .0001$), with sustained reductions in tender and swollen joints (17 and 10 vs. 6 and 3 at 12 months) ($p < .001$), self-reported pain ($p < .004$), fatigue ($p = .007$), and functional impairment (121 vs. 108, $p = .007$). The number of tender joints was lower in the prayed-for group (compared at 6 months with waitlist controls, $p = .016$). No effect was found for distant intercessory prayer.

Summary and Conclusions

Although there are many unanswered questions with regard to the pathogenesis and fluctuating course of autoimmune diseases, substantial data suggest a relationship with stress. By impairing immune function, psychosocial stressors may increase susceptibility to infection by viruses and other microbes; this may consequently increase susceptibility to autoimmune disease, perhaps by affecting the regulatory component of the immune system or by leading to cross-reactivity between microbial antigens and components of normal tissue. Thus, the effects of stress on increasing susceptibility to autoimmune phenomena may be indirect rather than direct and quite likely involve a number of different pathways.

Whatever the mechanisms that underlie this relationship, psychosocial factors that reduce stress may help prevent or ameliorate the course of disease. There is some evidence that religious practices may alter the course of autoimmune conditions like psoriasis and rheumatoid arthritis, as well as evidence that religious or spiritual beliefs may help persons with these disorders cope more effectively and experience better quality of life.

Religious beliefs may facilitate coping by providing patients with a greater "sense of coherence" that makes sense of or gives meaning to the pain and suffering that these people experience. We have only begun to scratch the surface of how psychosocial and spiritual factors affect autoimmune disease, making this a fertile ground for future study.

REFERENCES

Abraido-Lanza, A. F., Guier, C., & Revenson, T. A. (1996). Coping and social support resources among Latinas with arthritis. *Arthritis Care and Research* 9, 501–508.

Ackerman, K. D., Martino, M., Heyman, R., Moyna, N. M. & Rabin, B. S. (1996). Immunologic response to acute psychological stress in MS patients and controls. *Journal of Neuroimmunology* 68, 85–94.

Ackerman, K. D., Martino, M., Heyman, R., Moyna, N. M. & Rabin, B. S. (1998). Stressor-induced alteration of cytokine production in multiple sclerosis patients and controls. *Psychosomatic Medicine* 60, 484–491.

Aho, K. (1980). Autoantibodies and the risk of death. *Medical Biology* 58, 8–13.

Al'Abadie, M. S., Kent, G. G., & Gawkrodger, D. J. (1994). The relationship between stress and the onset and exacerbation of psoriasis and other skin conditions. *British Journal of Dermatology* 130, 199–203.

Antonovsky, A. (1979). *Health, stress and coping.* San Francisco: Jossey-Bass.

Arango, M.A., & Cano, P. O (1998). A potential moderating role of stress in the association of disease activity and psychological status among patients with rheumatoid arthritis. *Psychological Reports* 83, 147–157.

Barlow, J. H., Williams, B., & Wright, C. C. (1999). Instilling the strength to fight the pain and get on with life: Learning to become an arthritis self-manager through an adult education programme. *Health Education and Research* 14, 533–544.

Bennett, A. W., & Cambor, C. G. (1961). Clinical study of hyperthyroidism. *Archives of General Psychiatry* 4, 160–165.

Bradley, L. A., Young, L. D., Anderson, K. O., Turner, R. A., Agudelo, C. A., McDaniel, L. K., Pisko, E. J., Semble, E. L., & Morgan, T. M. (1987). Effects of psychological therapy on pain behavior of rheumatoid arthritis patients: Treatment outcome and six-month follow-up. *Arthritis and Rheumatism* 30, 1105–1114.

Calogero, A. E., Sternberg, E. M., Bagdy, G., Smith, C., Bernardini, R., Aksentijevich, S., Wilder, R. L., Gold, P. W., & Chrousos, G. P. (1992). Neurotransmitter-induced hypothalamic-pituitary-adrenal axis responsiveness is defective in inflammatory disease-susceptible Lewis rats: In vivo and in vitro studies suggesting globally defective hypothalamic secretion of corti-cotropin-releasing hormone. *Neuroendocrinology* 55, 600–608.

Chikanza, I. C., Petrou, P., Kingsley, G., Chrousos, U., & Panayi, G. S. (1992). Defective hypothalamic response to immune and inflammatory stimuli in patients with rheumatoid arthritis. *Arthritis and Rheumatism* 35, 1281–1288.

Cutolo, M., Masi, A. T., Bijlsma, J. W., Chikanza, I. C., Bradlow, H. L., & Castag-netta, L. (1999). Neuroendocrine immune basis of the rheumatic diseases. *Annals of the New York Academy of Sciences* 876, 11–15.

Elenkov, I. J., & Chrousos, G. P. (1999). Stress, cytokine patterns and susceptibil-ity to disease. *Best Practice and Research Clinical Endocrinology and Metabo-lism* 13, 583–595.

Elenkov, I. J., Webster, E. L., Torpy, D. J., & Chrousos, G. P. (1999). Stress, corti-cotropin-releasing hormone, glucocorticoids, and the immune/inflammatory response: Acute and chronic effects. *Annals of the New York Academy of Sci-ences* 876, 1–13.

Franklin, G. M., Nelson, L.M., & Keaton, R. K. (1988). Stress and its relationship to acute exacerbation in multiple sclerosis. *Journal of Neurological Rehabilita-tion* 2, 7–11.

Gaston, L., Crombez, J. C., Lassonde, M., Bernier-Buzzanga, J., & Hodgins, S. (1991). Psychological stress and psoriasis: Experimental and prospective correlational studies. *Acta Dermato-Venereologica* (Stockholm) 156, 37–43.

Geenen, R., Godaert, G. L. R., Jacobs, J. W. G., Peters, M. L., & Bijisma, J. W. J. (1996). Diminished autonomic nervous system responsiveness in rheuma-toid arthritis of recent onset. *Journal of Rheumatology* 23, 258–264.

Grant, I., Brown, G. W., Harris, T., McDonald, W. I., Patterson, T., & Trimble, M. R. (1989). Severely threatening events and marked life difficulties pre-ceding onset or exacerbation of multiple sclerosis. *Journal of Neurology, Neu-rosurgery, and Psychiatry* 52, 8–13.

Grey, M., Boland, E. A., Davidson, M., Li, J., & Tamborlane, W. V. (2000). Cop-ing skills training for youth with diabetes mellitus has long-lasting effects on metabolic control and quality of life. *Journal of Pediatrics* 137, 107–113.

Grey, M., Boland, E. A., Davidson, M., Yu, C., Sullivan-Bolyai, S., & Tamborlane, W. V. (1998). Short-term effects of coping skills training as adjunct to inten-sive therapy in adolescents. *Diabetes Care* 21, 902–908.

Grey, M., Boland, E. A., Davidson, M., Yu, C., & Tamborlane, W. V. (1999). Coping skills training for youths with diabetes on intensive therapy. *Applied Nursing Research* 12, 3–12.

Gupta, M. A., Gupta, A. K., & Watteel, G. N. (1996). Early onset (<40 years age) psoriasis is comorbid with greater psychopathology than late onset pso-riasis: A study of 137 patients. *Acta DermatoVenereologica* 76, 464–466.

Harbuz, M.S. (1999). Chronic inflammatory stress. *Best Practice and Research Clinical Endocrinology and Metabolism* 13, 555–565.

Harris, T., Creed, F., & Brugha, T. S. (1992). Stressful life events and Graves' disease. *British Journal of Psychiatry* 161, 535–541.

Harvima, R. I., Viinamaki, H., Harvima, I. T., Naukkarinen, A., Savolainen, L., Aalto, M. L., & Horsmanheimo, M. (1996). Association of psychic stress with clinical severity and symptoms of psoriatic patients. *Acta Dermato-Venereologica* 76, 467–471.

Istvan, B., Beatrix, F., Janos, H., & Zoltan, K. (1998). Experiences with group that do the treatment of psoriasis vulgaris. *Psychiatria Hungarica* 13, 591–596.

Kabat-Zinn, J., Wheeler, E., Light, T., Skillings, A., Scharf, M. J., Cropely, T. G., Hosmer, D., & Bernhard, J. D. (1998). Influence of mindfulness meditation-based stress reduction interventions on rates of skin clearing in patients with moderate to severe psoriasis undergoing phototherapy (UVB) and photochemotherapy (PUVA). *Psychosomatic Medicine* 60, 625–632.

Kark, J. D., Carmel, S., Sinnreich, R., Goldberger, N., & Friedlander, Y. (1996). Psychosocial factors among members of religious and secular kibbutzim. *Israel Journal of Medical Science* 32, 185–194.

Kelly, J. E., Lumley, M. A., & Leisen, J. C. (1997). Health effects of emotional disclosure in Roma toward arthritis patients. *Health Psychology* 16, 331–340.

Kubo, C., Gajar, A., Johnson, B. C., & Good, R. A. (1992). The effects of dietary restriction on immune function and development of autoimmune disease in BXSB mice. *Proceedings of the National Academy of Sciences* 89, 3145–3149.

Kung, A. W. (1995). Life events, daily stressors and coping in patients with Graves' disease. *Clinical Endocrinology* 42, 303–308.

Lidz, T. (1955). Emotional factors in theology of hyperthyroidism occurring in relationship to pregnancy. *Psychosomatic Medicine* 17, 420–427.

Mariotti, S., Sansoni, P., Barbesino, G., Caturegli, P., Monti, D., Cossarizza, A., Giacomelli, T., Passeri, G., Fagiolo, U., Pinchera, A., & Franceshi, C. (1992). Thyroid and other organ-specific autoantibodies in healthy centenarians. *Lancet* 339, 1506–1508.

Matthews, D. A., Marlowe, S. M., & MacNutt, F. S. (1999). Effects of intercessory prayer ministry on patients with rheumatoid arthritis. *Journal of General Internal Medicine* 13(suppl 1), 17.

Mendez, F. J, & Belendez, M. (1997). Effects of a behavioral intervention on treatment adherence and stress management in adolescents with IDDM. *Diabetes Care* 20, 1370–1375.

Mihara, M., Nakano, T., & Ohsugi, Y. (1987). An immunomodulating anti-rheumatic drug, lobenzarit disodium (CCA): Inhibition of polyclonal B-cell activation and prevention of autoimmune disease in *MRL/Mp-lpr/lpr* mice. *Clinical Immunology and Immunopathology* 45, 366–374.

Miller, J. F. (1985). Assessment of loneliness and spiritual well-being in chronically ill and healthy adults. *Journal of Professional Nursing* 1, 79–85.

Misiewicz, B., Poltorak, M., Raybourne, R.B., Gomez, M., Listwak, S., & Sternberg, E. M. (1997). Intracerebroventricular transplantation of embryonic neural tissue from inflammatory resistant into inflammatory susceptible rats suppresses specific components of inflammation. *Experimental Neurology* 146, 305–314.

Nisipeanu, P., & Korczyn, A. D. (1993). Psychological stress as a risk factor for exacerbations in multiple sclerosis. *Neurology* 43, 1311–1312.

Oro, A. S., Guarino, T. J., Driver, R., Steinman, L., & Umetsu, D. T. (1996). Regulation of disease susceptibility: Decreased prevalence of IgE mediated allergic disease in patients with multiple sclerosis. *Journal of Allergy and Clinical Immunology* 97, 1402–1408.

Panitch, E. S., Hirsch, R. L., Schindler, J., & Johnson, J. R. (1987). Treatment of multiple sclerosis with gamma-interferon: Exacerbations with activation of the immune system. *Neurology* 37, 97–102.

Parker, J. C., Smarr, K. L., Walker, S. E., Hagglund, K. J., Anderson, S. K., Hewett, X. E., Bridges, A. J., & Caldwell, C. W. (1991). Biopsychosocial parameters of disease activity in rheumatoid arthritis. *Arthritis Care and Research* 4, 73–80.

Polenghi, M., Gals, C., Citeri, A., Manca, G., Guzzi, R., Barcella, M., & Finzi, A. (1989). Psychoneurophysiological implications in the pathogenesis and treatment of psoriasis. *Acta Dermato-Venereologica* (Stockholm) 146, 84–86.

Potter, P. T., & Zautra, A. J. (1997). Stressful life events' effects on rheumatoid arthritis disease activity. *Journal of Consulting and Clinical Psychology* 65, 319–323.

Rabin, B. S. (1999). *Stress, immune function, and health: The connection.* New York: Wiley-Liss.

Rasmussen, J. E. (2000). The relationship between infection with group A beta hemolytic streptococci and the development of psoriasis. *Pediatric Infectious Disease Journal* 19, 153–154.

Rogers, M. P., Trentham, D. E, McCune, W. J., Ginsberg, B. I., Rennke, H. G., Reich, P., & David, J. R. (1980). Effect of psychological stress on the induction of arthritis in rats. *Arthritis and Rheumatism* 23, 1337–1342.

Schnyder, U., Buechi, S., Moergeli, H., Sensky, T., & Klaghofer, R. (1999). Sense of coherence: A mediator between disability and handicap? *Psychotherapy and Psychosomatics* 68, 102–110.

Schwartz, C. E., Foley, F. W., Rao, S. M., Bernardin, L. J., Lee, H., & Genderson, M. W. (1999). Stress and course of disease in multiple sclerosis. *Behavioral Medicine* 25, 110–116.

Servatius, R. J., Offenweller, J. E., & Natelson, B. H. (1994). A comparison of the effects of repeated stressor exposures and corticosterone injections on plasma cholesterol, thyroid hormones and corticosterone levels in rats. *Life Sciences* 55, 1611–1617.

Sinclair, V. G., Wallston, K. A., Dwyer, K. A., Blackburn, D. S., & Fuchs, H. (1998). Effects of a cognitive-behavioral intervention for women with rheumatoid arthritis. *Research in Nursing and Health* 21, 315–326.

Singh, L. K., Pan, X., Alexacos, N., Letourneau, R., & Theoharides, T. (1999). Acute immobilization stress triggers skin mast cell degranulation via corticotropin releasing hormone, neurotensin, and substance P: A link to neurogenic skin disorders. *Brain, Behavior, and Immunity* 13, 225–239.

Smyth, J., Stone, A., Hurwitz, A., & Kaell, A. (1999). Effects of writing about stressful experiences on symptom reduction in patients with asthma or rheumatoid arthritis: A randomized trial. *Journal of the American Medical Association* 281, 1304–1309.

Sonono, N., Girelli, M. E., Boscaro, M., Fallo, F., Busnardo, B., & Fava, G. A. (1993). Life events in the pathogenesis of Graves' disease. A controlled study. *Acta Endocrinologica* 128, 293–296.

Sternberg, E. M. (1995). Neuroendocrine factors in susceptibility to inflammatory disease: Focus on the hypothalamic-pituitary-adrenal axis. *Hormone Research* 43, 159–161.

Sternberg, E. M. (1997). Cytokines and the brain. *Journal of Clinical Investigation* 100, 1–7.

Sternberg, E. M., & Gold, P. W. (1997). The mind-body interaction in desease. *Scientific American* (Special Issue), 8–15.

Sternberg, E. M., Hill, J. M., Chrousos, G. P., Kamilaris, T., Listwak, S. J., Gold, P. W., & Wilder, R. L. (1989). Inflammatory mediator-induced hypothalamic-pituitary-adrenal axis activation is defective in streptococcal cell wall arthritis susceptible Lewis rats. *Proceedings of the National Academy of Sciences* 86, 2374–2378.

Stewart, M. W., Knight, R. G., Palmer, D. G., & Highton, J.(1994). Differential relationships between stress and disease activity for immunologically distinct subgroups of people with rheumatoid arthritis. *Journal of Abnormal Psychology* 103, 251–258.

Stip, E., & Truelle, I. L.(1994). Organic personality syndrome in multiple sclerosis and effect of stress on recurrent attacks. *Canadian Journal of Psychiatry* 39, 27–33.

Surwit, R. S., & Schneider, M. S. (1993). Role of stress in the etiology and treatment of diabetes mellitus. *Psychosomatic Medicine* 55, 380–393.

Tausk, F., & Whitmore, E.(1999). A pilot study of hypnosis in the treatment of patients with psoriasis. *Psychotherapy and Psychosomatics* 68, 221–225.

Valdimarsson, H., Sigmundsdottir, H., & Jonsdottir, I. (1997). Is psoriasis induced by streptococcal super-antigens and maintained by M-protein-specific
T cells that cross-react with keratin? *Clinical and Experimental Immunology*
107(suppl 1), 21–24.

Van Eden, W. (2000). Stress proteins as targets for anti-inflammatory therapies.
Drug Discovery Today 5, 115–120.

Van Noort, J. M., Bajramovic, J. J., Plomp, A. C., & Van Stipdonk, M. J. B.
(2000). Mistaken self, a novel model that links microbial infections with
myelin-directed autoimmunity in multiple sclerosis. *Journal of Neuro-
Immunology* 105, 46–57.

Volpe, R. (1977). The role autoimmunity in hypoendocrine and hyperen-
docrine function: With special emphasis on autoimmune thyroid disease.
Annals of Internal Medicine 87, 86–99.

Volpe, R. (1993). Suppressor T lymphocyte dysfunction is important in the
pathogenesis of autoimmune thyroid disease-A perspective. *Thyroid* 3,
345–352.

Warren, S., Greenhill, S., & Warren, K. G. (1982). Emotional stress and the development of multiple sclerosis: Case control evidence of a relationship.
Journal of Chronic Diseases 35, 821–831.

Winchell, S. A., & Wafts, R. A. (1988). Relaxation therapies in the treatment of
psoriasis and possible psychologic mechanisms. *Journal of the American
Academy of Dermatology* 18, 101–104.

Winsa, B., Adami, H. O., Bergstrom, R., Gamstedt, A., Dahlberg, P. A., Adam-
son, U., Jansson, R., & Karlsson, A. (1991). Stressful life events and Graves'
disease. *Lancet* 338, 1475–1479.

Wofsy, D. & Seaman, W. E. (1985). Successful treatment of autoimmunity in
NZB/NZW F1 mice with monoclonal antibody to L3T4. *Journal of Experimental Medicine* 161, 378–391.

Yoshiuchi, K., Kumano, H., Nomura, S., Yoshimura, H., Ito, K., Kanaji, Y.,
Ohashi, Y., Kuboki, T., & Suematsu, H. (1998). Stressful life events and
smoking were associated with Graves' disease in women, but not in men.
Psychosomatic Medicine 60, 182–185.

Young, L. D. (1993). Rheumatoid arthritis. In R. J. Gatchel & E. B. Blanchard
(Eds.), *Psychophysiological disorders*. Washington, DC: American Psychological Association.

Young, L. D., Bradley, L. A., & Turner, R. A. (1995). Decreases in health care resource utilization in patients with rheumatoid arthritis following a cognitive
behavioral intervention. *Biofeedback and Self Regulation* 20, 259–268.

Zachariae, R., Oster, H., Bjerring, P., & Kragballe, K. (1996). Effects of psychologic intervention on psoriasis: A preliminary report. *Journal of the American
Academy of Dermatology* 34, 1008–1015.

Zautra, A. J., Hamilton, N. A., Potter, P., & Smith, B. (1999). Field research on the relationship between stress and disease activity in rheumatoid arthritis. *Annals of the New York Academy of Sciences* 876, 397–412.

Zautra, A. J., Hoffman, J., Potter, P., Matt, K. S., Yocum, D., & Castro, L. (1997). Examination of changes in interpersonal stress as a factor in disease exacerbations among women with rheumatoid arthritis. *Annals of Behavioral Medicine* 19, 279–286.

11

Immune, Neuroendocrine, and Religious Measures

BRUCE S. RABIN & HAROLD G. KOENIG

In this chapter, we describe measures of immune and neuroendocrine function that investigators can use to explore the possible interaction between religion and the mind-body-health axis. We also describe measures of religious belief, practice, and commitment that can be used to assess the religious variable. In each section, we try to identify those measures that are most sensitive to change and most likely to detect relationships between independent and dependent variables. The particular measure used may depend on a number of factors, including the type of population studied and the study design (cross-sectional vs. longitudinal vs. interventional). We also suggest other variables that must be controlled when studying these relationships. Finally, we discuss the *meaning* of associations that may occur between immune, neuroendocrine and religious variables. Further details and references for the following discussion may be found in Rabin (1999).

Overview of Immune Structure and Function

A number of solid organs, cellular components, and soluble proteins make up the immune system. These include the lymphoid tissues, lymphocytes and other immune cells, and immunoglobulins and cytokines. The following offers a brief overview of these immune components. Lymphoid tissues are divided into two classes: (1) the *primary lymphoid tissues*, which are the bone marrow and thymus, and (2) the *secondary lymphoid tissues*, which are the spleen, lymph nodes, and lymphoid tissues of the gastroin-testinal tract and pulmonary system.

Primary Lymphoid Tissues

Bone Marrow

The bone marrow is where white blood cells originate. White blood cells are collectively referred to as leukocytes. *Leukocyte* is translated as "pale cell." The cells that comprise the leukocytes are the neutrophils, eosino-phils, basophils, monocytes, and lymphocytes. There are immature cells in the bone marrow, termed *stem cells*, that are the progenitors of all classes of white blood cells. The maturation of the cells of the bone marrow is under the influence of hormonal factors called *colony-stimulating factors* (CSFs). CSFs act upon the progenitor cells in the marrow and induce them to be-come either a granulocyte (of which there are several types: the neutro-phil, the eosinophil, and the basophil), a monocyte, a lymphocyte, or a megakaryocyte.

Thymus Gland

The thymus gland is a lymphoid organ located just above the heart. It is re-sponsible for the maturation of the T class of lymphocytes that originate in the bone marrow. The thymus is filled with a meshwork of epithelial cells, macrophages, and dendritic cells. The remaining space is filled with lym-phocytes. When the immature T cells leave the bone marrow and enter the thymus, they lack the CD4 and CD8 markers (discussed later). How-ever, both markers appear on the T cells once they are in the thymus and the cells undergo cell division. Most of these double positive cells will die, however, with a small proportion (approximately 5%) surviving and leav-ing the thymus as "single positive" cells with either the CD4 (helper) or CD8 (cytotoxic) marker.

The epithelial cells of the thymus produce hormones, called *thymic hor-mones*. These thymus-derived hormones act on the immature T cells in the thymus and help them mature into T cells that can become functional ef-fector cells. The concentration of thymic hormones in the blood begins to decrease at approximately 60 years of age. A question of concern to psy-choneuroimmunology research will be whether individuals who experi-ence high levels of stressors during their lifetimes are more likely to

undergo earlier decreases in the ability of the thymus to promote maturation of T lymphocytes than individuals who experience lower lifetime levels of stress. It is possible that behaviors and coping skills that lower stress
levels will have a beneficial effect on the long-term production of thymic
hormones.

There is also a nerve supply to the thymus with both sympathetic and
parasympathetic nerve fibers. In rats, there is a dense innervation of sympathetic nerve fibers at the corticomedullary junction, whereas in humans
the medulla may have more sympathetic innervation. The sympathetic
and parasympathetic nervous systems have been shown to influence T-cell
maturation and emigration from the thymus. The role of the thymic innervation in modifying thymic hormone production has not been defined.
The thymus gland increases in size from birth to puberty and then slowly
undergoes involution, but it is often still functionally active, producing
thymic hormones, into the seventh decade of life. Unfortunately, there are
no data bearing on the appearance of the thymus in individuals who have
effective stress-coping skills or who have low levels of stress in their lives.

The thymus also participates in the elimination of immature bone marrow–derived T lymphocytes that (1) have a receptor for "self-antigens"
that are constituents of the individual or (2) are functionally useless.

Secondary Lymphoid Tissues

Spleen

The spleen filters blood and removes antigens and old or damaged erythrocytes. A single artery splits into six branches as it enters the spleen, and
then each branches further. Each arterial branch becomes covered with a
mass of lymphocytes, which are called the *periarteriolar lymphocyte sheath*
(PALS). Because the artery is in the center of the lymphoid tissue, it is
called the *central artery*. The portion of the PALS nearest the artery is rich
in T lymphocytes, and the outer portion of the PALS is a mixture of T and
B lymphocytes. As in the lymph nodes, accumulations of B lymphocytes
are grouped into follicles.

The central arteries in the spleen send off perpendicular branches that
open into spaces called the *marginal sinuses*. The marginal sinuses contain
dendritic cells, macrophages, and T and B lymphocytes. Surrounding the
marginal sinus is the "marginal zone" that covers the PALS. At its termination, the central artery discharges into a venous sinus or ends in a space

between the venous sinuses called a *splenic cord*. The venous sinuses are lined by endothelial cells. The splenic cords consist of erythrocytes, macrophages, monocytes, and lymphocytes. Cells pass between the sinuses and cords. The cords and sinuses are called the *red pulp* because of the large number of erythrocytes. The venous sinuses coalesce and form veins that leave the spleen at the hilus.

Although there are no lymphatic vessels that empty into the spleen, there are efferent lymphatics that leave the spleen. They originate as closed-ended tubes in the follicles of the PALS, merge together, and drain as a single lymphatic to a lymph node located in the hilus of the spleen. Antigen (e.g., bacteria, viruses) in the bloodstream will pass into the spleen, where it is ingested by dendritic cells in the marginal zone and venous sinuses. The dendritic cells move to the PALS of the white pulp. In the PALS, the dendritic cells interact with naive T cells, which then move to the B-cell follicles. Antibody production is initiated, and the antibody-producing B lymphocytes leave the spleen by moving to the red pulp or marginal sinuses, or through the efferent lymphatics. Activated T lymphocytes probably migrate to the venous sinus and then to the circulation.

Lymphatic Vessels

Thin-walled porous lymphatic capillaries (which often travel alongside the thicker-walled blood capillaries) form a dense network within all tissues. The capillaries merge together to eventually form two large "lymphatic vessels" that empty back into the bloodstream and return the plasma (which is called *lymphatic fluid* when in the lymphatic system) to the blood. There are two places that the lymphatic fluid returns to the bloodstream: the *right lymphatic duct* (which drains the upper right part of the body and empties into the right subclavian vein) and the *thoracic duct* (which drains the rest of the body and empties into the left sub-clavian vein).

Lymph Nodes

Along the path that the lymphatic fluid takes to the subclavian veins are accumulations of lymphocytes that form into nodules called *lymph nodes*. The lymph nodes are located along the pathway of the flow of lymph fluid from the periphery to the vasculature. Several lymph nodes are located along the lymphatic vessels, so that the fluid passes through a sequence of nodes as it moves from the periphery to the vasculature. As the lymph fluid passes through the lymph nodes, it accumulates lymphocytes from the nodes. Eventually, the lymphocytes are passed into the bloodstream.

Diffuse Lymphoid Tissue

The connective and parenchymal tissue of the body contains large numbers of effector/memory lymphocytes in its meshwork. Where these accumulations are particularly dense, they are referred to as *diffuse lymphoid tissue*. The lungs, gastrointestinal tract, and skin areas are particularly rich in such lymphocyte accumulations. It makes sense for lymphocytes to be in these locations, which are where foreign antigens are most likely to gain access to the body.

Solitary Lymphoid Follicles

B and T lymphocytes that aggregate into a dense sphere containing dendritic cells mixed with the B lymphocytes surrounded by T lymphocytes are called *solitary lymphoid follicles*. They do not occur in fixed sites but are transiently present. They occur in the same tissue locations as the diffuse lymphoid tissue, and their presence may indicate an active immune response within the tissue.

Aggregated Lymphoid Follicles

In the body, there also are accumulations of several solitary lymphoid follicles. Examples are the tonsils, found at the posterior part of the nasopharynx; bronchiole-associated lymphoid tissue (BALT) in the lungs; Peyer's patches, which are aggregated lymphoid follicles in the wall of the small intestine; and the appendix.

Mucosa-Associated Lymphoid Tissue

Mucosa-associated lymphoid tissue (MALT) protects the mucosal surfaces of the body and provides immunity to the respiratory tract (BALT) and the gastrointestinal tract (gut-associated lymphoid tissue [GALT], also known as Peyer's patches). These areas of the body receive the highest volume of exposure to foreign antigens (e.g., food, microorganisms, environmental pollutants, parasites, allergens). The mucosal immune system can produce cell-mediated immune reactions and a specialized antibody-mediated immunity that consists of secretory immunoglobulin A (IgA). This IgA antibody is synthesized by B lymphocytes in submucosal sites and then transported across the epithelium to the lumen. Secretory IgA binds to foreign antigens and prevents them from adhering to the mucosal surface.

Once a B lymphocyte has reacted with an antigen and has received the necessary help to begin to produce antibody, it leaves the MALT in efferent lymphatics and goes to the mesenteric lymph nodes, where it matures to a plasma cell or becomes a B memory cell. These cells then leave the node through the efferent lymphatic, enter the lymphatic system, go to the bloodstream, and then through specific adhesion molecules reenter the mucosal tissue. It is possible that B lymphocytes derived from mucosal sites produce all classes of immunoglobulin and that only the cells that produce IgA go back to the mucosal sites, but this has not been determined. Regardless of the mechanism, the predominant class of immunoglobulin produced in mucosal sites is IgA.

Lymphocytes and Other Immune Cells

Lymphocytes are white blood cells responsible for the immune response. Different types of lymphocytes originate from a common stem cell in the bone marrow. There are several types of lymphocytes, each with a different function.

B and T Lymphocytes

Lymphocytes that complete their maturation in the bone marrow become B lymphocytes, which function by producing antibody. Lymphocytes that migrate from the bone marrow to the thymus gland for their maturation become T lymphocytes, which are able to identify tissue cells that have an infectious agent within the cell. B lymphocytes release antibodies into the plasma and tissue fluids (humors) that bind to the antigen and "mark" it for elimination by T lymphocytes. T lymphocytes identify an infected cell and initiate reactions that will kill the infected cell. Thus, B lymphocytes act through what is commonly referred to as "humoral" immunity, whereas T lymphocytes act through "cell-mediated" immunity.

A lymphocyte that has never interacted with an antigen is called a *naive lymphocyte*. Naive cells are not found in tissues; they are found only in the

blood and secondary lymphoid tissues. Naive lymphocytes are not activated at the site of antigen entry into the body but rather in lymph nodes
and spleen. Once a lymphocyte has been activated by an antigen, it is
termed an *effector lymphocyte*. Effector lymphocytes are activated to carry
out processes that will rid the body of infectious agents.

The activation of a lymphocyte requires at least two different types of
interaction with an antigen-presenting cell. One of the events is related to
the specificity of the lymphocyte receptor molecule for antigen. When the
lymphocyte's antigen receptor recognizes its specific antigen, a reaction
occurs that allows that particular lymphocyte to become activated. Actual
activation requires an interaction between a second molecule on the lymphocyte surface and a molecule on the surface of another cell. This second
interaction, which has no specificity for antigen, is called *costimulation*.

Each lymphocyte is capable of responding to a single antigen. This
means that each lymphocyte has a different receptor specificity. The selective activation by an antigen of those lymphocytes that can respond to the
antigen is referred to as *clonal selection*. A clone of lymphocytes is the expansion (by cell division) of exact copies of the single lymphocyte that first
responded to the antigen.

During early maturation, T cells begin to express the surface markers
CD1, CD2, CD4, CD5, and CD8. The "CD" nomenclature is a standardized system that is used to designate a specific substance that is present on
the surface of a cell. Many of the CD markers have been well characterized, both as to the cells they are present on and as to what they do on that
cell. For example, all T lymphocytes have CD3 on their surfaces. Some
T lymphocytes also have CD4 and are termed CD4+; others are CD8+.
Regardless of whether they have CD4 or CD8, they also have CD3. The
CD3 participates in signaling the T cell that the T cell receptor (TCR) has
bound an antigenic peptide.

Thus, several different CD markers are present on the surface of the
same cell. CD markers are commonly detected by reacting the cells with
an antibody that is specific for the CD marker. Thus, to determine if a
cell is CD3+, the cells would be incubated with an antibody that is reactive to CD3. To detect whether the antibody is bound to the cells, the antibody has a dye attached to it. If the color product of the dye is visual-
ized on the cell, it would be known to be CD3+. A common procedure to
detect CD markers on lymphocytes is termed *flow cytometry* (discussed
later in this chapter). We now describe the function of CD4+ and CD8+
T lymphocytes.

CD4 T Lymphocytes

Effector CD4 T lymphocytes are capable of binding to an antigen presented in MHC class II molecules on the surface of a tissue cell and then releasing cytokines (discussed later in this chapter), which attract inflammatory cells (neutrophils, eosinophils, monocytes, and macrophages) to the tissue site where the CD4 lymphocyte has bound. The inflammatory cells release enzymes to kill infectious agents in tissue. The phagocytic cells then ingest the killed or damaged tissue. Cytokines released from effector CD4 T lymphocytes will activate a macrophage that has ingested an infectious agent, inducing the macrophage to kill the infectious agent.

The CD4 lymphocyte population has two functional components: Th1 cells and Th2 cells. Each population has important functional differences. When an activated Th1 lymphocyte binds to a B lymphocyte that has processed an antigen, the Th1 cell releases cytokines that cause the B lymphocyte to release the IgG-1, IgG-2, and IgG-3 classes of immunoglobulin (discussed later in this chapter). These immunoglobulin classes participate in the removal of bacteria from the body by enhancing the ability of the bacteria to be ingested by neutrophils. In addition, the Th1 cells are responsible for reactions called *cell-mediated immunity* or *delayed hypersensitivity*, which produces an inflammatory response at the site of later infection by the same infectious agent (discussed later in this chapter).

The Th2 cells produce different cytokines than the Th1 cells. The Th2-derived cytokines stimulate B lymphocytes to produce the IgA, IgE, and IgG-4 classes of immunoglobulin. Th2 cells do not participate in cell-mediated immune reactions.

There is a down-regulating interaction between Th1 and Th2 cells. Cytokines released by either Th1 or Th2 cells will decrease the activity of the other cell population. Thus, increased activity of one of the cell populations is associated with decreased activity of the other population.

CD8 T Lymphocytes

The CD8 class of T lymphocytes is capable of binding to an antigen being presented in major histocompatibility complex (MHC) class I molecules on the surface of a tissue cell and then killing the tissue cell. These are commonly called *cytotoxic* lymphocytes. CD8 lymphocytes have the capability of binding to a foreign antigenic peptide in the groove of a class I MHC molecule and of releasing an enzyme that will kill the cell displaying the foreign peptide. The influence of hormones that are increased in concentration by stress on the functional activity of the CD8 cells is an important and needed area of investigation. As CD8 cells are important for the elimination of virally infected cells, a decrease in their activity may contribute to an increased susceptibility to viral infection.

Monocytes

Monocytes, like lymphocytes, have a round nucleus and are not granular. These cells are collectively called *mononuclear cells*. Monocytes are phagocytic cells, meaning they ingest foreign materials that get into the body. When the monocyte enters tissue, it enlarges in size and is called a *macrophage*. Monocytes also play a role in making and releasing cytokines.

Neutrophils

Neutrophils are granular leukocytes possessing a nucleus with three to five lobes. The granules in their cytoplasm contain enzymes that can digest bacteria. Neutrophils are involved in ingestion (phagocytosis) of solid particles such as bacteria. Neutrophils have the properties of being attracted to areas where they are needed by the mechanism of *chemotaxis*. Chemotactic cytokines (see later in this chapter) such as interleukin-8 (IL-8) act primarily on neutrophils and function as mediators of acute inflammation. Neutrophils, thus, have the capability of binding foreign particles (e.g., bacteria) to their surface so that the particles can be ingested and killed. Antibodies produced by the immune system participate by helping neutrophils ingest bacteria. Neutrophils do not present antigen to lymphocytes as part of the process by which an immune reaction is initiated, however.

Basophils and Mast Cells

Basophils arise from the bone marrow and circulate in the blood. The granules in basophils absorb blue dye, which has a basic pH (greater than 7.0) value. Hence, these "blue-stained" leukocytes are referred to as *basophils*. They have granules containing histamine and surface receptors for the Fc portion of the IgE antibody molecule. Basophils usually do not enter tissue.

A cell with a similar morphology to basophils is the *mast cell.* Like basophils, mast cells also have histamine-containing granules and surface receptors for IgE. Mast cells do not circulate. Chemical factors released from mast cells mediate many allergic reactions. IgE binds to tissue mast cells and circulating basophils. The binding of IgE to mast cells and basophils has no effect on the cells. However, when the antibody interacts with specific antigen, a programmed sequence of events starts. The antigen must be capable of binding to adjacent molecules of IgE. This cross-linking causes an aggregation of Fc receptors. Changes occur in the cytoplasmic cytoskeleton to which the receptors are attached, and a signal is given that leads to release of the contents of the granules of the basophils and mast cells.

In addition to degranulation, there is increased synthesis and release of prostaglandins (chemicals that inhibit effects of heparin on smooth-muscle cells and vascular endothelial cells and increase platelet aggregation) and leukotrienes (chemicals that increase vascular permeability and contract pulmonary smooth muscle). The release of the various mediators produces smooth-muscle contraction, vascular leakage, hypotension, mucus secretion, wheal and flare (swelling and redness of skin), itching, and pain. These events occur within minutes of exposure to the antigen (the first exposure initiates IgE synthesis), and by 60 minutes they are over. This is termed the *immediate hypersensitivity reaction,* which is followed in 2 to 8 hours by a late-phase response that lasts for 1 to 2 days. The late-phase response is an inflammatory reaction mediated by synthesized mediators and consists of lymphocytes, neutrophils, eosinophils, monocytes, and a few basophils. The late-phase reaction results in a localized burning sensation, tenderness, erythema, and induration.

Eosinophils

Like basophils and mast cells, eosinophils are granulocytes that help protect against infections with some parasitic worms by releasing proteins that are toxic to the worms. They migrate to sites of allergic reactions that lead to damage of normal tissue. Granules of eosinophils take up red (eosin) dye, hence the name *eosinophils.*

MHC Molecules

Lymphoid cells and tissue cells express molecules on their surfaces, called *major histocompatibility complex* molecules. The term *major histocompatibility complex* (MHC) is derived from the initial identification of molecules on the surface of tissue cells that were found to be important in stimulating the immune reaction that produced rejection of transplanted tissue. Thus, these molecules were called *major* because they were important, *histocompatibility* because they were involved in determining if transplanted tissue would be compatible when taken from an organ donor and given to an organ recipient, and *complex* because there are many different molecules that are coded for by several genetic loci (locations on a chromosome) with multiple alleles (alternate choices of a gene from the total population).

In addition to their role in organ transplantation, the MHC molecules are important because they are located on the surfaces of cells (e.g., monocytes, macrophages, B lymphocytes, and dendritic cells) that present antigens to lymphocytes as part of the process of a lymphocyte being converted from a naive state to an effector state. There are two major groupings of MHC molecules, designated MHC I and MHC II molecules. Monocytes, macrophages, B lymphocytes, and dendritic cells express both class I and class II MHC molecules. Tissue cells primarily express MHC class I molecules. Infectious agents that are ingested by monocytes and macrophages are often killed when the monocyte or macrophage is activated by a T lymphocyte. The T lymphocyte recognizes a portion of the infectious agent in MHC II molecules on the membrane of the monocyte or macrophage. Infectious agents that are ingested by monocytes and macrophages are then killed when the monocyte or macrophage is activated by the T lymphocyte.

Immunoglobulins and Cytokines

Immunoglobulins

Immunoglobulins are a family closely related (though not identical) to proteins commonly called *antibodies*. Immunoglobulins have *specificity* in that they combine most strongly with the particular antigen that stimulated their production. Immunoglobulins are produced by B lymphocytes, and each B lymphocyte can produce only a single type of immunoglobulin (e.g., IgE). The B lymphocyte will produce thousands of that particular immunoglobulin molecule each second. Immunoglobulins bind to antigens located outside tissue cells.

There are five classes of immunoglobulin: IgG, IgA, IgM, IgD, and IgE. Each class of immunoglobulin has its own characteristic and identifiable heavy chain. It is the heavy chain that allows for the identification of each class as the light chains are common to all classes (there are only two classes of light chains: κ and λ). The term applied to the class differentiation of immunoglobulin is *isotype*. Thus, there are five isotypes of immunoglobulin.

It can be deduced that the portion of the antibody molecule that combines with antigen must have a structure that depends on the antigen for which the antibody has specificity. Thus, the terminal end that combines with antigen is termed the *variable* portion of the immunoglobulin molecule. The remaining portions of the protein are called *constant* regions.

Cytokines

Cytokines are one of numerous proteins made by immune cells that can influence the activity of other cells. Cytokines bind to cytokine receptors on cells, with different receptors binding different cytokines. Lymphocytes and antigen-presenting cells produce cytokines that, depending on the particular cytokine and the cell that it binds to, may either upregulate or downregulate the activity of other immune cells. Cytokines are also involved in the regulation of endocrine hormone production and contribute to the modulation of activity of the central nervous system. A variety of cells, other than cells of the immune system, produce cytokines. The nomenclature used to identify cytokines is interleukin (IL), followed by a number, Greek letter, or both (see chapter 3). For example, interleukin-2 (IL-2) is a cytokine produced by CD4 lymphocytes with the biological property of promoting division of T lymphocytes.

Several cytokines stimulate the growth and differentiation of bone marrow progenitor cells. Cytokines that stimulate growth and differentiation of bone marrow progenitor cells are termed *colony-stimulating factors* (CSFs). The names given to CSFs reflect the types of colonies that they stimulate when bone marrow cells are cultured in agar.

Measures of Immune Function

A variety of laboratory tests are used to determine the number of different types of immune cells or chemicals released by immune cells present in blood or other tissues. Many of these tests have been mentioned in this chapter. The remainder of this section presents information about the tests—how the test is performed and what is learned from each. The list is not comprehensive but represents the tests most commonly used in research of the interrelationship between mind, body, and health.

Lymphocytes Subsets: Quantifying T and B Lymphocytes

One method often used is flow cytometry, which involves combining lymphocytes with an antibody carrying a colored label that will bind to a receptor on the lymphocyte surface. When the lymphocyte with the colored antibody molecule is exposed to an ultraviolet (UV) light source, the dye emits a visible light that can be measured. Flow cytometry can be used to quantify different populations of lymphocytes. For example, one antibody directed to the CD3 marker, which is present on all T lymphocytes, can be labeled with a red dye, whereas an antibody directed to the CD4 marker, present on all T-helper lymphocytes, can be labeled with green dye. Once illuminated with UV light, photodetectors count the number of cells that have each dye attached to them.

As noted, all T lymphocytes have the CD3 marker, all B lymphocytes have the CD19 marker, and NK lymphocytes have the CD56 marker. Additional surface markers are used to identify subgroups of the different populations. For example, CD3 cells can be identified as helper (CD4+) or cytotoxic (CD8+). Surface markers to identify T-helper cells as Th1 or Th2 are not yet available, however.

Lymphocyte Response to Mitogens

Another way to examine lymphocytes is to measure their activity levels. This often is done by incubating lymphocytes with either nonspecific mitogens (which stimulate most T or B cells to divide) or specific mitogens (which stimulate division in only those cells that have previously reacted with an antigen). Activity is measured by the amount of cell division that is induced in the lymphocytes. Nonspecific mitogens are usually derived from plants and induce mitosis without the lymphocytes having to make an immune response to the plant substance. Specific mitogens are antigens that will induce mitosis only if the lymphocytes are derived from an individual who has previously made an immune response to the antigen.

Although a positive response to a specific mitogen (e.g., a fungal antigen) indicates that exposure has previously occurred to that mitogen, the ability of lymphocytes to respond to a nonspecific mitogen is often difficult to relate to biological significance. Indeed, although the response to nonspecific mitogenic stimulation can be altered by stress, there is a lack of basic immunological information that allows the investigator to determine if the changes have meaning in regard to altering susceptibility to infection or on the course of an immune-mediated disease. Then again, if the lymphocytes have, for example, less than 10% of the "normal" response to a nonspecific mitogen, it might indicate the presence of an immune deficiency syndrome (e.g., AIDS). In that case, the individual would be susceptible to the infectious disease(s) against which those lymphocytes provide protection.

Natural Killer (NK) Cells

The NK cells are part of the innate host defense system. To measure their activity, a cell that is susceptible to being killed by NK cells is prepared and labeled with radioactive chromium. The radioactive compound remains within the cytoplasm of the cell but is released when the cell dies. When the target cells are incubated with NK cells, the amount of radioactivity released is determined. The ability of NK cells to kill radioactively labeled target cells indicates that the cells are functional and that they should be able to contribute to resistance to viral infections and react against cells that become malignant. However, as with other immune functional assays, it is unclear as to how little or how much function is enough. Certainly, the lack of NK function is significant, but a reduction from normal is difficult to interpret in regard to biological meaning. Alterations of NK function subsequent to a stressor are frequently reported in the research literature, and NK cell activity is a commonly used indicator of stressor effects on a component of the immune system.

Immunoglobulins

The usual procedure to quantify the amount of the major classes of immunoglobulin (e.g., IgG, IgA, 1gM) is called *nephelometry*. In this procedure, a known amount of antibody that binds to the heavy chain of the immunoglobulin class that is being measured is added. This forms an immune complex (with the antigen component of the complex being the antibody class that is being measured). The amount of precipitate that is formed relates to the concentration of the immunoglobulin class being measured. The amount of precipitate is compared with the amount produced by known concentrations of the antigen being measured. The results are usually reported as milligrams of immunoglobulin in 100 ml of blood (mg/dl). Normal values are determined by quantifying the amount of each class of immunoglobulin in large numbers of normal individuals. The range of normal for adults for IgG, IgA, and IgM is broad. Children under the age of 16 have lower levels of immunoglobulin than adults. Therefore, when evaluating immunoglobulin levels in children, an age-related norm must be used.

There are differences between the normal concentration determined statistically and the normal physiological concentration—that is, the physiological normal is lower than the normal determined from measuring immunoglobulin levels in large populations and determining the mean and standard deviation. Thus, a single number at a point in time provides little information regarding biological significance for immunoglobulins, unless the amount detected is extremely low. Changes in immunoglobulin levels occur slowly and may be due to inadequate nutrition. If stress or depression interferes with an individual's obtaining adequate nutrition, low immunoglobulin levels could ensue. Quantifying immunoglobulins does not provide information regarding what antigens the antibodies can react to and how much antibody is present to a given antigen.

Cytokines

The production of cytokines by lymphocytes is an important indication of their function. The method currently used to compare Th1 and Th2 cell function (e.g., Th1 cells produce IFN-γ and Th2 cells produce IL-4) has two parts. The first is the generation of cytokines. The procedure is similar to a lymphocyte response to mitogens with the culture medium being collected after stimulation of the lymphocytes. The second part of the procedure involves quantifying the cytokines in the supernatant. The ELISA procedure is commonly used for this.

Cytokine production before and after exposure to an acute laboratory stressor has been shown to change. Again, as in other immune assays, there are limitations in regard to the biological interpretation of the data. The effect of stress on altering cytokine production by a specific lymphocyte population can be determined.

Measures of Neuroendocrine Function

A number of brain areas, endocrine organs, and hormones interact to form the neuroendocrine system. The major components that make up this system are illustrated and described in chapter 3.

Tables 11.1 and 11.2 present a variety of immune and neuroendocrine research studies with findings relevant to the study of the effects of stress on stress-related immune system function and hormone production. They also present information relevant to the study of the potential effects of behaviors and activities as buffers of stressor-induced immune alteration.

Measuring Religious Variables

There are an enormous number of measures to choose from to assess religious beliefs, practices, motivation, and commitment. Peter Hill and Ralph Hood have compiled more than 125 such instruments in their recent publication, *Measures of Religiosity* (1999). We have discussed elsewhere those measures most often used in studies of the religion-health relationship (Koenig, McCullough, et al., 2001). Here we explore measures of religiosity and spirituality that might be used in studying the religion-psychoneuroimmunology relationship.

At least 10 major religious dimensions require consideration: denomination/affiliation, religious belief, religious attitudes, organizational or social religious activity, nonorganizational or private religious activity, religious salience or importance, religious orientation or motivation, religious coping, religious history, religious experience, and religious development or maturity. Finally, there are the wider domains of spirituality and spiritual experience.

Denomination/Affiliation

For years, denomination or affiliation was often the only religious measure used in studies of the religion-health relationship (Larson et al., 1986). Although not sufficient, assessing a subject's religious affiliation is necessary.

First, it is important to determine if the person is Christian, Jewish, Muslim, Hindu, Buddhist, Confucian, Taoist, or unaffiliated. Second, it is important to know the particular subgroup to which the person is affiliated.

For example, if the subject is Christian, the investigator must determine if the person is Catholic, Protestant, or of other Christian affiliation. If the subject is Protestant, the investigator may wish to know if he or she is affiliated with a liberal, moderate, conservative, or fundamentalist denomination (Roof & McKinney, 1987). The finest level of detail is the subject's specific denomination (there are well over 50 major Christian denominations in the United States alone). In our studies at Duke, we ask subjects to place themselves into one of 54 categories (available from authors on request).

If the subject is Jewish, it is important to determine whether the person is ultra-Orthodox, Orthodox, Conservative, Reform, Reconstructionist, or Messianic. Similar subclassifications exist for Muslims (Sunni, Shiah, Wahhabis, Amidiyya, Babism), Buddhists (Hinayana, Mahayana, Vajrayana), Confucianists (traditional Confucianism, neo-Confucianism), and Hindus (Jainism, classical Hinduism, Sikhism, modern Hinduism) (Fellows, 1979).

Because beliefs, practices, and rituals vary tremendously between these different religious groups, it is likely that effects on health and on neuroendocrine and immune functioning also will vary. Then again, level of religious devotion may have effects that transcend the particular belief system. No research has yet compared differences in endocrine or immune functioning between members of different religious groups. Such research, while challenging and expensive, is not impossible, although comparisons should probably be made between subjects living in their native country/cultures (i.e., Jews in Israel, Christians in Western countries, Hindus in India, Buddhists in Tibet, Confucians and Taoists in China, and Muslims in Saudi Arabia). Otherwise, effects of immigrant or minority status may bias results, given the greater psychosocial stress often experienced by such groups.

Religious Belief

A simple question asking about belief in the existence of God or a Universal Spirit is unlikely to yield much useful information in a country like the United States, where 96% of the population would assent to such a belief (Princeton Religion Research Center, 1996). Perhaps more valid is the assessment of *certainty* of belief. In fact, one of the first religiosity measures ever published assessed this dimension of religiousness (Thouless, 1935). The Thouless beliefs scale asks the subject to rate 25 religious belief statements (e.g., "There is a personal God") on a 7-point scale from complete certainty of the statement's truth to complete certainty of its falsehood. Related to but not the same as certainty of belief is religious *orthodoxy*. A number of religious orthodoxy scales exist that measure the extent to which the person's beliefs conform to the established, original doctrines of the religious tradition (Brown & Lowe, 1951; Glock & Stark, 1966; Lenski, 1963; Martin & Westie, 1959). Most assess Christian orthodoxy, although the first six items of the Ben-Meir and Kedem (1979) scale can be used as an index of Jewish orthodoxy.

If one believes in God, then it may also be important to determine exactly what type of God is believed in. Is the image of God one that is loving, kind, controlling, vindictive, stern, impersonal, or distant? Studies have shown that self-esteem is significantly related to one's image of God—greater self-esteem if the image is that of a loving or kind God, but lower self-esteem if God is seen as vindictive, impersonal, distant, controlling, or stern (Benson & Spilka, 1973; Pollner, 1989).

Religious Attitudes

Religious attitudes may be defined as "*evaluative* reactions"—positive or negative feelings—toward religion or religious experiences (Hill & Hood, 1999). There is some overlap with belief in that many of the attitude scales include items assessing belief. Examples of such scales include the Religious Attitude Inventory (Ausubel & Schpoont, 1957), Religious Attitude Scale (Poppleton & Pilkington, 1963), Religious Doubts Scale (Hunsberger et al., 1993), and Religious Values Scale (Morrow et al., 1993).

Involvement in Religious Community

Genuineness of belief should be reflected in behavior. Religious behaviors are divided into organizational religious activities and nonorganizational or private religious activity. Frequency of religious attendance is the most widely used measure of involvement in religious community. This may be asked as a single question such as "How often do you attend Sunday worship services?" (Glock & Stark, 1966) or "How often do you attend church or other religious meetings?" (Koenig, Meador, & Parkerson, 1997). Response options typically range from never to more than once per week, although investigators frequently compare those who attend religious services at least once a week with those who attend less often.

Other investigators have used multi-item scales to measure religious community involvement, including such items as religious service attendance, participation in other activities at church, frequency of taking Communion, number of offices or special jobs held, proportion of income given to church, and number of closest friends who are members of their church (Idler, 1999; King & Hunt, 1967; Koenig, Smiley, & Gonzales, 1988). A related concept is the amount of religious support received from one's church congregation. Krause (1999) has developed an eight-item measure that assesses emotional support received from others, emotional support provided to others, negative interactions, and anticipated support likely to be received if needed.

Private Religious Activities

Some religious activities may be performed alone, in private. Such activities are not as dependent on support or reinforcement by the group and depend more on personal motivations. A single question that taps this dimension is "How often do you spend time in private religious activities, such as prayer, meditation, or Bible study?" (with six response options ranging from "more than once a day" to "rarely or never") (Koenig, Meador, & Parkerson, 1997). Other investigators have developed multi-item "devotionalism" subscales that measure activities like prayer, frequency of consulting God in making everyday decisions, reading religious literature, and watching or listening to religious programs on television or radio (Glock & Stark, 1966; Koenig, Smiley, & Gonzales, 1988; Lenski, 1963).

Summing public and private religious activities to obtain an "overall" religious activities score is probably unwise because these two dimensions of religious activity may have very different relationships to health, especially cross-sectionally. For example, severe physical disability may limit attendance at formal religious services but may promote private religious activities as a way of coping with disabling illness.

Religious Salience

Level of personal religiousness is often assessed with a single question such as "How important is religion to you?" Because response options are usually limited (very important, somewhat important, not important) and 80% of subjects in most areas of United States indicate "very" or "somewhat" important, this item yields relatively little information. One way to increase the sensitivity of such an item is to have the subject rate on a 0 to 10 visual analog scale how important religion is to his or her life. Multi-item scales of religious importance, however, do exist (Putney & Middleton, 1961).

Religious Orientation

Religious orientation scales attempt to assess the person's true motivation for being religious. To what extent do religious beliefs and teachings affect the person's day-to-day decisions and lifestyle? Gordon Allport, a psychologist at Harvard in the 1950s and 1960s, developed important concepts concerning religious motivation in his study of religious prejudice (Allport, 1954). He separated religious people into those who were "intrinsically" religious versus those who were "extrinsically" religious and defined each as follows:

> Persons with this orientation [intrinsic] find their master motive in religion. Other needs, strong as they may be, are regarded as of less ultimate significance, and they are, so far as possible, brought into harmony with the religious beliefs and prescriptions. Having embraced a creed, the individual endeavors to internalize it and follow it fully. It is in this sense that he lives his religion. (Allport & Ross, 1967, p. 434)

> Persons with this orientation [extrinsic] may find religion useful in a variety of ways—to provide security and solace, sociability and distraction, status and self-justification. The embraced creed is lightly held or else selectively shaped to fit more primary needs. In theological terms the extrinsic type turns to God, but without turning away from self. (Allport & Ross, 1967, p. 434)

Allport developed a 20-item intrinsic-extrinsic scale to distinguish the two types of religious motivation and administered it to 309 church members (Allport & Ross, 1967). He discovered that prejudice was related to extrinsic but not intrinsic religiosity. Examples of extrinsic items included statements such as "One reason for my being a church member is that such membership helps to establish a person in the community" and "The church is most important as a place to formulate good social relationships. Examples of intrinsic items included statements such as "I try hard to carry my religion over into all my other dealings in life" and "My religious beliefs are what really lie behind my whole approach to life." Several other investigators have now developed other versions of the scale, and the number of questions now ranges from 3 to 21 (Feagin, 1964; Gorsuch & McPherson, 1989; Hoge, 1972).

Religious Experience

A number of measures assess religious experience (Edwards, 1976; Glock & Stark, 1966; Hood, 1970). Glock and Stark's (1966) measure inquires about the following five Christian experiences: "A feeling that you were somehow in the presence of God," "A sense of being saved in Christ," "A feeling of being afraid of God," "A feeling of being punished by God for something you had done," and "A feeling of being tempted by the Devil." Single items from a variety of other religiosity scales also tap religious experience. For example, the religious well-being subscale of Paloutzian and Ellison's (1982) Spiritual Well-Being Scale has the item, "I experience God's love and care for me in my relationship with him" (response options ranging from 1, strongly disagree, to 6, strongly agree). Hoge's (1972) intrinsic religiosity scale includes the item, "In my life I experience the presence of the Divine" (response options ranging from "definitely not true" to "definitely true").

Religious Coping

Religion often is turned to as a source of comfort during severe stress, especially when the stress is out of the person's control. Although it may be argued that "use" of religion in this way is an extrinsic form of religiousness, religious coping tends to be more strongly related to intrinsic religiousness (Bjorck & Cohen, 1993; Koenig, 1998; Pargament, 1997). Many devoutly religious people turn to their faith during times of stress, whether that stress is major or minor. Repeated use of religion as a coping behavior throughout life may increase its effectiveness when it is needed in more difficult situations.

A number of approaches have been used to measure religious coping. One approach is a global one that assesses overall likelihood of depending on religion when stressed. A three-item religious coping index has been developed and validated for use in persons experiencing physical health problems (Koenig, 1994; Koenig, Cohen, Blazer, et al., 1992). This instrument includes open-ended questions about how people cope with stress and the extent to which they use religion in this regard. A second approach uses a multi-item measure to assess specific religious coping styles. Pargament and Koenig have developed the RCOPE scale, which assesses 21 methods of religious coping by using 63 items (Koenig, Pargament, & Nielsen, 1998; Pargament, Koenig, & Perez, 2000). A 14-item brief RCOPE has also been developed (Pargament, Smith, et al., 1998) that assesses "negative" and "positive" forms of religious coping, which tend to be related to mental and physical health in opposite directions.

Religious History

Most of these measures (and those discussed later in this chapter) assess religiousness in the present. In other words, these instruments assess the current level of religious belief, activity, or commitment. However, recent efforts have attempted to assess religious activity and "turning points" across the life span and then relate health outcomes to total exposure to religion. Although such assessment depends on subject recall, which is heavily influenced by present religiousness, it tends to give a more longitudinal picture of religious involvement that is not usually captured with traditional measures. Taking this perspective may help determine the direction of causality when a relationship is found between religion and a health outcome. Using traditional measures of religiousness, it is often difficult to determine whether better or worse health followed or preceded the increase in religiousness. A number of efforts are now under way to measure religious history, although no single instrument has been used consistently (George, 1999; Hays et al. 1998).

Religious Maturity and Development

Religious belief and practice may exist in mature and immature forms. James Fowler (1981) has written a book called *Stages of Faith*. In this book, he describes the various stages of religious faith as they develop from infancy to old age: intuitive-projective (ages 2–7), mythic-literal (ages 7–12), synthetic-conventional (adolescence onward), individuative-reflective (mid-20s and beyond), conjunctive (midlife and beyond), and universalizing faith (late life). Although this theory of faith development is not without critique (Koenig, 1994), it conveys the idea that religious faith may proceed from immature to mature forms over time and with experience.

Because the "content" of religious faith is important to the definition of "maturity," it is best to measure religious maturity within each major religious tradition separately (Christianity, Judaism, Islam, Buddhism, Hinduism, etc.). Most instruments available today have been developed to assess Christian spiritual maturity. An example is Ellison's (1983) 30-item Spiritual Maturity Index. This index assesses a person's need for institutional structure for expression of religious involvement, participation in religious practices as a spontaneous part of everyday life, absence of need for social support to bolster religious belief and practice, and expression of generosity, forgiveness, and compassion toward others. Other measures of religious development include the Faith Maturity Scale (Benson et al., 1993) and the Religious Status Interview (Malony, 1988).

Jewish Religiosity Scales

To our knowledge, there exist at least two scales designed specifically to measure Jewish religiousness. One instrument developed by Ben-Meir and Kedem (1979) assesses six religious beliefs (God, the soul after death, Torah, etc.) and 20 religious practices (Shabbat, synagogue attendance, making kiddush, etc.). Ressler (1997) has developed a 10-item "Jewishness" scale for use in epidemiological studies. Ressler examined relationships between Jewish identification (Jewishness) and sense of belonging, optimism, and self-acceptance in 177 American Jews, age 22 to 40 years. Two aspects of Jewish identification in particular—activism in mainstream Jewish organizations and religiosity—significantly predicted well-being scores, accounting for 7% to 11% of the variance.

Hindu Religiosity Scales

Again, few scales have been developed to capture the essence of Hindu religious beliefs and practice—although some attempts have been made. Studying fear of death and religiosity among college students in northern India, Dhawan and Sripat (1986) used a 36-item religiosity scale developed by Bhushan (1970) to assess Hindu belief and practice. Measured in this way, however, religiosity did not serve to reduce fear of death or subsequently to influence affiliation behavior in this experimental study. Using a different scale, Hassan and Khalique (1981) examined the relationship between religiosity and personality characteristics of 480 students from colleges in India (320 Hindus and 160 Muslims). Investigators used a 10-item religiosity scale that assessed faith in God and religion, acceptance of religious values, traditions, conventions, and observance of religious rituals and prayers—using questions that were apparently both acceptable and relevant to Hindus and Muslims. The scale's validity was documented in part by its high correlation with the Bhushan scale.

Muslim Religiosity Scales

We know of no scales developed specifically for use with Muslims, although Shams and Jackson (1993) used the Allport-Vernon Scale of Values (Allport et al., 1968) to assess religiosity and well-being among employed and unemployed male Muslims living in Great Britain (finding a significant correlation in the unemployed group). Likewise, Thorson (1998) used the Hoge (1972) intrinsic religiosity scale to examine the relationship between religiosity and fear of death among 249 Muslims in Egypt and among 172 Christians in America. Interestingly, intrinsic religious commitment was significantly higher in Muslims than in Christians for all 10 items on the Hoge scale.

Buddhist Belief Scales

To our knowledge, only one such scale exists, the Buddhist Beliefs and Practices Scale (Emavardhana & Tori, 1997). This scale was used in a study of self-concept, ego defense mechanisms, and religiosity following a 7-day meditation retreat. Other investigators, however, have studied intrinsic and extrinsic religiousness as a predictor of anxiety in Buddhists.

Tapanya et al. (1997) used the 20-item Gorsuch-Venable I-E [Intrinsic=Extrinsic] scale to examine worry and intrinsic-extrinsic religious orientation among elderly Buddhists in Thailand and elderly Christians in Canada. The words *church*, *God*, and *Bible* were modified for the Buddhist version. Investigators found that intrinsic religiosity was inversely related to worry in both groups but especially in Buddhists, and extrinsic religiosity was positively related to worry, but only in Buddhists.

Among things that each group worried about, church/temple was ranked second among Buddhists but sixth among Christians.

Recommended Religiosity Scales

Although all scales have deficiencies in one way or another, certain measures may be better than others. As far as religious beliefs are concerned, it is probably more important to assess what kind of God one believes in (kind, loving, merciful vs. distant, uninvolved, punishing) than simply whether one believes in God (Benson & Spilka, 1973). Private religious activities such as frequency of prayer and scripture reading are important to measure, but response options should provide a wide range to enhance dispersion across categories (i.e., at least 1–6 ranging from not at all to several times per day). Organizational religious activity and support obtained from religion are likewise important variables to measure for all studies in psychoneuroimmunology. A single item on religious attendance will often suffice (but again, with a wide range of response options), and religious support is measured best by using Krause's (1999) instrument. Intrinsic religiousness is an essential variable to assess religious motivation and depth of religious commitment. We recommend the 10-item Hoge scale (1972) or the 20-item Allport and Ross (1967) I-E scale. For religious coping, the 14-item RCOPE assesses both positive and negative religious behaviors (Pargament, Smith, et al., 1998).

For those wishing a brief instrument that assesses the three most widely recognized dimensions of religious involvement, the five-item Duke University Religion Index (DUREL) is recommended. It measures organizational religiousness (1 item), nonorganizational religiousness (1 item), and intrinsic religiosity (3 items) (Koenig, Meador, & Parkerson, 1997). This instrument is useful in large epidemiological surveys of population-based samples where only a few items can be included to assess religiosity. For studies involving smaller clinical samples, where more items tapping religious dimensions can be included, we recommend multi-item, multidimensional scales to obtain a more comprehensive picture of subjects' religiousness. In statistically examining associations, it is essential to examine each dimension of religiousness separately as a predictor, rather than combining scores for the different dimensions; likewise, more than one dimension of religiousness should not be included together in regression models because of multiple co-linearity.

Measuring Spirituality

Because *spirituality* has become a more popular term than *religiosity*, investigators frequently seek to assess this construct. Unfortunately, spirituality has become so broadly defined that it has lost its distinctiveness (Koenig, McCullough, & Larson, 2001). Under the term *spirituality* have been included many other psychological yearnings and experiences—including meaning and purpose in life; forgiveness; gratefulness; a sense of beauty, wonder, or awe; even well-being itself. This makes studying the relationship between spirituality and mental health outcomes difficult because tautology (a single underlying construct predicting itself) becomes a real problem. Included in many measures of spirituality today, then, are items asking about well-being, satisfaction, and a sense of purpose or meaning in life. The remaining questions typically tap traditional religious beliefs, practices, and experiences. Again, this mixture of items will contaminate assessments of the relationship between spirituality and health outcomes. In the authors' opinion, the term *spirituality* is distinctive only if it involves a relationship with or search for the *transcendent*—however one defines the transcendent. We now examine a variety of spirituality scales.

Spiritual Well-Being Scale

The best-known and most widely used spirituality scale is Paloutzian and Ellison's (1982) 20-item Spiritual Well-Being (SWB) scale. The SWB scale consists of two 10-item sections, a religious well-being (RWB) subscale and an existential well-being (EWB) subscale. Many studies have found SWB related to better mental health and greater well-being. Most of the variance in well-being, however, is predicted by the EWB subscale—which itself directly measures psychological well-being. It is not surprising, then, that existential well-being predicts well-being—an expected and clearly tautological association. More meaningful is the relationship between the RWB subscale and mental health—although the items in this subscale have a traditionally religious content (i.e., examine relationships with God).

Index of Spiritual Orientation

Based on Sorokin's theory of cultural values, Glik (1990) developed a 19-item scale designed to assess "nontraditional religious group orientations."

It contains ideational belief, salience of religion, purpose in life, and mysticism subscales. Regular participation in healing groups is used instead of participation in religious services. The scale has not been used widely.

INSPIRIT Scale

Kass et al. (1991) have developed a scale called the Index of Core Spiritual Experiences (INSPIRIT). They used this scale to assess 83 medically ill adults as part of a 10-week study of Benson's (1975) relaxation response. The stated purpose of the scale is to assess "the occurrence of experience that convinces a person God exists and evokes feelings of closeness with God, including the perception that God dwells within." The scale includes seven items: self-rated religiousness/spiritual orientation, frequency of religious/spiritual practices, feeling close to a powerful spiritual force, feeling close to God, having an experience convincing the person that God exists, agreeing that God dwells within the person, and a rating of other spiritual experiences. The scale has a relatively strong correlation with the intrinsic religiosity subscale of Allport and Ross's (1967) I-E scale ($r = 0.69, p < .0001$). INSPIRIT has been used widely in a variety of studies and has the advantage of tapping both religious and spiritual beliefs and practices. In particular, it is not contaminated by items that measure mental health per se.

FACIT Spiritual Well-Being Scale

The Spiritual Well-Being (SpWB) scale is is a subscale of the Functional Assessment of Chronic Illness Therapy (FACIT) scale developed by Cella and colleagues at Rush Presbyterian Medical Center in Chicago (Cella, 1996; Cella & Webster, 1997). There is also a new 24-item version of the scale (Version 4) (FACIT Sp-Ex) (Brady et al., 1999). The measure consists of two parts: a Faith/Assurance subscale and a Meaning/Purpose subscale. The scale is heavily contaminated with items that measure mental health and well-being, making tautology a serious concern.

Systems of Belief Inventory

Jimmie Holland from the Sloan-Kettering Cancer Center in New York has developed a 15-item Systems of Belief Inventory (SBI-15) for patients who are experiencing severe life-threatening illness (Holland et al., 1998, 1999). This measure assesses religious beliefs, feelings, and experiences and the support received from one's religious congregation. According to the authors, this scale is correlated with the Allport-Ross I-E scale ($r = .60$) and the INSPIRIT scale ($r = .74$). Again, spirituality is largely operationalized in terms of religious beliefs and practices, but the scale also attends to broader issues, as INSPIRIT does. Of particular importance is its inclusion of items that assess support received from one's religious community, which is particularly relevant for patients with serious medical illness.

Fetzer Institute's Measure of Religiousness and Spirituality

A multidimensional measure of religion and spirituality was developed by a team of scientists who were convened by the Fetzer Institute (Idler et al., 1999; Fetzer Institute, October 1999). The Fetzer scale assesses a broad range of religious and spiritual dimensions, including denomination, organizational religiousness, private spiritual practices, religious social support, religious coping, religious belief, moral values, religious commitment/intrinsic religiosity, financial contributions, time spent working in the church, forgiveness, spiritual experience, and self-ratings of religiousness and spiritual salience. Although overall this is a fine instrument, like the FACIT, some of its subscales are contaminated by items that directly assess mental health and well-being. Several studies have now used this measure, and psychometric information has been included with the most recent version of the instrument (Fetzer Institute, October 1999).

Spiritual Involvement and Beliefs Scale

Family physician Robert Hatch and colleagues (1998) developed a 26-item scale based on a study of 50 medical patients and 33 family practice educators. It demonstrates a strong correlation with Paloutzian and Ellison's SWB scale ($r = .80$). Many of the items, however, have little or no relationship to the sacred or transcendent, and contamination with items that assess mental health are present (tapping the consequences of spirituality, but not spirituality itself).

Recommended Spirituality Scales

For a brief spirituality measure that is not contaminated with mental health items and assesses spirituality more broadly than traditional measures of religiousness, the 7-item INSPIRIT is a good instrument. Nevertheless, INSPIRIT focuses primarily on spiritual or religious experience and less so on level of spiritual commitment, intrinsic motivation, and involvement in religious or spiritual community. Holland's 15-item SBI is also useful as a broad measure of spirituality, particularly because it includes support received from one's religious or spiritual community. Use of the scale in clinical samples—particularly those with cancer—may be especially appropriate. Finally, for a comprehensive measure of spiritual and religious beliefs and practices, the Fetzer Institute's instrument is preferred—if items on mental health, well-being, meaning in life, and forgiveness are removed to avoid tautology.

Conclusions

Measures used to assess immune and neuroendocrine function must be carefully chosen, considering the study design (cross-sectional, longitudinal, or interventional), the population being studied (e.g., high or low life stress, physically fit or sedentary, high or low in optimism, with or without social support network, young or elderly, high or low religiosity, with or without diseases that affect the sympathetic nervous system), and type of stress involved (acute vs. chronic). Immune and neuroendocrine measures should be those affected by psychological stress or social support as determined in other PNI studies. However, it is especially important to understand how the hormonal and immune alterations influence susceptibility to or exacerbations of *disease*.

Unfortunately, studies of the mechanism of how stressor-induced immune alterations affect the quality of an individual's health are only just beginning. This is not to suggest that important associations with stress and disease do not exist. Indeed, they do. Exactly how stressor-induced immune alteration occurs and susceptibility to disease is altered still needs to be determined. It is possible that individuals who are experiencing high levels of stress may alter their diets and sleep patterns, increase their use of cigarettes and/or alcohol, or decrease their adherence to personal hygiene, all of which can affect their immune systems.

With regard to religious or spiritual measures, choice of instrument should be guided by the mechanism by which religion or spirituality is hypothesized to influence immune or neuroendocrine functioning. For example, if an immune measure is influenced particularly strongly by social support, then religious measures that assess the social dimension of religiousness (organizational religious activities and support received from the religious congregation) should be chosen. Religious or spiritual measures must also be sensitive enough to distinguish relatively small differences in religiousness or spirituality, depending on the population studied. For example, more sensitive measures are needed in elderly African-American women than in studies of young Norwegian males. Having a religious measure that captures a wide range of responses (maximizes variance) will increase the likelihood that associations between religious/spiritual, immune, and neuroendocrine variables will be detected. Finally, instruments should be chosen that identify religious or spiritual changes that result from illness, as well as those that precede it.

REFERENCES

Allport, G. W. (1954). *The nature of prejudice*. New York: Addison-Wesley.

Allport, G. W., & Ross, J. M. (1967). Personal religious orientation and prejudice. *Journal of Personality and Social Psychology* 5, 432–443.

Allport, G. W., Vernon, P. E., & Linzey, G. (1968). *Study of values*, 3rd ed. Boston: Houghton Mifflin.

Andersen, B. L., Farrar, W. B., Golden-Kreutz, D., Kutz, L. A., MacCallum, R., Courtney, J. E., & Glaser, R. (1998). Stress and immune responses after surgical treatment for regional breast cancer. *Journal of the National Cancer Institute* 90, 30–38.

Ausubel, D. P., & Schpoont, S. H. (1957). Prediction of group opinion as a function of extremist of predictor attitudes. *Journal of Social Psychology* 46, 19–29.

Baron, R. S., Cutrona, C. E., Hicklin, D., Russell, D. W., & Lubaroff, D. M. (1990). Social support and immune function among spouses of cancer patients. *Journal of Personality and Social Psychology* 59, 344–352.

Bartrop, R. W., Luckhurst, E., Lazarus, L., Kiloh, L. G., & Penny, R. (1977). Depressed lymphocyte function after bereavement. *Lancet* 1(8016), 834–836.

Ben-Eliyahu, S., Yirmiya, R., Liebeskind, J., Taylor, A. M., & Gale, R. P. (1991). Stress increases metastatic spread of a mammary tumor in rats: Evidence for mediation by the immune system. *Brain, Behavior, and Immunology* 5, 193–205.

Ben-Meir, Y., & Kedem, P. (1979). Index of religiosity of the Jewish population of Israel. *Megamot* 24, 353–362 (translated from Hebrew into English by Rabbi Dayle A. Friedman, chaplain at the Philadelphia Geriatric Center).

Benson, H. (1975). *The relaxation response*. New York: William Morrow.

Benson, P. L., Donahue, M. J., & Erickson, J. A. (1993). The faith maturity scale: Conceptualization, measurement, and empirical validation. In M. Lynn, & D. Moberg (Eds.), *Research in the social scientific study of religion*, vol. 5, Greenwich, CT: JAI.

Benson, P. L., & Spilka, B. P. (1973). God image as a function of self-esteem and locus of control. *Journal for the Scientific Study of Religion* 12, 297–310.

Bhushan, L. I. (1970). Religiosity scale. *Indian Journal of Psychology* 45, 335–342.

Bjorck, J. P., & Cohen, L. H. (1993). Coping with threats, losses, and challenges. *Journal of Social and Clinical Psychology* 12, 36–72.

Boccia, M. L., Scanlan, J. M., Laudenslager, M. L., Berger, C. L., Hijazi, A. S., & Reite, M. L. (1997). Juvenile friends, behavior, and immune responses to separation in bonnet macaque infants. *Physiology and Behavior* 61, 191–198.

Bonneau, R. H. (1996). Stress-induced effects on integral immune components in herpes simple simplex virus (HSV) specific memory cytotoxic T lymphocyte activation. *Brain, Behavior, and Immunity* 10, 139–163.

Brady, M. J., Peterman, A. H., Fitchett, G., & Cella, D. (March 1999). The expanded version of the functional assessment of chronic illness therapy-spiritual well-being scale (FACIT Sp-Ex): Initial report of psychometric properties. Paper presented at the twentieth annual meeting of the Society of Behavioral Medicine, San Francisco.

Brown, D., & Lowe, W. (1951). Religious beliefs and personality characteristics of college students. *Journal of Social Psychology* 33, 103–129.

Cabot, P. J., Carter, L., Gaiddon, C., Zhang, Q., Schafer, M., Loeffler, J. P., & Stein, C. (1997). Immune cell derived beta-endorphin. Production, release, and control of inflammatory pain in rats. *Journal of Clinical Investigation* 100, 142–148.

Cacioppo, J. T., Malarkey, W. B., Kiecolt-Glaser, J. K., Uchino, B. N., Sgoutas-Emch, S. A., Sheridan, J. F., Berntson, G. G., & Glaser, R. (1995). Heterogeneity in neuroendocrine and immune responses to brief psychological stressors as a function of autonomic cardiac activation. *Psychosomatic Medicine* 57, 154–164.

Cella, D. (1996). Quality of life outcomes: Measurement and validation. *Oncology* 10(Supplement), 233–246.

Cella, D., & Webster, K. (1997). Linking outcomes management to quality-of-life measurement. *Oncology* 11, 232–235.

Dhawan, N., & Sripat, K. (1986). Fear of death and religiosity as related to need for affiliation. *Psychological Studies* 31, 35–38.

Edwards, K. J. (1976). Sex-role behavior and religious experience. In W. J. Donaldson Jr. (Ed.), Research in mental health and religious behavior: An introduction to research in the integration of Christianity and the behavioral sciences. Atlanta: Psychological Studies Institute.

Ellison, C. W. (1983). Spiritual Maturity Index. Unpublished manuscript. (Contact Craig W. Ellison, Alliance Theological Seminary, Nyack, New York, for a copy.)

Emavardhana, T.,& Tori, C. D. (1997). Changes in self concept, ego defense mechanisms, and religiosity following seven-day Vipassana meditation retreats. *Journal for the Scientific Study of Religion* 36, 194–206.

Esterling, B. A., Kiecolt-Glaser, J. K., Bodnar, J. C., & Glaser, R. (1994). Chronic stress, social support, and persistent alterations in the natural killer cell response to cytokines in older adults. *Health Psychology* 13, 291–299.

Esterling, B. A., Kiecolt-Glaser, J. K., & Glaser, R. (1996). Psychosocial modulation of cytokine-induced natural killer cell activity in older adults. *Psychosomatic Medicine* 58, 264–272.

Fawzy, F. I., Kemeny, M. E., Fawzy, N. W., Elashoff, R., Morton, D., Cousins, N., & Fahey, J. L. (1990). A structured psychiatric intervention for cancer patients. II: Changes over time in immunological measures. *Archives of General Psychiatry* 47, 729–735.

Feagin, J. (1964). Prejudice and religious types: A focused study of southern fundamentalists. *Journal for the Scientific Study of Religion* 4, 3–13.

Fellows, W. J. (1979). *Religions: East and West.* New York: Holt, Rinehart and Winston.

Fetzer Institute (October 1999). *Multidimensional measurement of religiousness/spirituality for use and health research.* A report of the Fetzer Institute/National Institute on Aging working group (with additional psychometric data). Kalamazoo, MI: John E. Fetzer Institute.

Fowler, J. W. (1981). *Stages of faith.* San Francisco: Harper and Row.

George, L. K. (1999). Religious/spiritual history. In *Multidimensional measurement of religiousness/spirituality for use in health research.* Kalamazoo, MI: John E. Fetzer Institute.

Glaser, R., Kennedy, S., Lafuse, W. P., Bonneau, R. H., Speicher, C. E., Hillhouse, J., & Kiecolt-Glaser, J. K. (1990). Psychological stress-induced modulation of interleukin 2 receptor gene expression and interleukin 2 production in peripheral blood leukocytes. *Archives of General Psychiatry* 47, 707–712.

Glaser, R., Kiecolt-Glaser, J. K., Bonneau, R. H., Malarkey, W., Kennedy, S., & Hughes, J. (1992). Stress-induced modulation of the immune response to recombinant hepatitis B vaccine. *Psychosomatic Medicine* 54, 22–29.

Glik, D. C. (1990). Participation in spiritual healing, religiosity, and mental health. *Sociological Inquiry* 60, 158–176.

Glock, C. Y., & Stark, R. (1966). *Christian beliefs and anti-Semitism.* New York: Harper and Row.

Goodkin, K., Blaney, N. T., Feaster, D., Fletcher, M. A., Baum, M. K., Mantero-Atienza, E., Klimas, N. G., Millon, C., Szapocznik, J., & Eisdorfer, C. (1992). Active coping style is associated with natural killer cell cytotoxicity in symptomatic HIV-1 seropositive homosexual men. *Journal of Psychosomatic Research* 36, 635–650.

Gorsuch, R. L., & McPherson, S. E. (1989). Intrinsic/extrinsic measurement: I/E-revised and single-item scales. *Journal for the Scientific Study of Religion* 28, 348–354.

Gunnar, M. R., Larson, M. C., & Hertsgaard, L. (1992). The stressfulness of separation among nine-month-old infants: Effects of social context and infant temperament. *Child Development* 63, 290–303.

Gust, D. A., Gordon, T. P., Brody, A. R., & McClure, H. M. (1996). Effect of companions in modulated stress associated with new group formation in juvenile rhesus macaques. *Physiology and Behavior* 59, 941–945.

Hadid, R., Spinedi, E., Giovambattista, A., Chautard, T., & Gaillard, R. C. (1996). Decreased hypothalamo-pituitary-adrenal axis response to neuroendocrine challenged under repeated endotoxemia. *Neuroimmunomodulation* 3, 62–68.

Hassan, M. K., & Khalique, A. (1981). Religiosity and its correlates in college students. *Journal of Psychological Research* 25, 129–136.

Hatch, R. L., Burg, M. A., Naberhasu, D. S., & Hellmich, L. K. (1998). The Spiritual Involvement and Beliefs Scale: Development and testing of a new instrument. *Journal of Family Practice* 46, 476–486.

Hays, J. C., Meador, K. G., & George, L. K. (1998). *Developing a major of religious history*. Durham, NC: Center for Aging and Human Development, Duke University Medical Center.

Hill, P. C., & Hood, R. (1999). *Measures of religiosity*. Chattanooga, TN: Religious Education Press.

Hoge, D. R. (1972). A validated intrinsic religious motivation scale. *Journal for the Scientific Study of Religion* 11, 369–376.

Holland, J. C., Kash, K. M., Passik, S., Gronert, M. K., Sison, A., Lederberg, M., Russak, S. M., Baider, L., & Fox, B. (1998). A brief spiritual beliefs inventory for use in quality of life research in life-threatening illness. *Psycho-oncology* 7, 460–469.

Holland, J. C., Passik, S., Kash, K. M., Russak, S. M., Gronert, M. K., Sison, A., Lederberg, M., Fox, B., & Baider, L. (1999). The role of religious and spiritual beliefs in coping with malignant melanoma. *Psycho-oncology* 8, 14–26.

Hood, R. W. (1970). Religious orientation and the report of religious experience. *Journal for the Scientific Study of Religion* 9, 285–291.

Hunsberger, B., McKenzie, B., Pratt, M., & Pancer, S. M. (1993). Religious doubt: A social psychological analysis. In M. Lynn & D. Moberg (Eds.), *Research in the social scientific study of religion*, vol. 5, Greenwich, CT: JAI.

Idler, E. L. (1999). Organizational religiousness. In *Multidimensional measurement of religiousness/spirituality for use in health research*. Kalamazoo, MI: John E. Fetzer Institute.

Idler, E. L., Ellison, C. G., George, L. K., Krause, N., Levin, J. S., Ory, M., Pargament, K. I., Powell, L. H., Williams, D. R., & Underwood-Gordon, L. (1999).
Brief measure of religiousness and spirituality: Conceptual development. *Research on Aging,* in submission.

Irwin, M., Brown, M., Patterson, T., Hauger, R., Mascovich, A., & Grant, I
(1991). Neuropeptide Y and natural killer cell activity: Findings in
depression and Alzheimer caregiver stress. *FASEB Journal* 5, 3100–3107.

Kaplan, J. R., Heise, E. R., Mannuck, S. P., Shively, C. A., Cohen, S., Rabin, B. S., &
Kasprowics, A. L. (1991). The relationship of agonistic and affiliative behavior
patterns to cellular immune function among Cynomolgus monkeys living in
stable and unstable social groups. *American Journal of Primatology* 25, 157–173.

Kass, J. D., Friedman, R., Leserman, J., Zuttermeister, P. C., & Benson, H.
(1991). Health outcomes and a new index of spiritual experience (IN-
SPIRIT). *Journal for the Scientific Study of Religion* 30, 203–211.

Katz, J., Weiner, H., Gallagher, T., & Hellman, L. (1970). Stress, distress, and ego
defenses. *Archives of General Psychiatry* 23, 131–142.

Kemp, V. H., & Hatmaker, D. D. (1989). Stress and social support in high-risk
pregnancy. *Research in Nursing Health* 12, 331–336.

Kiecolt-Glaser, J. K., Glaser, R., Cacioppo, J. T., MacCallum, R. C., Snydersmith,
M., Kim, C., & Malarkey, W. B. (1997). Marital conflict in older adults: Endocrinological and immunological correlates. *Psychosomatic Medicine* 49,
339–349.

Kiecolt-Glaser, J. K., Glaser, R., Gravenstein, S., Malarkey, W. B., & Sheridan, J.
(1996). Chronic stress alters the immune response to influenza virus vaccine
in older adults. *Proceedings of the National Academy of Sciences of the United
States of America* 93, 3043–3047.

Kiecolt-Glaser, J. K., Malarkey, W. B., Chee, M., Newton, T., Cacioppo, J. T.,
Mao, H. Y., & Glaser, R. (1993). Negative behavior during marital conflict is
associated with immunological down-regulation. *Psychosomatic Medicine* 55
395–409.

Kiecolt-Glaser, J. K., Marucha, P. T., Malarkey, W. B., Mercado, A. M., & Glaser,
R. (1996). Slowing of wound healing by psychological stress. *Lancet*
346(8984), 1194–1196.

Kiecolt-Glaser, J. K., Newton, T., Cacioppo, J. T., MacCallum, R. C., Glaser, R.,
& Malarkey, W. B. (1996). Marital conflict and endocrine function: Are men
really more physiologically affected than women? *Journal of Consulting and
Clinical Psychology* 64, 324–332.

King, M., & Hunt, R. (1967). Dimensions of religiosity in "measuring the religious variable." *Journal for the Scientific Study of Religion* 6, 173–190.

Kirschbaum, C., Klauer, T., Filipp, S. H., & Hellhammer, D. H. (1995). Sex-spe-
cific effects of social support on cortisol in subjective responses to acute psychological stress. *Psychosomatic Medicine* 57, 23–31.

Kirschbaum, C., Prussner, J. C., Stone, A. A., Federenko, I., Gaab, J., Lintz, D., Schommer, N., & Hellhammer, D. H. (1995). Persistent high cortisol responses to repeated psychological stress in a subpopulation of healthy men. *Psychosomatic Medicine* 57, 468–474.

Koenig, H. G. (1994). *Aging and God*. Binghamton, NY: Haworth.

Koenig, H. G. (1998). Religious beliefs and practices of hospitalized medically ill older adults. *International Journal of Geriatric Psychiatry* 13, 213–224.

Koenig, H. G., Cohen, H. J., Blazer, D. G., Pieper, C., Meador, K. G., Shelp, F., Goli, V., & DiPasquale, R. (1992). Religious coping and depression in elderly hospitalized medically ill men. *American Journal of Psychiatry* 149, 1693–1700.

Koenig, H. G., Cohen, H. J., George, L. K., Hays, J. C., Larson, D. B., & Blazer, D. G. (1997). Attendance at religious services, interleukin-6, and other biological indicators of immune function in older adults. *International Journal of Psychiatry in Medicine* 27, 233–250.

Koenig, H. G., McCullough, M., & Larson, D. B. (2001). *Handbook of religion and health*. New York: Oxford University Press.

Koenig, H. G., Meador, K. G., & Parkerson, G. (1997). Religion index for psychiatric research. *American Journal of Psychiatry* 154, 885–886.

Koenig, H. G., Pargament, K. I., & Nielsen, J. (1998). Religious coping and health status in medically ill hospitalized older adults. *Journal of Nervous and Mental Disorders* 186, 513–521.

Koenig, H. G., Smiley, M., & Gonzales J. (1988). *Religion, health, and aging*. Westport, CT: Greenwood.

Krause, N. (1999). Religious support. In Multidimensional measurement of religiousness/spirituality for use in health research. Kalamazoo, MI: John E. Fetzer Institute.

Larson, D. B., Pattison, E. M., Blazer, D. G., Omran, A. R., & Kaplan, B. H. (1986). Systematic analysis of research on religious variables in four major psychiatric journals, 1978–1982. *American Journal of Psychiatry* 143, 329–334.

Lenski, G. (1963). *The religious factor*. Garden City, NY: Doubleday.

Levine, S., Coe, C., & Wiener, S. G. (1989). Psychoneuroendocrinology of stress: A psychobiological perspective. In F. R. Brush & S. Levine (Eds.), *Psychoendocrinology*. New York: Academic.

Levy, S., Lippman, M., & d'Angelo, T. (1987). Correlation of stress factors with sustained suppression of natural killer cell activity and predictive prognosis in patients with breast cancer. *Journal of Clinical Oncology* 5, 348–353.

Levy, S. M., Herberman, R. B., Whiteside, T., Sanzo, K., Lee, J., & Kirkwood, J. (1990). Perceived social support and tumor estrogen/progesterone receptor status as predictors of natural kill cell activity in breast cancer patients. *Psychosomatic Medicine* 52, 73–85.

Linn, B. S., Linn, B. W., & Klimas, N. G. (1988). Effects of psychophysical stress on surgical outcomes. *Psychosomatic Medicine* 50, 230–244.

Lutgendorf, S. (1997). *IL-6 level, stress, and spiritual support in older adults.* Ames: Psychology Department, University of Iowa.

Malarkey, W., Kiecolt-Glaser, J. K., Pearl, D., & Glaser, R. (1994). Hostile behavior during marital conflict alters pituitary and adrenal hormones. *Psychosomatic Medicine* 56, 41–51.

Malony, H. N. (1988). The clinical assessment of optimal religious functioning. *Review of Religious Research* 30, 3–17.

Martin, J., & Westie, F. (1959). Religious fundamentalism scale in "the tolerant personality." *American Sociological Review* 24, 521–528.

Menzies, R., Phelps, C., Wiranowska, M., Oliver, J., Chen, L., Horvath, E.,& Hall, N. (1996). The effect of interferon-alpha on the pituitary-adrenal axis. *Journal of Interferon and Cytokine Research* 16, 619–629.

Morrow, D., Worthington, E. L., & McCullough, M. E. (1993). Observers' perceptions of a counselors treatment of a religious issue. *Journal of Counseling and Development* 71, 452–456.

Paloutzian, R., & Ellison, C. W. (1982). Loneliness, spiritual well-being and quality of life. In L. Peplau & D. Perlman (Ed.), *Loneliness: A sourcebook of current theory, research, and therapy.* New York: Wiley.

Pargament, K. I. (1997). *The psychology of religion and coping: Theory, research, practice.* New York: Guilford.

Pargament, K. I., Koenig, H. G., & Perez, L. M. (2000). A comprehensive measure of religious coping: Development and initial validation of the RCOPE. *Journal of Clinical Psychology* 56, 519–543.

Pargament, K. I., Smith, B. W., Koenig, H. G., & Perez, L. (1998). Patterns of positive and negative religious coping with major life stressors. *Journal for the Scientific Study of Religion* 37, 710–724.

Perry, S., Fishman, B., Jacobsberg, L., & Frances, A. (1992). Relationships over 1 year between lymphocyte subset and psychosocial variables among adults with infection by human immunodeficiency virus. *Archives of General Psychiatry* 49, 396–401.

Persson, L., Gullberg, B., Hanson, B. S., Moestrup, T., & Ostergren, P. O. (1994). HIV infection: Social network, social support, and CD4 lymphocyte values in infected homosexual men in Malmo, Sweden. *Journal of Epidemiology and Community Health* 48, 580–585.

Pollner, M. (1989). Divine relations, social relations, and well-being. *Journal of Health and Social Behavior* 30, 92–104.

Poppleton, P. K., & Pilkington, G. W. (1963). The measurement of religious attitudes in a university population. *British Journal of the Society of Clinical Psychology* 2, 20–36.

Princeton Religion Research Center. (1996). *Religion in America: Will the vitality of the church be the surprise of the 21st century?* Princeton, NJ: Gallup.

Pruessner, J. C., Hellhammer, D. H., & Kirschbaum, C. (1999). Burnout, perceived stress, and cortisol responses to awakening. *Psychosomatic Medicine* 61, 197–204.

Putney, S., & Middleton, R. (1961). Dimensions and correlates of religious ideologies. *Social Forces* 39, 285–291.

Rabin, B., Cunnick, J., & Lysle, D. (1990). Stress-induced alteration of immune function. *Progress in Neuroendoimmunology* 3, 116–124.

Rabin, B. S. (1999). *Stress, immune function, and health: The connection.* New York: Wiley-Liss.

Ressler, W. H. (1997). Jewishness and well-being: Specific identification and general psychological adjustment. *Psychological Reports* 81, 515–518.

Roof, W. C., & McKinney, W. M. (1987). *American mainline religion.* New Brunswick, NJ: Rutgers University Press.

Schaal, M. D., Sephton, S. E., Thoreson, C., Koopman, C., & Spiegel, D. (August 1998). Religious expression and immune competence in women with advanced cancer. Paper presented at the meeting of the American Psychological Association, San Francisco.

Schulkin, J., McEwen, B. S., & Gold, P. W. (1994). Allostasis, amygdala, and anticipatory angst. *Neuroscience and Biobehavior Review* 18, 385–386.

Seeman, T. E., Berkman, L. F., & Blazer, D. B. (1994). Social ties and support and neuroendocrine function, MacArthur Studies of Successful Aging. *Annals of Behavioral Medicine* 16, 95–106.

Seeman, T. E., & McEwen, B. S. (1996). Impact of social environment characteristics on neuroendocrine regulation. *Psychosomatic Medicine* 58, 459–471.

Shams, M., & Jackson, P. R. (1993). Religiosity as a predictor of well-being and moderator of the psychological impact of unemployment. *Journal of Medical Psychology* 66, 341–352.

Sonnenfeld, G., Cunnick, J. E., Armfield, A. V., Wood, P. G., & Rabin, BS (1992). Stress-induced alterations in interferon production in class II MHC histocompatibility antigen expression. *Brain, Behavior, and Immunity* 6, 170–178.

Stanisz, A. M., Befus, D., & Bienenstock, J. (1986). Differential effects of vasoactive intestinal peptide, substance P, and somatostatin on immunoglobulin synthesis and proliferation by lymphocytes from Peyer's patches, mesenteric lymph nodes, and spleen. *Journal of Immunology* 136, 152–156.

Takada, Y., Ihara, H., Urano, T., & Takada, A. (1995). Changes in blood and plasma serotonergic measurements in rats: Effect of nicotine and/or exposure to different stresses. *Thrombosis Research* 80, 307–316.

Tapanya, S., Nicki, R., & Jarusawad, O. (1997). Worry and intrinsic/extrinsic religious orientation among Buddhist (Thai) and Christian (Canadian) elderly persons. *International Journal of Aging and Human Development* 44, 73–83.

Theorell, T., Blomkvist, V., Jonsson, H., Schulman, S., Berntorp, E., & Stigendal, L. (1995). Social support and the development of the immune function in human immunodeficiency virus infection. *Psychosomatic Medicine* 57, 32–36.

Thomas, T. D., Goodwin, J. M., & Goodwin, J. S. (1985). Effects of social support on stress-related changes in cholesterol level, uric acid level, and immune function in an elderly sample. *American Journal of Psychiatry* 142, 735–737.

Thorson, J. A. (1998). Religion and anxiety: Which anxiety? Which religion? In H. G. Koenig (Ed.), *Handbook of religion and mental health*. San Diego: Academic.

Thouless, R. (1935). The tendency to certainty in religious beliefs. *British Journal of Psychology* 6, 16–31.

Wichmann, M. W., Zellweger, R., DeMaso, R., Ayala, A., & Chaudry, I H. (1996). Melatonin administration attenuates depressed immune functions following trauma-hemorrhage. *Journal of Surgical Research* 63, 256–262.

Woods, T. E., Antoni, M. H., Ironson, G. H., & Kling, D. W. (1999). Religiosity is associated with affective and immune status in symptomatic HIV-infected gay men. *Journal of Psychosomatic Research* 46, 165–176.

Table 11.1.   Immune Measures

Measure	Publication/ Parameter/ Species	Relevant Finding
Immune response to vaccination		
Hepatitis B	Glaser et al., 1992 Social support/stress Human	Study of medical students given three immunizations with hepatitis B vaccine during times of examination stress; students reporting higher levels of stress and greater loneliness had weaker responses to the vaccine (lower levels of antibody produced). Stress interferes with primary antibody response.
Influenza	Kiecolt-Glaser, Glaser, et al., 1996 Social support/stress Human	Compared antibody response to vaccination between 32 family caregivers of patients with dementia (stressed) and 32 sex-, age-, and socioeconomically matched controls; caregivers showed poorer antibody response following influenza vaccination than control subjects as measured by two independent methods; in addition, caregivers also had decreased in vitro virus-specific-induced interleukin-2 levels and interleukin-1 beta.
White blood cell quantities		
Neutrophils and lymphocytes	Kiecolt-Glaser, Glaser, et al., 1996 Anxiety/stress Human	Compared 32 family caregivers of patients with dementia (stressed) and 32 sex-, age-, and socioeconomically matched controls; there were no significant differences between caregivers and controls on percentages of monocytes, CD3, CD4, or CD8 lymphocytes.
	Schaal et al., 1998 Anxiety Religion Human	Study of 112 women with metastatic breast cancer. Religious expression (but not church attendance) was positively associated with total lymphocytes ($r = .15, p = .05$), natural killer (NK) cell numbers (Spearman $r = .19, p = .02$), and T-helper cell (CD4+) counts ($r = .16, p = .05$).

(*continued*)

Table 11.1. (*continued*)

Measure	Publication/ Parameter/ Species	Relevant Finding
Neutrophils and lymphocytes (*continued*)	Koenig et al., 1997 Religious attendance Human	Study of 1,718 older adults examining association between church attendance (in 1986, 1989, and 1992) and lymphocyte and neutrophil counts (measured in 1992). Religious attendance in 1989 and 1992 was inversely related to total lymphocyte and neutrophil counts, respectively, in 1992 (after controlling for age, sex, race, education, chronic illness, physical functioning, depressive symptoms, and negative life events).
	Cacioppo et al., 1995 Stress Human	Among 22 older women, an experimentally induced, brief psychological stressor resulted in a decreased percentage of CD4+ helper cells, although absolute cell numbers determined were unaffected by the stressor. Total leukocyte numbers, lymphocytes, and total T cells all increased. The percentage and number of CD8+ cytotoxic cells also increased, and there was a reduced ratio of CD4+:CD8+ cells.
	Kiecolt-Glaser et al., 1993 Anxiety/stress Human	Study of 90 newlywed couples, finding subjects who displayed high negative/ hostile behaviors during a 30-minute discussion of marital problems showed larger increases in numbers of total T lymphocytes and helper-T lymphocytes.
	Bartrop et al., 1977 Bereavement Human	Study of 26 bereaved spouses assessed in a prospective fashion, compared with 26 hospital staff members matched for age, sex, and race; there were no differences in T and B cell numbers between bereaved group and controls.

(*continued*)

Table 11.1. (*continued*)

Measure	Publication/ Parameter/ Species	Relevant Finding
Neutrophils and lymphocytes (*continued*)	Fawzy et al., 1990 Stress/coping Human	Studied effects of a 6-week structured social-psychological group intervention in 61 patients with malignant melanoma (35 in intervention and 26 in control groups); subjects in test group experienced a small decrease in % of CD4+ T lymphocytes ($p =.042$) compared with controls and an increase in natural killer (NK) cells ($p =.022$).
	Woods et al., 1999 Religion/HIV Human	Study of 106 HIV+ gay men. Religious activities—prayer, religious attendance, spiritual discussions, reading religious/spiritual literature—correlated with significantly higher CD4+ counts and CD4+ percentages; not confounded by disease progression.
	Perry et al., 1992 HIV/social support Human	Study of 221 HIV+ patients without AIDS (93% men), finding that total perceived social support was unrelated to CD4+ counts or percentages at baseline, 6-month, and 12-month follow-up. Total perceived social support unrelated to CD8+ counts and unrelated to CD4+ to CD8+ ratio.
	Persson et al., 1994 HIV/social support Human	Study of 47 HIV+ men (hemophiliac patients in Sweden), finding that low social participation, low satisfaction with social participation, low material support, and low emotional support were associated with lower CD4+ counts.
	Theorell et al., 1995 HIV/social support Human	In a prospective 5-year study of 48 HIV+ men, social support was associated with different changes in CD4 counts over time from 1986 to 1990: +2%, −9%, −22%, −24%, −37% for high social support vs. 0%, −4%, −26%, −46%, −64% for low support.

(*continued*)

Table 11.1. (*continued*)

Measure	Publication/ Parameter/ Species	Relevant Finding
Neutrophils and lymphocytes (*continued*)	Gust et al., 1996 Companionship Nonhuman primate	This study found that monkeys transferred from their home to a new group of monkeys experienced a significant suppression of CD4 lymphocyte count; however, if the monkey was transferred with one other monkey from the home group, CD4 suppression was significantly less.
	Kiecolt-Glaser et al., 1991 Anxiety/stress Human	Two-year prospective study of 69 caregivers under chronic stress and 69 non-stressed controls found that stressed caregivers did not differ significantly from controls in percent NK cells, percent helper T cells (CD4+) and percent cytotoxic T cells (CD8+), nor did significant differences emerge during follow-up.
NK cell function	Fawzy et al., 1990 Stress/coping Human	Studied effects of a 6-week structured social-psychological group intervention in 61 patients with malignant melanoma (35 in intervention and 26 in control groups); subjects in test group experienced an increase in NK cytotoxic activity ($p = .034$). Anxiety and depression were significantly negatively correlated with interferon-augmented NK cell activity (anxiety: $r = -.37$, $p < .04$; depression: $r = -.33$, $p < .06$). Anger was significantly and positively correlated with interferon-augmented NK cell activity ($r = .45$, $p < .008$).
	Esterling et al., 1996 Stress/social support Human	Compared 28 current and former spousal caregivers of Alzheimer's patients and 29 control subjects; NK cell cytotoxicity was significantly decreased in both current and former spousal caregivers, compared with controls (but did not differ from each other); NK cell cytotoxicity was also positively related to positive emotional and tangible social support (independent of depression).

(*continued*)

Table 11.1. (*continued*)

Measure	Publication/ Parameter/ Species	Relevant Finding
NK cell function (*continued*)	Levy et al., 1987, 1990 Stress/social support Human	Three-month prospective study of 75 women with stage I–II breast cancer; both at baseline and at 3-month follow-up, there was a similar cross-sectional correlation between fatigue and perception of family support and NK cell activity; those reporting depressive, fatiguelike symptoms and who complained about lack of family support at baseline tended to show a decrease in NK activity levels at 3 months.
	Andersen et al., 1998 Stress Human	Studying 116 breast cancer patients, found that stress levels significantly predicted lower NK cell lysis and diminished response of NK cell recombinant interferon-gamma.
	Ben-Eliyahu et al., 1991 Stress Rodents	Studying mammary tumor in rats, found that reductions in natural killer cell activity produced by stress are sufficient to allow tumor metastasis.
	Kaplan et al., 1991 Affiliation Nonhuman primate	In a study of nonhuman primates, found that monkeys who exhibited the highest affiliation behavior had the highest NK cell activity, when compared with less affiliating monkeys.
	Goodkin et al., 1992 HIV/stress/social support Human	Study of 62 HIV+ gay men, finding that total perceived social support had no overall effect on NK cell activity; in persons with low life stress (but not high life stress), social support was associated with greater NK cell activity ($p = .06$).
	Kiecolt-Glaser et al., 1985 Stress/social support Human	Studying a sample of 45 men and women, found no effect of social contact (students visited subjects for 3 days/week for 45 minutes/visit for 1 month) on NK cell activity.

(*continued*)

Table 11.1. (*continued*)

Measure	Publication/ Parameter/ Species	Relevant Finding
NK cell function (*continued*)	Esterling et al., 1994 Stress/social support Human	Studied 14 current caregivers and 17 bereaved caregivers; caregivers with high social support (emotional, tangible support and closeness of relationships) had greater NK cell activity in response to both rIL-2 and rIFN-γ.
	Kiecolt-Glaser et al., 1993 Stress Human	Study of 90 newlywed couples, finding subjects who displayed high negative/ hostile behaviors during a 30-minute discussion of marital problems showed greater decreases (relative to low-negative S's) in NK cell lysis.
	Baron et al., 1990 Stress/social support Human	Studying 23 spouses of cancer patients, found that total social support and all components were positively related to NK cell activity, even after controlling for life events and depression.
Lymphocyte function	Kiecolt-Glaser et al., 1991 Anxiety/stress Human	In a 2-year prospective study of 69 care-givers under chronic stress and 69 non-stressed controls, found that stressed care-givers had significantly lower blastogenic T-lymphocyte response to Con A and PHA mitogens compared to controls. Lower social support at baseline predicted greater worsening of immune function, and these effects were more pronounced in care-givers than in controls.
	Andersen et al. 1998 Anxiety/stress Human	Studying 116 breast cancer patients, found that stress levels significantly predicted decreased proliferative response of periph-eral blood lymphocytes to plant lectins and to a monoclonal antibody directed against the T-cell receptor.

(*continued*)

Table 11.1. (*continued*)

Measure	Publication/ Parameter/ Species	Relevant Finding
Lymphocyte function (*continued*)	Kiecolt-Glaser et al., 1993 Anxiety/stress Human	Study of 90 newlywed couples, finding subjects who displayed high negative/ hostile behaviors during a 30-minute discussion of marital problems showed greater decreases (relative to low-negative S's) on blastogenic response to two mitogens, and proliferative response to a monoclonal antibody to the T3 receptor.
	Bartrop et al., 1977 Bereavement Human	Study of 26 bereaved spouses assessed in a prospective fashion, compared with 26 hospital staff members matched for age, sex, and race; response to phytohemagglutinin was significantly depressed in the bereaved group at 6 weeks, as was response to concanavalin A.
	Kiecolt-Glaser et al., 1997 Anxiety/stress Human	Study of 31 older couples married an average 42 years, who underwent 30-minute conflict session; both men and women with negative behavior during conflict showed poorer blastogenic response to two T-cell mitogens.
	Baron et al., 1990 Companionship Human	Studying 23 spouses of cancer patients, found that total social support and all components were positively related to PHA stimulation (but not Con A stimulation), even after controlling for life events and depression.
	Thomas et al., 1985 Social support Human	Study of 256 healthy older adults. Women (54% of the sample) with high social support had stronger proliferative responses to PHA than women with low social support.
	Linn et al., 1988 Social support Human	Studying 24 men experiencing first-time hernia repair, found that social support was consistently related to stronger proliferative responses to Con A, PHA, and PWM at pre- and postoperative assessments; difference was statistically significant, however, only for the postoperative PHA assessment.

(*continued*)

Table 11.1. *(continued)*

Measure	Publication/ Parameter/ Species	Relevant Finding
Lymphocyte function *(continued)*	Boccia et al., 1997 Social support Nonhuman primate	Study of bonnet macaque monkeys, found that when juvenile monkeys were separated from their mother, if separated without friends showed more depression and suppression of lymphocyte function (compared with those who were separated but together with a peer).
Antibody titers to latent herpesvirus (EBV)	Kiecolt-Glaser et al. 1991 Anxiety/stress Human	In a 2-year prospective study of 69 caregivers under chronic stress and 69 non-stressed controls, found significant increase in EBV antibody in caregivers compared with controls (antibody titers tripled between baseline and follow-up in caregivers). This was considered consistent with viral activation due to decreased cellular immune function. Lower social support at baseline predicted worsening of cellular immune function, and these effects were more pronounced in caregivers than in controls.
	Kiecolt-Glaser et al., 1993 Anxiety/stress Human	Study of 90 newlywed couples, finding subjects who displayed high negative/hostile behaviors during a 30-minute discussion of marital problems showed higher antibody titers to latent Epstein-Barr virus (consistent with downregulated cellular immune function).
	Kiecolt-Glaser et al., 1997 Anxiety/stress Human	Study of 31 older couples married an average 42 years, who underwent 30-minute conflict session. Both men and women with negative behavior during conflict again showed higher antibody titers to latent EB virus.
Delayed hypersensitivity	Schaal et al., 1998 Anxiety Religion Human	Study of immune function in 112 women with metastatic breast cancer, finding that religious expression and church attendance were unrelated to delayed-type hypersensitivity responses to skin test antigens.

(continued)

Table 11.1.   (*continued*)

Measure	Publication/ Parameter/ Species	Relevant Finding
Cytokine production	Kiecolt-Glaser, Glaser, et al., 1996 Anxiety/stress Human	Compared 32 family caregivers of patients with dementia (stressed) and 32 sex-, age-, and socioeconomically matched controls; caregivers had significantly lower levels of virus-specific-induced IL-2 levels and IL-1β; there was no difference, however, in IL-6 production.
	Glaser et al., 1990 Anxiety/stress Human	Study of medical students undergoing stressful examinations, found fewer cells expressing IL-2 and lower amounts of IL-2 mRNA during times of high stress. (Here, IL-2 is that released from lymphocyte and monocytes in vitro.)
	Kiecolt-Glaser, Marucha, et al., 1996 Anxiety/stress Human	Study of 13 older women caring for demented relatives compared with 13 controls matched for age and family in-come; subjects in caregivers (stressed) and control groups underwent 3.5 mm punch biopsy. Wounds in caregivers took signifi-cantly longer to heal (48.7 vs. 39.3 days, $p <.05$); in particular, peripheral blood leukocytes of caregivers produced signifi-cantly less IL-1β mRNA in response to lipopolysaccharide stimulation.
	Marucha et al., 1998 Anxiety/stress Human	Study of 11 dental students who under-went an experimental wound on their buc-cal mucosa at two points in time, one dur-ing the summer and the other just prior to a major examination. During the stressful period, wounds took 40% longer to heal. Again, production of IL-1b declined by 68% during the stressful period.
	Kiecolt-Glaser et al., 1993 Anxiety/stress Human	Study of 90 newlywed couples, finding subjects who displayed high negative/ hostile behaviors during a 30-minute dis-cussion of marital problems did not show a difference in INFγ (gamma inter-feron) production by lymphocytes stimu-lated with Con A.

(*continued*)

Table 11.1. (*continued*)

Measure	Publication/ Parameter/ Species	Relevant Finding
Cytokine production (*continued*)	Koenig et al., 1997 Religion Human	Study of 1,718 older adults examining association between church attendance measured in 1986, 1989, and 1992, and plasma interleukin-6 (IL-6) levels measured in 1992; frequent religious attendance in 1986, 1989, and 1992 predicted lower plasma IL-6 levels in 1992; strongest effect was noted for the cross-sectional association in 1992, where the likelihood of having high IL-6 levels (>5 pg/ml) among church attenders was only about half that of nonattenders (OR 0.51, 0.35–0.73, p <.001 uncontrolled; OR 0.58, 0.40–0.84, p <.005, controlled for age, sex, race, education, chronic illness, physical functioning).
	Lutgendorf, 1997 Religion Human	Examined religious coping and plasma IL-6 in 55 older adults, half of whom were voluntarily moving from their own homes to senior housing (stressed group). Independent of stress level, greater use of religious/spiritual coping (i. e., in times of stress, do you pray to God for help, use meditation, etc.) was associated with lower IL-6 levels (partial $r = -.26$, $p =.075$).
	Hadid et al., 1996 Stress Rodents	Study showing that repeated stress in laboratory animals leads to endotoxemia, which decreases reactivity of HPA axis and decreases production of TNFα.
	Sonnenfeld et al., 1992; Bonneau, 1996 Stress Rodents	Studies showing that stress is capable of inhibiting the production of INFγ by lymphocytes.
	Menzies et al., 1996 Stress Rodent	Study showing that IFNα and INFβ are capable of elevating plasma cortisol concentrations.

Table 11.2.   Neuroendocrine Measures

Measure	Publication/ Parameter/ Species	Relevant Finding
HPA axis		
Cortisol or ACTH	Katz et al., 1970 Anxiety/stress Religion Human	Thirty women undergoing breast biopsy for possible malignancy (22 were positive). Correlated urine cortisol levels with psychological defenses used. Those who employed prayer and faith ($n = 4$) appeared to have lower cortisol levels than those depending on projection or displacement.
	Schaal et al., 1998 Anxiety/stress Religion Human	Among 112 women with metastatic breast cancer, correlated salivary cortisol levels with religious attendance and religious expression. Evening (5 P.M.) cortisol levels were lower among women reporting higher religious expression ($r = .22, p = .01$), but not with religious attendance.
	Seeman & McEwen, 1996 Review	Reviews research showing a link between increased social support and neuroendocrine function.
	Levine et al., 1989 Companionship Nonhuman primate	Squirrel monkeys exposed to stressful stimuli experienced half the elevations in serum cortisol if they had another squirrel monkey with them. Effects of social support.
	Kirschbaum, Prussner, et al., 1995 Personality characteristics Human	Correlated personality characteristics with hormonal response to stress. Healthy men were exposed to the same psychological stress on 5 consecutive days. Two patterns of response were observed: (1) lower cortisol levels on day 2 in comparison to day 1 with no further decline of cortisol subsequently, or (2) elevation of cortisol on each of the 5 days. Subjects in the second group had lower self-esteem, negative self-concept, depressed mood, and more health problems than subjects in the first group.

(continued)

Table 11.2. (*continued*)

Measure	Publication/ Parameter/ Species	Relevant Finding
Cortisol or ACTH (*continued*)	Kirschbaum, Klauer, et al., 1995 Companionship Human	Study demonstrated that the presence of a socially supportive companion (either a friend or a stranger) was associated with a reduced serum cortisol response during the anticipatory period before public speaking. Effect was seen only in men, not women.
	Kiecolt-Glaser, Newton, et al., 1996 Anxiety/stress Human	Among 90 newlywed couples on days experiencing conflict, examined endocrine measures. For wives, husband's withdrawal in response to wife's negative behavior was associated with higher serum cortisol levels; husbands' endocrine data were not associated with behavioral data. No relationship was found between ACTH levels and negative behaviors in wives or husbands.
	Kiecolt-Glaser et al., 1997 Anxiety/stress Human	Among 31 older couples married an average 42 years, experimentally induced a 30-minute conflict session followed by 15-minute recovery; among wives, escalation of negative behavior during conflict and marital satisfaction showed strong relationships to endocrine changes, explaining 16% to 21% of variance in rates of change of cortisol, ACTH, and norepinephrine (but not epinephrine); husbands' endocrine data did not show relationships with negative behavior or marital quality.
	Seeman et al., 1994 Companionship Human	In a sample of high-functioning older men and women, found that among men 12-hour overnight measure of urinary cortisol was lower among those with high emotional support or instrumental support. Similar effects were not seen in women.
	Schulkin et al., 1994 Anxiety/stress Human	Study demonstrating that anticipatory worry or anxiety can drive up serum ACTH and cortisol levels.

(*continued*)

Table 11.2. (*continued*)

Measure	Publication/Parameter/Species	Relevant Finding
Cortisol or ACTH (*continued*)	Cacioppo et al., 1995 Stress Human	Among 22 older women, individuals characterized by high cardiac sympathetic reactivity showed higher stress-related changes in ACTH and plasma cortisol level.
	Gunnar et al., 1992 Stress/companionship Human	Study of children showing that experimentally induced maternal separation increased cortisol levels, responses that were attenuated in the presence of a warm, responsive caregiver.
Catecholamines	Kiecolt-Glaser, Newton, et al., 1996 Anxiety/stress Human	Among 90 newlywed couples on days experiencing conflict, no relationship was found between serum epinephrine and negative behaviors in wives or husbands. Husband's withdrawal in response to wife's negative behavior was associated with higher serum norepinephrine levels in wives. Husbands' endocrine data were not associated with behavioral data.
	Kiecolt-Glaser et al., 1997 Anxiety/stress Human	Among 31 older couples, a 30-minute conflict session was experimentally induced; for wives and husbands, escalation of negative behavior during conflict and level of marital satisfaction were not related to serum levels of epinephrine. Among wives, escalation of negative behavior during conflict and low marital satisfaction were associated with increased levels of serum norepinephrine; this was not true in husbands.
	Schulkin et al., 1994 Anxiety Human	Study demonstrating that anticipatory worry or anxiety can drive up serum epinephrine levels.
	Cacioppo et al., 1995 Stress Human	Among 22 older women, experimentally induced brief psychological stressors elevated plasma epinephrine and norepinephrine levels significantly.

(*continued*)

Table 11.2. (*continued*)

Measure	Publication/ Parameter/ Species	Relevant Finding
Catecholamines (*continued*)	Seeman et al., 1994 Emotional support Human	In a sample of high-functioning older men and women, found that among men 12-hour overnight measure of urinary epinephrine and norepinephrine was lower among those with high emotional support. Similar effects were not seen in women (except in married women).
	Kemp & Hatmaker, 1989 Social support Human	Study showing high levels of social support among men were associated with lower levels of urinary norepinephrine than individuals with less social support. Effect not found in women.
Other anterior pituitary hormones		
Prolactin and Somatotropin	Kiecolt-Glaser Newton, et al., 1996 Anxiety/stress Human	Assessed 90 newlywed couples on days experiencing conflict; among wives, negative behavior was associated with lower serum prolactin levels, and positive behaviors by husband were associated with higher levels; husbands' prolactin levels were not associated with behavioral data (although prolactin was inversely related to negative affect in men). (Prolactin tends to enhance immune function.) Negative and positive behaviors by wives and husbands were largely unrelated to serum somatotropin levels. (Somatotropin tends to enhance immune function.)
	Malarkey et al., 1994 Negative behavior Human	Study showing that among women, lower frequency of negative behaviors is associated with higher prolactin levels.
Somatostatin	Stanisz et al., 1986 Hormone supplementation Rodents	Study showing that natural killer cell function and immunoglobulin synthesis are decreased by somatostatin.

(*continued*)

Table 11.2. (*continued*)

Measure	Publication/ Parameter/ Species	Relevant Finding
Melatonin	Wichmann et al., 1996 Experimental hypovolemia Rodents	Study showing that suppression of non-specific lymphocyte function by trauma was reversed by melatonin.
Substance P	Rabin et al., 1990	Receptors for SP are found on the membranes of both T and B cells, mononuclear phagocytic cells, and mast cells. It is released from sensory nerve fibers and contributes to the induction of localized inflammatory reactions.
Neuropeptide Y	Irwin et al., 1991	Study showing that NPY plasma levels are negatively correlated with NK cell activity.
Vasoactive intestinal peptide	Rabin et al., 1990	Cytokine production by T lymphocytes is modified by VIP. Both Th1-derived (IL-2) and Th2-derived (IL-4 and IL-10) cytokine production can be modified by VIP, with the concentration of VIP possibly influencing whether enhancement (low VIP concentrations) or inhibition (high VIP concentrations) will occur.
Enkephalins, endorphins	Cabot et al., 1997	Study showing that opioids are produced and released in response to stress (endorphins from the pituitary and enkephalins from adrenal medulla).
Serotonin transporter genotype	Takada et al., 1995 Rats	Shows that stress can increase levels of serotonin in plasma.

12

Psychoneuroimmunology and Eastern Religious Traditions

PAUL J. GRIFFITHS

When we speak of "Eastern religions," we are talking about religions that originated, roughly, east of Baghdad. Religions from this part of the world have contributed significantly to the development of Western religious thought and practice. Christianity, for instance, owes a debt to religious movements from Persia and India: the first mention of the Buddha in a Christian text is from the second century ce. Indeed, the Mediterranean area always has been a place where East meets West: during some periods, the West was markedly influenced by the East (e.g., during the later days of the Alexander the Great's empire, there was much contact and influence with Persia; during the Crusades, there was Muslim influence as far west as Spain). Some of the most important of the Eastern religions are Hinduism, Buddhism, Daoism (also known as Taoism), Confucianism, and Shintoism. These five religious traditions together command the devotion of a significant proportion of the human race (Littleton, 1996, p. 6).

Hinduism,[1] which is most easily thought of as India's traditional religion or family of religions, a family to which perhaps 70% of contemporary Indians would say they belong, can be traced back almost 5,000 years (to the third millennium BCE) and has profoundly influenced the religious and philosophical traditions of almost every civilization in Asia. Indeed, although the large-scale practice of Hinduism is confined largely to the Indian subcontinent and to emigrant communities of Indians elsewhere, Buddhism, the "daughter religion" of Hinduism, spread the fundamental ideas of Hinduism—profoundly modified, of course—in much the same way that Christianity has spread the fundamental ideas of its parent religion, Judaism, to almost every corner of the globe.

Buddhism was founded by the Buddha, or the Enlightened One (born, according to legend, Prince Siddhartha Gautama sometime in the sixth century BCE), in part as a reform movement in protest against some ritual and philosophical aspects of Hinduism in India; a distant analogy can be drawn with the formation of Christian Protestant movements in Europe that arose in protest against the doctrines and practices of the Catholic church. Early on, however, the Buddhist community split into two major factions, which are sometimes known, polemically, as the "Greater Vehicle" (Mahayana) and the "Lesser Vehicle" (Hinayana). One of the so-called Hinayana traditions, the Theravada ("doctrine of the elders"), which emphasizes meditation and monasticism, has become the primary religion of Southeast Asia, from Burma to Cambodia, and, in premodern times, of Indonesia as well; the Mahayana, which emphasizes universal salvation and a host of quasi divinities called *bodhisattvas*, spread north and east, first to China and then to Korea, Japan, and Tibet (Smith, 1991). In the process of expansion, Buddhism has become a transcultural religion that has managed to coexist with indigenous beliefs and practices throughout the regions it has penetrated, especially in East Asia.

Buddhists in large numbers are found in China, Sri Lanka, Burma, Thailand, Indochina, Korea, sections of the former Soviet Union, and Japan. In China, Buddhism has competed and/or coexisted with both Confucianism, which is a body of moral and ritual teachings that originated in China in the sixth and fifth centuries BCE, and Daoism, a religion that urges followers to emulate the way of nature, as encapsulated in the *Dao* ("way" or "path"). In Japan, rather than competing, Buddhism has become fully integrated with Shintoism, the indigenous religion in which natural objects, such as mountains, rivers, and heavenly bodies, are worshiped and personified. Indeed, many Japanese practice both Shintoism and Buddhism because the beliefs of Shintoism do not conflict with those of other faiths (Littleton, 1996).

Besides the commonality of either incorporation of and/or competition with Hindu-derived beliefs, another common thread running through Eastern religious traditions is a focus on achieving balance within the realm of nature between humankind and the divine—a balance in which each element supports the other for the good of the whole. This focus of seeking balance in everyday life is epitomized in concepts such as yin and yang (the two opposing forces in the universe) in Daoism, and karma (a Sanskrit word meaning "action": every action or deed "ripens" into a certain kind of result) in Buddhism and Hinduism. Most of these Eastern religions also emphasize the "internal" being versus the external being. Indeed, in Hinduism, Buddhism, Daoism, and Shintoism, adherents are advised to free themselves from their bodily form so that they can experience the infinite. For example, an aim of some kinds of Daoist meditation is to empty the mind of thoughts that are distorted by an individual's consciousness (Littleton, 1996, p. 129). Daoists believe that the individual human being and cosmos share three life forces—spirit (*shen*), breath (*qi*), and vital essence (*jing*)—and in meditation the practitioner strives to join the macrocosm (the universe) and microcosm (the individual human being) into one. Similarly, in Hindu meditation, chanting the word *Om* during meditation is believed to give the individual access to the universe (macrocosm) and lead to enlightenment and immortality (Littleton, 1996, p. 21). Shintoism, Buddhism, and Confucianism all have similar internal aspects.

Nevertheless, there are many differences and variations between and among these religions, just as there are between and among the people who practice them in various Asian countries. For example, in Japan there are two forms of Zen Buddhism. One is Rinzai Zen, which is best known for the use of the *koan*, or riddle, to train the mind to teach enlightenment (*satori*) in a sudden flash. The koan guides a person into seeking new interpretations for seemingly unsolvable problems, and it is said that solving a koan involves a mental "leap" (Littleton, 1996, p. 88). "What is the sound of one hand clapping?" is an example of a koan that has no apparent sensible answer. The other form of Zen in Japan is Soto Zen, which is a more traditional form of Buddhism that teaches a gradual approach to enlightenment through self-discipline, self-control, and meditative practices. Thus, even within the same religion practiced in a relatively small geographical region, there are significant differences and variations that defy stereotypical classifications.

In recent years, a variety of Eastern religious beliefs and practices have been adopted by groups in the West and promoted as beneficial for health and spiritual well-being. Few of these, however, have been studied empirically, with the exception of meditative and related practices derived from the Hindu and Buddhist religious traditions. Therefore, the remainder of this chapter will focus on the research relating to Hindu- and Buddhist-based meditative practices. It also discusses the problems and obstacles involved in attempting to relate such research back to the religions from which they have come.

Meditation and Health

Meditation, as understood by those Western scholars who have undertaken empirical research on it, is a self-directed practice in which the meditator makes a concentrated effort to focus on a single thought, physical experience, sound, or memorized passage (Easwaran, 1989; Goleman, 1988). A variety of meditative methods reflect different spiritual-religious and philosophical-scientific beliefs, assumptions, and practices. Examples include transcendental meditation (TM) (a Hindu-based meditation) and mindfulness meditation (a kind of Buddhist meditation). However, meditation with a religious-spiritual orientation is deeply rooted and extensively practiced in almost all Eastern religions and in some Western religions as well (Benson, 1993; Goleman, 1988, Schopen & Freeman, 1992).

Although a highly cognitive activity, meditation involves the whole person in a psychophysiological experience, which has been characterized as "active passivity" (e.g., sitting quietly while being inwardly alert and focused) and "creative quiescence" (e.g., inwardly calm while being open to expanded awareness) (Shafi, 1985, pp. 90–91). This calm but alert attentiveness is practiced in two basic forms (Carrington, 1993; Goleman, 1988; Odajnyk, 1993). One is *concentration*, or fixed meditation, in which the meditator fixes his or her mind on an internal or external object (e.g., sound, word, bodily sensation, statue) while minimizing distractions and bringing the wandering mind back to attention on the chosen object. The second meditative practice is known as *mindfulness*, in which the meditator, rather than concentrating on a fixed object, focuses alertly but nonjudgmentally on everything passing through the mind (Goleman, 1988; Kabat-Zinn, 1993).

Since the early 1960s, there has been a growing interest in the use of meditation as an intervention for various types of physical and mental problems. More recently, many of these studies have focused on the use of meditation as an adjunct to the conventional therapy model for the treatment of alcohol and substance abuse, as well as the alleviation of pain, depression, and the symptoms of heart disease (see Craven, 1989; Ornish, 1990; Shapiro & Walsh, 1984; Smith, 1975, for reviews of the literature on this topic). Many of these studies suggest a positive effect for various types of meditation on such conditions. The following offers a brief overview of the research literature on the relationship of meditation and stress.

Meditation and Stress Reduction

During the past 20 years, meditation has been extensively studied as a way of reducing physiological and psychosocial stress (e.g., Benson, 1996). For example, Lehrer et al. (1980) taught either of three relaxation techniques —(1) clinically standardized meditation (CSM), (2) respiratory one-method meditation (ROM), or (3) progressive relaxation (PMR)—to a group of New York Telephone employees who were self-selected for stress. In addition to the three relaxation groups, another group served as a control (they did not learn a meditation technique or PMR). This study found that at 5.5 months after the relaxation training, the three treatment groups showed clinical improvement in self-reported symptoms of stress, but only the two meditation groups (not the PMR group) showed significantly more symptom reduction than the controls. The meditation groups had a lowering of self-perceived stress at 5.5 months, whether they meditated frequently or just occasionally.

Similarly, Miller et al. (1995) conducted a 3-year study of 22 patients with DSM-III-R–defined anxiety disorders who had been given an 8-week stress-reduction intervention based on mindfulness meditation. At 3-month follow-up, 20 of the patients demonstrated significant reductions in Hamilton and Beck Anxiety and Depression scores after intervention; in a 3-year follow-up of 18 of the original 22 patients, the gains observed in the original study on the Hamilton and Beck anxiety scales were maintained. In addition, at the 3-year follow-up, the patients displayed consistent improvements in depression scales, panic scores, the number and severity of panic attacks, and generalized fear.

Astin (1997) examined the effects of an 8-week stress-reduction program based on training in mindfulness meditation. In this study, 28 volunteers were randomized into either an experimental group (mindfulness meditation) or a nonintervention control group. Following participation, experimental subjects, when compared with controls, had significantly greater (1) reductions in overall psychological problems, (2) increases in overall domain-specific sense of control and utilization of an accepting or yielding mode of control in their lives, and (3) scores on a measure of spiritual experiences. Based on these results, Astin concluded that mindfulness meditation, with its emphasis on developing detached observation and awareness of the contents of consciousness, "may represent a powerful cognitive behavioral coping strategy for transforming the ways in which we respond to life events."

In a similar study, Shapiro et al. (1998) examined the short-term effects of an 8-week meditation-based stress-reduction intervention on premedical and medical students. This study found that the meditation intervention effectively (1) reduced self-reported state and trait anxiety, (2) reduced reports of overall psychological distress including depression, (3) increased scores on overall empathy levels, and (4) increased scores on a measure of spiritual experiences assessed at termination of intervention. These results, which were replicated in the waitlist control group, held across different experiments and were observed even during exam periods.

Meditation and Stress Hormones

Several studies also have found corresponding changes in stress hormones as a result of meditation. For example, Jevning et al. (1978) studied acute plasma cortisol and testosterone concentration changes during transcendental meditation (TM) among a group of normal, young adult volunteers. In addition to studying a group of regular TM practitioners (3 to 5 years of practice), the investigators also took blood samples from a group of controls (nonmeditators), who were reexamined after 3 to 4 months of TM practice. This study found no changes in cortisol or testosterone in controls and only a small decline in cortisol after they had meditated for several months. However, cortisol decreased significantly in long-term practitioners during meditation and remained somewhat low afterward. No change in testosterone concentration was noted during either rest or TM. According to the researchers, "The practice of TM becomes associated with psychophysiologic response(s) which acutely inhibit pituitary-adrenal activity" (p. 54).

In a more recent and extensive experiment, Walton and colleagues (1995) examined endocrine differences between high-stress but otherwise healthy students not practicing a systematic stress-reduction technique and a similar group of low-stress students who had practiced TM on average for 8.5 years. The two groups of students, matched for age and area of study, performed timed collections of urine that included (separately) the entire waking and sleeping portions of 1 day. They also completed the

Profile of Mood States and the State-Trait Anxiety Inventory, self-report instruments sensitive to subjective level of stress. This study found that the two groups differed significantly on most measures. Specifically, the low-stress group was lower in cortisol and aldosterone and higher in dehydroepiandrosterone sulfate and the serotonin metabolite, 5-hydroxyindoleacetic acid. In women practicing TM, cortisol correlated inversely and dehydroepiandrosterone sulfate directly with number of months of TM practice.

Perhaps the most definitive evidence of a reduction of stress hormones as a result of practicing meditation comes from a randomized, prospective trial by MacLean and colleagues (1997), who measured changes in four hormones—(1) cortisol, (2) growth hormone, (3) thyroid-stimulating hormone, and (4) testosterone—before and after 4 months of either the TM technique or a stress education control condition. This study found significantly different changes between the two groups for each hormone over the 4 months. In the TM group, but not in the controls, baseline (before) cortisol levels and average cortisol levels across the stress session decreased from pretest to posttest. Cortisol responsiveness to stressors, however, increased in the TM group compared with controls. The baselines and/or stress responsiveness for TSH and GH changed in opposite directions for the groups, as did the testosterone baseline. According to the investigators, "The cortisol and testosterone results appear to support previous data suggesting that repeated practice of the TM technique reverses effects of chronic stress."

In summary, there is increasing evidence that the meditative practices derived from both Hindu and Buddhist belief systems can be used as interventions to affect clinical outcomes. In particular, there is evidence that certain types of meditation may reduce or protect against stress. The lower levels of stress hormones found among those who regularly practice meditative techniques are particularly noteworthy and have many important implications for PNI research.

It has been suggested that the therapeutic benefits of meditation are mainly a result of the "relaxation response," which was first characterized in the 1970s by cardiologist Herbert Benson as one of the effects of various types of meditation (Benson, 1975). It is now well established that elicitation of the relaxation response can produce reductions in muscle tension, activity of the sympathetic branch of the autonomic nervous system, activity of the anterior pituitary-adrenocortical axis, blood pressure and heart rate, and oxygen consumption. The relaxation response also has been shown to correlate with changes in brain wave activity and wave function (see Benson, 1996; Delmonte, 1985, for reviews of this literature). The relaxation response also is associated with improvement in many acute and chronic illnesses and conditions (e.g., acute and chronic pain) (see Benson, 1996; Benson & Stuart, 1993, for a review of this research).

Thus, the relaxation response as a component of meditation may have important psychological and physiological effects. There is evidence that the relaxation response is also common not only to meditation but also possibly to other Eastern religion–derived practices, such as meditative prayer (Schopen & Freeman, 1992), yoga (Vedanthan et al., 1998), and guided imagery (Richardson et al., 1997; Walker et al., 1999).

Problems and Obstacles to Studying Eastern Religious Practices from a PNI Perspective

Despite these promising results on the ability of meditation and related approaches to reduce or protect against stress, it is still difficult to make generalizations about the use of religious-based interventions for health problems. This is because many of the studies in this area involve variables that are divorced from the context that gave them religious meaning and purpose in the first place. For example, the type of yoga that is practiced in the United States and Europe is typically a derivation of "hatha" yoga, which is mainly physical exercise and postures (asanas). In traditional Hinduism, however, the use of asanas is only a single step in an eight-step path, and they are supposed to be used as a stepping-stone for the higher paths (Littleton, 1996). Similarly, according to the teachings of the Theravada tradition, the practice of mindfulness meditation is simply one element in a complex set of religious practices (including adherence to a set of ethical principles) and can have its proper effect only when placed in that context. When yoga asanas or the techniques of mindfulness meditation are separated from these contexts of meaning, it is doubtful whether they can usefully any longer be identified as the same practices: something essential to their identity and efficacy has been removed, and as a result they have been transformed into something very different.

Furthermore, many sincere or orthodox religious people do not practice their religion with practical benefits in mind. If such benefits occur, that is often seen as a side effect and not as the main point of the practice.

For example, Buddhist and Hindu religious philosophies discourage attachment to physical health and the use of religious practices for material gain (Littleton, 1996). Some Hindu thinkers would say that using yoga for the purpose of merely working on the beauty and welfare of an impermanent object (the body) is a waste of time and effort. Indeed, all serious yogis agree in disapproving of the use of yogic methods for worldly purposes. It is possible, then, that the health benefits evident in Westerners who practice yoga with such benefits as their main goal are produced as much by their expectations as by the practices. But it is also possible that the benefits are directly related, causally, to the practice of yoga, and that they are at least as evident in those who practice yoga without interest in health benefits as in those who practice it with such interests. The present state of research does not permit clear conclusions on such matters.

Then again, in some Buddhist traditions, especially in contemporary Japan, some practices are precisely aimed at material or physical benefit, or at least are concerned with it as one important element among others. This is especially clear in some of the new Buddhist movements in Japan, such as the Soka Gakkai. So, again, much depends on particulars. This is one more example of the difficulty of using broad categories such as "Eastern" or "Western" religion.

Another problem associated with studying isolated practices outside the broader context of a religion is that "suffering," including physical suffering, is seen as inevitable in many Eastern (and Western) religious philosophies and is judged to be a proper means of attaining some higher spiritual result. For example, Buddha set forth four noble truths for his followers: (1) the truth of suffering, (2) the cause of suffering, (3) the cessation of suffering, and (4) the means of overcoming suffering. The ultimate aim of experiencing and then overcoming suffering in Buddhism is a radical transformation of one's personality (Smith, 1991), and an exit, as a result, from the endless round of rebirth and redeath. However, in Western medicine, suffering is usually understood very differently as something that is to be avoided at all costs and that has no meaning or use. Indeed, a major aim of Western medicine is to reduce or completely relieve suffering.

Buddhists might agree that, finally, suffering is to be removed: Nirvana is often understood precisely as a condition in which there is no more suffering. But suffering is nonetheless often understood as an essential condition for attainment of the religious goals of Buddhism. Buddhists say that, for example, the semidivine beings who inhabit the heavenly realms cannot reach Nirvana precisely because they do not suffer enough to understand that their condition is finally unsatisfactory. From a Buddhist point of view, then, Western medicine might be understood as an attempt to make us all like those semidivine beings, an attempt that, if successful, would prevent our attainment of Nirvana.

Other such differences could be sketched. The point of mentioning them is to underscore the fact that Western medicine, just as much as the philosophies and theologies of the religions of the East, is committed to an understanding of what human beings are like and what is good for them and that its understanding is often at odds with that of the religions. This leads to difficulties of a conceptual and practical kind in any attempt to adopt Eastern religious practices for their potential PNI benefits.

Finally, there is evidence that for a religious practice to result in a health benefit, there may need to be an element of "true belief." For example, research on Western religions has demonstrated that "extrinsic" religiousness (using religion for one's own needs, such as gaining social status or for social convention) may be related to poorer health outcomes, whereas "intrinsic" religiousness (using religion as a fundamentally trustworthy guide for one's everyday decisions) may be related to better health outcomes (Batson & Ventis, 1982; Donahue, 1985). A number of studies also have shown that intrinsic religiousness tends to decrease one's level of anxiety and personal distress on a daily basis, whereas extrinsic religiousness tends to increase one's everyday level of anxiety (Genia, 1996; Tapanya et al., 1997). Thus, the failure to find a beneficial effect of a religious practice on health does not necessarily indicate that the particular practice is not healthy, but rather that the individual does not truly believe that the religious practice is important to his or her everyday life.

REFERENCES

Astin, J. A. (1997). Stress reduction through mindfulness meditation: Effects on psychological symptomatology, sense of control, and spiritual experiences. *Psychotherapy and Psychosomatics* 66, 97–106.

Batson, C. D., & Ventis, W. L. (1982). *The religious experience*. New York: Oxford University Press.

Benson, H. (1975). *The relaxation response*. New York: Morrow.

Benson, H. (1993). The relaxation response. In D. Goleman & J. Gurin (Eds.), *Mind-body medicine: How to use your mind for better health*. Yonkers, NY: Consumer Report Books.

Benson, H. (1996). *Timeless healing.* New York: Scribner.

Benson, H., & Stuart, E. M. (1993). *The wellness book: A comprehensive guide to maintaining health and treating stress-related illness.* New York: Fireside.

Carrington, P. (1993). Modern forms of meditation. In P. M. Lehter & R. Woolfolk (Eds.), *Principles and practices of stress management.* New York: Guilford.

Craven, J. L. (1989). Meditation and psychotherapy. *Canadian Journal of Psychiatry* 34, 648–653.

Delmonte, M. M. (1985). Biochemical indices associated with meditation practice: A literature review. *Neuroscience and Biobehavioral Reviews* 9, 557–561.

Donahue, M. J. (1985). Intrinsic and extrinsic religiousness: A review and meta-analysis. *Journal of Personality and Social Psychology* 48, 400–419.

Easwaran, E. (1991). *Meditation.* Tomales, CA: Nilgiri Press.

Genia, V. (1996). I, E, quest, and fundamentalism as predictors of psychological and spiritual well-being. *Journal for the Scientific Study of Religion* 35, 56–64.

Goleman, D. (1988). *The meditative mind.* Los Angeles: Thatcher.

Haskins, J. (1991). *Religions of the world,* rev. ed. New York: Hippocrene.

Jevning, R., Wilson, A. F., & Davidson, J. M. (1978). Adrenocortical activity during meditation. *Hormones and Behavior* 10, 54–60.

Kabat-Zinn, J. (1993). Mindfulness meditation: Health benefits of an ancient Buddhist practice. In D. Goleman & J. Gurin (Eds.), *Mind-body medicine: How to use your mind for better health.* Yonkers, NY: Consumer Report Books.

Lehrer, P. M., Schoicket, S., Carrington, P., & Woolfolk, R. L. (1980). Psychophysiological and cognitive responses to stressful stimuli in subjects practicing progressive relaxation and clinically standardized meditation. *Behaviour Research and Therapy* 18, 293–303.

Littleton, C. S. (1996). *Eastern wisdom.* New York: Henry Holt.

MacLean, C. R., Walton, K. G., Wenneberg, S. R., Levitsky, D. K., Mandarino, J. P., Waziri, R., Hillis, S. L., & Schneider, R. H. (1997). Effects of the Transcendental Meditation program on adaptive mechanisms: Changes in hormone levels and responses to stress after 4 months of practice. *Psychoneuroendocrinology* 22, 277–295.

Miller, J. J., Fletcher, K., & Kabat-Zinn, J. (1995). Three-year follow-up and clinical implications of mindfulness meditation–based stress reduction intervention in the treatment of anxiety disorders. *General Hospital Psychiatry* 17, 192–200.

Odajnyk, V. W. (1993). *Gathering the light: A psychology of meditation.* Boston: Shambhala.

Ornish, D. (1990). *Dr. Dean Ornish's program for reversing heart disease.* New York: Random House.

Richardson, M. A., Post-White, J., Grimm, E. A., Moye, L. A., Singletary, S. E., & Justice, B. (1997). Coping, life attitudes, and immune responses to imagery and group support after breast cancer treatment. *Alternative Therapies in Health and Medicine* 3, 62–70.

Schopen, A., & Freeman, B. (1992). Meditation: The forgotten Western tradition. *Counseling and Values* 36, 123–134.

Shafi, M. (1985). *Freedom from self: Sufism, meditation, and psychotherapy*. New York: Human Sciences Press.

Shapiro, D. H., & Walsh, R. N. (Eds.). (1984). *Meditation: Classic and contemporary perspectives*. New York: Aldine.

Shapiro, S. L., Schwartz, G. E., & Bonner, G. (1998). Effects of mindfulness-based stress reduction on medical and premedical students. *Journal of Behavioral Medicine* 21, 581–599.

Smith, H. J. (1991). *The illustrated world's religions: A guide to our wisdom traditions*. San Francisco: HarperCollins.

Smith, J. C. (1975). Meditation as psychotherapy: A review of the literature. *Psychological Bulletin* 82, 558–564.

Tapanya, S., Nicki, R., & Jarusawad, O. (1997). Worry and intrinsic/extrinsic religious orientation among Buddhist (Thai) and Christian (Canadian) elderly persons. *International Journal of Aging and Human Development* 44, 73–83.

Vedanthan, P. K., Kesavalu, L. N., Murthy, K. C., Duval,l K., Hall, M. J., Baker, S., & Nagarathna, S. (1998). Clinical study of yoga techniques in university students with asthma: A controlled study. *Allergy and Asthma Proceedings* 19, 3–9.

Walker, L. G., Walker, M. B., Ogston, K., Heys, S. D., Ah-See, A. K., Miller, I. D., Hutcheon, A. W., Sarkar, T. K., & Eremin, O. (1999). Psychological, clinical and pathological effects of relaxation training and guided imagery during primary chemotherapy. *British Journal of Cancer* 80, 262–268.

Walton, K. G., Pugh, N. D., Gelderloos, P. & Macrae, P. (1995). Stress reduction and preventing hypertension: Preliminary support for a psychoneuroendocrine mechanism. *Journal of Alternative and Complementary Medicine* 1, 263–283.

13

Psychoneuroimmunology and Western Religious Traditions

WARREN S. BROWN

A fundamental and often referred to distinction in descriptions of the world's major religions is between "Eastern" and "Western." But what is the nature of this difference, particularly with respect to developing and understanding the relationship between psychoneuroimmunology (PNI) and religion?

The terms *Eastern* and *Western religions* do not really correspond to the Eastern and Western Hemispheres of the earth but rather to the religious traditions born in the Near East, North Africa, and Europe (Western) versus those born in countries of the Far East (Eastern). However, this difference is not wholly geographic. The terms *Eastern* and *Western* also refer to a fundamental difference in an individual's view of life, of God, and of his or her relationship to both.

Hinduism and Buddhism (Eastern religions) both arose in India, although Buddhism moved out of India and is practiced chiefly in Southeast Asia (see chapter 12). Hindus and Buddhists believe that there is no real meaning to human existence and that the life of the individual is not important (Haskins, 1991). Hindus' greatest fear, therefore, is that life may continue on in an endless cycle of births and rebirths on earth. Their greatest hope is that they will find a way to escape this eternal earthly life and unite with a universal spirit that is above meaninglessness and meaning and is therefore impersonal.

By contrast, the Western religions—Judaism, Christianity, and Islam—have a common origin and therefore share fundamental beliefs regarding the nature of God and the meaning of human life. All three religions trace their origins back to the Book of Genesis and the stories of Abraham (Haskins, 1991). These religious traditions all stress belief in one God, who has human characteristics and with whom it is possible to communicate directly. There also is the prevailing belief in Western religious traditions that God cares about humankind and will reward believers by providing them with greater well-being and meaning in their lives here on earth and with immortality after they die (Haskins, 1991).

Western religious traditions, therefore, promote the belief that there is a "personal" God who listens to one's prayers and actively intervenes in one's affairs. Western religions also employ many aides to enhance feelings of a personal God. In Catholicism, for example, this sense of closeness to God is facilitated by confessionals; various images of Jesus, Mary, and the saints; and the use of incense and other sacred objects, rituals, or texts. Similarly, evangelical Protestants have a strong concept of the spiritual in-dwelling of the Holy Spirit, which is the concept of a God in the form of a supernatural spirit that is close enough to be continually in and around one's life (Haskins, 1991).

Although the aforementioned distinction between Eastern and Western religions represents a valuable "rule of thumb," it does not always hold. As all of these religions have moved outside their country of origin and changed over the centuries, they have evolved into a great variety of mix-tures and amalgams. Nevertheless, several questions elicit critical distinc-tions: "How personal is God presumed to be?" "Do followers believe that God hears one's prayers?" "Is God concerned about the events of one's life?" It is the thesis of this chapter that these questions also are important in grasping the power of religion to engage the processes described in the research on PNI. Indeed, if God is presumed by the religious person to be a "supernatural" person who hears, cares about, and responds to prayer, then it is possible that praying to God will engage the interpersonal processes that are known to enhance immune function (e.g., social support, benefits of disclosure, and other positive consequences of interpersonal contact).

This chapter discusses briefly the research linking Western religious practices and beliefs to physical health, using the model of the benefits of personal relatedness, social support, and disclosure of distress that have been described in the PNI literature. In addition, this chapter discusses the metaphysical and theological status of a PNI model of religion and health, pointing out the inherent shortcomings of attempting to study the reli-gion-health association solely from a PNI perspective.

Research on Western Religiousness and Health

A long history and continued tradition of sociological research on the association between religion and mortality dates back to Durkheim's (1897–1951) pioneering work, which demonstrated that people who were more religious were less likely to commit suicide. Only in recent years, however, have the medical, sociology, and public health communities become interested in this association in a more general sense. Most of these studies have investigated the association between Western religious denominational membership and two outcomes: mortality (death rates) and morbidity (the rate of illness and disease). Because this topic is covered in detail in the first chapter of this book, it is covered only briefly here.

Religion and Mortality

In general, research over the past several decades has demonstrated that people who belong to behaviorally strict denominations have lower mortality risks than people who belong to less strict religious groups or who have no religious affiliation at all (Dwyer et al., 1990; Goldstein, 1996; Kark et al., 1996; Lyon et al., 1976; Phillips et al., 1980). Furthermore, investigations have shown that those who are the most conscientious adherents to the stricter religious traditions (e.g., Mormons) tend to exhibit lower mortality than those who are tied more loosely to the same groups (Gardner & Lyon, 1982).

Using the Alameda County Study data, Wingard (1982) demonstrated that church membership was related to lower mortality for both women and men but that socioeconomic and behavioral controls eliminated the association. However, a more recent analysis of these same data found that frequent religious attendance reported at the baseline assessment was associated with lower mortality over a 28-year follow-up period (Strawbridge et al., 1997). In this latter study, the lower mortality rates for frequent religious attenders were only partly explained by improved health practices, increased social contacts, and more stable marriages occurring in conjunction with attendance. In other words, some other factor involved in being religious played a role in lower mortality in this group. In addition, both the Alameda County Study and the Tecumseh Community Health Study found a beneficial effect on mortality of a social network index, one component of which was church membership (Berkman & Syme, 1979; House et al., 1982; Seeman et al., 1987). More recently, in an analysis of nationally representative data from the National Health Interview Survey-Multiple Cause of Death survey, Hummer and colleagues (1999) found that people who never attend church exhibited 1.87 times the risk of death in the follow-up period compared with people who attended more than once a week. Indeed, this translated into a 7-year difference in life expectancy at age 20 between those who never attend church and those who attend more than once a week. This study also found that health selectivity was responsible for a portion of this "religious attendance effect"—that is, people who do not attend church or religious services were more likely to be unhealthy and, consequently, to die. However, it was also found that religious attendance affects health, at least partially, through increased social ties and behavioral factors that decrease the risks of death.

Therefore, there does appear to be a strong association between frequent attendance at religious services and reduced mortality. Part of this effect is due to social and behavioral factors that decrease one's likelihood of engaging in life-threatening behaviors. However, greater social interactions and better health behaviors account for only part of this association. Indeed, Oman and Reed (1998) recently found that mortality was 24% lower among frequent religious service attenders than among nonattenders, even after controlling for a variety of factors, including social support and physical functioning. Furthermore, Koenig and colleagues (1999) also demonstrated a 28% decrease in relative hazard of dying, for frequent church attenders compared with infrequent attenders, that was independent of demographics, health conditions, social connections, and health practices.

Religion and Morbidity

A larger body of literature has investigated the association between religion and morbidity—that is, the risk of illness in a specified population (e.g., Ellison, 1991; Idler, 1987; Levin & Markides, 1986; Levin & Vanderpool, 1989; Musick, 1996). For example, a number of studies in a variety of populations have found that religious commitment is associated with lower blood pressure (see Levin & Vanderpool, 1989, for a review of this literature). Additionally, Larson et al. (1989) found that persons who attend church frequently and for whom religion is of "major importance" to their lives have lower blood pressure than those who attend church infrequently and for whom religion is of less importance.

In attempting to identify which aspects of religion are responsible for its beneficial effects on morbidity, studies have shown that church attendance often is associated with greater social support (Bradley, 1995; Ellison & George, 1994), which is related to lower morbidity and mortality (Blazer, 1982). Additionally, some religious beliefs and practices appear to be associated with higher self-esteem (Krause, 1992; Krause & Van Tran, 1989; Nelson, 1989), which, in turn, may promote a healthier lifestyle and/or reduce stress. Religious factors also have been shown to significantly and positively affect quality of life (Hadaway & Roof, 1978; Koenig et al., 1997), which, in turn, affects compliance with medical treatments and health outcomes.

Thus, the relationship between religion and morbidity mirrors that of religion and mortality. Some of this relationship can be explained in terms of religion's ability to increase social support, reduce health-damaging behaviors, and enhance compliance with treatment. However, these factors do not entirely explain this beneficial relationship. For example, Koenig and Larson (1998) recently found, in a consecutive sample of medical patients age 60 or older who had been admitted to Duke University Medical Center, that elderly individuals who attended church weekly or more often were significantly less likely in the previous year to have been admitted to the hospital, had fewer total hospital admissions, and spent fewer days in the hospital than those who attended less often. Furthermore, these associations retained their significance after controlling for age, sex, race, education, social support, depressive symptoms, level of physical functioning, and severity of medical illness. Additionally, this study found that patients who were not affiliated with a religious community, while not using more acute hospital services in the year before admission, had significantly longer hospital stays than those who were affiliated with a religious community. Unaffiliated patients spent an average of 25 days in the hospital, compared with 11 days for affiliated patients; this association strengthened when physical health and other covariates were controlled.

Models for Examining the PNI Influence of Religion in Health

How might the field of PNI approach the study of the impact of religious beliefs, behaviors, and practices on physical health? As already mentioned, religion's effect on morbidity and mortality may be due to encouragement of better health behaviors, or to the fact that religious communities often provide social support and relief from loneliness (Ellison & George, 1994; Walton et al., 1991). Such perceived social support may aid in coping with serious illness and, thus, aid in recovery, particularly when people require extensive medical care.However, increased social support and coping skills do not account for all of this relationship. Thus, religious activities, beliefs, and practices also exert their beneficial effects on morbidity and mortality via some other, more direct mechanism(s).

What might be the nature of this (these) other mechanism(s), and might PNI shed light on such effects? Evidence of at least one more direct psychological influence of religion on health is provided by the work of James Pennebaker and colleagues at Southern Methodist University. Although these studies did not involve religiousness per se, they demonstrated a strong link between *emotional disclosure (confession)* and autonomic and immune activation. In one study, Pennebaker, Hughes, and O'Heeronet (1987) investigated the short-term autonomic correlates of disclosing personal and traumatic experiences among two samples of healthy undergraduate college students: one group that disclosed past traumatic events and another group that merely talked about upcoming plans. This study found that having students talk about traumatic events was associated with decreased behavioral inhibition, as measured by lower skin conductance levels among high disclosers, as well as with increased cardiovascular activity. In contrast, students who merely thought or talked about plans for the day had higher skin conductance levels and lower cardiovascular reactivity. Interestingly, the presence of an interactive confessor, versus a silent confessor who sat behind a curtain, inhibited subjects' ability to talk about traumatic events

In another study, Pennebaker, Barger, and Tiebout (1989) asked 33 Holocaust survivors to talk on videotape for 1 to 2 hours about their personal experiences during World War II. During the interview, the researchers continuously monitored each subject's skin conductance level and heart rate. Approximately 14 months after the interview, self-reports of the subjects' health were collected. Controlling for pre-interview health problems, the study found that the degree of disclosure during the interview was positively correlated with long-term health after the interview.

In attempting to relate emotional disclosure to immune indices, Pennebaker, Kiecolt-Glaser, and Glaser (1988) randomly assigned 50 undergraduate college students to write either about "trivial" or emotionally traumatic experiences for 20 minutes on 4 consecutive days. The investigators collected blood samples on the day before beginning the experiments, on the last day of writing, and again 6 weeks later and assayed the blood samples for immune response to two common mitogens (i.e., substances that stimulate immune cells to divide). This study found that the students who were assigned to write about emotionally traumatic events had significant improvement in immune system functioning from the beginning to the end of the experiment compared with the control (trivia writing) students, and these differences tended to persist 6 weeks later. Furthermore, those students in the trauma writing group visited the student health center for illnesses significantly less often after the experiment than before, compared with the students in the trivia writing group.

A later study by Pennebaker and others (Petrie et al., 1995) investigated whether emotional expression of traumatic experiences influenced the immune response to a hepatitis B vaccination. In this study, 40 medical students who tested negative for hepatitis B antibodies were randomly assigned to write about personal traumatic events or control topics (time usage during the day) during four consecutive daily sessions. The day after completion of the writing, participants were given their first hepatitis B vaccination, with booster injections at 1 and 4 months after the writing. Blood was collected before each vaccination and at a 6-month follow-up. Compared with the control group, participants in the "emotional expression" group showed significantly higher antibody levels against hepatitis B at the 4- and 6-month follow-up periods. The emotional expression group also had other significant immune changes immediately after writing, including significantly lower numbers of circulating T helper lymphocytes and basophils. The finding that a writing intervention can influence immune response provides further support for a link between emotional disclosure and health.

How does disclosure benefit health and immune indices? In a review of the literature, Pennebaker and Susman (1988) found that surveys and experiments indicate that (1) childhood traumatic experiences, particularly those never discussed, are highly correlated with current health problems; (2) recent traumas that are not discussed are linked with increased health problems and ruminations about the traumas; (3) requiring individuals to confront earlier traumas in writing improves health and immune system functioning; and (4) actively talking about upsetting experiences is associated with immediate reductions in selected autonomic activity.

Thus, disclosure of traumatic events and other emotionally disturbing problems enhances both autonomic and immune function. These findings suggest that a novel approach to investigating the PNI aspects of religion may be to examine the confessional aspects of Western religious practices. Indeed, many aspects of religious practices, such as confession and prayer (whether personal or communal), involve self-disclosure. This brings us back to our discussion of the distinction between Western and Eastern religions with respect to the degree to which God is presumed to be personal and the religious life formulated in terms of a personal relationship. If prayer is understood to be communication with a God who is there and who is personally responsive, then prayer will maximally engage those psychoneuroimmune responses that are known to be modulated by interpersonal interactions. If, in addition, this relationship encourages disclosure (confession and repentance), then additional psychoneuroimmune interactions will be engaged. Thus, it is along the lines of the perception of an interpersonal interaction that one can evaluate the differential engagement of PNI processes by various religious traditions and by various religious individuals.

The beneficial effects of disclosure could explain the appeal of institutions that prescribe disclosure practices (confessions or public self-criticisms). In the course of satisfying basic human motivation, however, institutionalized prescriptions for disclosure also may serve a second gratifying purpose: social integration. For example, pleading guilty to wrongdoing (i.e., confession to sin) with the church or family may force the individual to reconcile personal views with those of the institution requiring confession. Additionally, shared secrets often serve to cement interpersonal intimacy and, thus, shore up social support.

Finally, it must be appreciated that all forms of religiousness are psychologically, behaviorally, and culturally complex. The religiousness of an individual or group involves such dimensions as:

- Religious experiences (ecstatic, meditative, emotions, awe)
- Behaviors and practices, such as prayer and behavioral disciplines
- Verbal statements of belief
- Affective evaluations of situations (usually operating in the preconscious or unconscious)
- Structures for relating to others (ethics, compassion, altruism)
- Worldviews
- Belief in, and response to, a personal relationship with God

The specific effects of each of these dimensions is deserving of further study in attempting to understand the positive impact of religiousness on health and the potential role of PNI.

A Caveat regarding PNI, Spirituality, and Healing

And yet, it is important to avoid "nothing buttery" metaphysics. Indeed, if one finds a natural mechanism that explains the effects of religion on health, this does not presuppose the exclusion of theological explanations. For example, it is argued in this book that many of the effects of religion on health may be attributed to placebo effects. In the history of medical research, the term *placebo* has been a pejorative word referring to changes in symptoms or medical conditions that are "only in the head." Of course, the now voluminous research in PNI makes it clear that "placebo effects" refer to the impact of important top-down natural mechanisms (i.e., causal processes operating from cognitive to neurological to immune systems). Theologically, it is coherent to consider the mechanism of PNI as a manifestation of intent or design in which humans have been created to respond in a positive way physiologically to the operation of faith, hope, joy, belief, confession, and love.

Theologically, to understand the complexity of the relationship between religion and physical health, one must distinguish between religion and health as a natural event (i.e., a common, frequently occurring process understood within natural theology) and as a manifestation of supernatural healing, which would be, by definition, not subject to scientific study. Indeed, in the case of supernatural healing, one cannot scientifically control the major variable (i.e., God). Natural theology, by contrast, rests on the manifestation of design and intent (although complicated by human willfulness and sin) within the natural world. It is logically incoherent to say, on the basis of scientific investigation, that there *is* nothing more, when the "something more" is not subject to study by scientific methods and procedures.

Relatedness, Soulishness, and PNI

I recently joined with a number of colleagues in an attempt to create a Christian but nondualist account of human nature—that is, an account of human religiousness and spirituality without recourse to a distinction between body and soul but nevertheless consistent with biblical Christianity (see Brown, Murphy, & Malony, *Whatever Happened to the Soul? Scientific and Theological Portraits of Human Nature*). In attempting to bring together the dimensions of human persons traditionally termed *body*, *mind*, and *soul* into a singularity, one must be concerned about preserving the critical properties and attributes of human nature and potentials for human experience that have been traditionally assigned to the "soul." To be theologically adequate, this portrait of human persons needed to allow for those soulish capacities and experiences that are assumed or described in Western religious teachings.

In this context, I argued that there is a fundamental core capacity running through descriptions of human soulful experiences and attributes— the capacities for, and experiences of, personal relatedness. For example, the Bible presumes a unique depth and scope of human relatedness that is not presumed for the rest of the animal kingdom. The term *personal* captures this uniqueness (in quality or quantity). The term *relatedness* is meant to encompass three important dimensions: (1) subjective processes of self-relatedness and self-representation, (2) inter-individual relatedness, and (3) relatedness to God. In this view, it is experiences of relatedness to others, to the self, and most particularly to God that endow a person with the attributes that have been attached to the concept of "soul."

We have seen that PNI demonstrates that healthy interpersonal relatedness and support has a positive impact on the immune system. Thus, according to this view of the nature of human soulishness, it is the exercise of our "soulishness" that enhances immune function. Our experiences of relatedness to other individuals and to God (when understood as a personal relationship)—experiences that I would designate as *soulish*—are also those that modulate (positively or negatively) the activation of our immune systems and influence our health.

REFERENCES

Berkman, L. F., & Syme, S. L. (1979). Social networks, host resistance, and mortality: A nine-year follow-up study of Alameda County residents. *American Journal of Epidemiology* 109, 186–204.

Blazer, D. (1982). Social support and mortality in an elderly community population. *American Journal of Epidemiology* 115, 684–694.

Bradley, D. E. (1995). Religious involvement and social resources: Evidence from the data set, "Americans' Changing Lives." *Journal of the Scientific Study of Religion* 34, 259–267.

Brown, W. S., Murphy, N., & Malony, H. N. (Eds.) *Whatever happened to the soul? Scientific and theological portraits of human nature*. Minneapolis: Fortress, 1998.

Durkheim, E. [1897] 1951. *Suicide: A study in sociology.* New York: Free Press.

Dwyer, J. W., Clarke, L.L., & Miller, M. K. 1990. The effect of religious concentration and affiliation on county cancer mortality rates. *Journal of Health and Social Behavior* 31, 185–202.

Ellison, C. G. (1991). Religious involvement and subjective well-being. *Journal of Health and Social Behavior* 32, 80–99.

Ellison, C. G., & George, L. K. (1994). Religious involvement, social ties, and social support in a southeastern community. *Journal of the Scientific Study of Religion* 33, 46–60.

Gardner, J. W., & Lyon, J. L. (1982). Cancer in Utah Mormon men by lay priesthood level. *American Journal of Epidemiology* 116, 243–257.

Goldstein, S. (1996). Changes in Jewish mortality and survival, 1963–1987. *Social Biology* 43, 72–97.

Hadaway, C. K., & Roof, W. C. (1978). Religious commitment and the quality of life in American Society. *Review of Religious Research* 19, 295–307.

Haskins, J. (1991). *Religions of the world,* rev. ed. New York: Hippocrene.

House, J. S., Robbins, C., & Metzner, H. L. (1982). The association of social relationships and activities with mortality: Prospective evidence from the Tecumseh Community Health Study. *American Journal of Epidemiology* 116, 123–140.

Hummer, R. A., Rogers, R. G., Nam, C. B., & Ellison, C. G. (1999). Religious involvement and U.S. adult mortality. *Demography* 36, 273–285.

Idler, E. (1987). Religious involvement and the health of the elderly: Some hypotheses and an initial test. *Social Forces* 66, 226–238.

Kark, J. D., Shemi, G., Friedlander, Y., Martin, O., Manor, O., & Blondheim, S. H. (1996). Does religious observance promote health? Mortality in secular vs. religious kibbutz in Israel. *American Journal of Public Health* 86, 341–346.

Koenig, H. G., Cohen, H. J., George, L. K., Hays, J. C., Larson, D. B., & Blazer, D. G. (1997). Attendance at religious services, interleukin-6, and other biological indicators of immune function in older adults. *International Journal of Psychiatry in Medicine* 27, 233–250.

Koenig, H. G., George, L. K., Hays, J. C., Larson, D. B., Cohen, H. J., & Blazer, D. G. (1998). The relationship between religious activities and blood pressure in older adults. *International Journal of Psychiatry in Medicine* 28, 189.

Koenig, H. G., Hays, J. C., Larson, D. B., George, L. K., Cohen, H. J., McCullough, M. E., Meador, K. G., & Blazer, D. G. (1999). Does religious attendance prolong survival? A six-year follow-up study of 3,968 older adults. *Journals of Gerontology: Series A, Biological Sciences and Medical Sciences* 54, M370-M376.

Koenig, H. G., & Larson, D. B. (1998). Use of hospital services, religious attendance, and religious affiliation. *Southern Medical Journal* 91, 925–932.

Krause, N. (1992). Stress, religiosity, and psychological well-being among older blacks. *Journal of Aging and Health* 4, 412–439.

Krause, N., & Van Tran, T. (1989). Stress and religious involvement among older blacks. *Journal of Gerontology* 44, S4–13.

Larson, D. B., Koenig, H. G., Kaplan, B. H., Greenberg, R. S., Logue, E., & Tyroler, H. A. (1989). The impact of religion on men's blood pressure. *Journal of Religion and Health* 28, 265–278.

Levin, J. S., & Markides, K. S. (1986). Religious attendance and subjective health. *Journal of the Scientific Study of Religion* 25, 31–39.

Levin, J. S., & Vanderpool, H. Y. (1989). Is religion therapeutically significant for hypertension? *Social Science and Medicine* 29, 69–78.

Lyon, J. L., Klauber, M. R., Gardner, J. W., & Smart, C. R. (1976). Cancer incidence in Mormons and non-Mormons in Utah, 1966–1970. *New England Journal of Medicine* 294, 129–133.

Musick, M. A. (1996). Religion and subjective health among black and white elders. *Journal of Health and Social Behavior* 37, 221–237.

Nelson, P. B. (1989). Ethnic differences in intrinsic/extrinsic religious orientation and depression in the elderly. *Archives of Psychiatric Nursing* 3, 199–204.

Oman, D., & Reed, D. (1998). Religion and mortality among the community-dwelling elderly. *American Journal of Public Health* 88, 1469–1475.

Pennebaker, J. W., Barger, S. D., & Tiebout, J. (1989). Disclosure of traumas and health among Holocaust survivors. *Psychosomatic Medicine* 51, 577–589.

Pennebaker, J. W., Hughes, C. F., & O'Heeron, R. C. (1987). The psychophysiology of confession: Linking inhibitory and psychosomatic processes. *Journal of Personality and Social Psychology* 52, 781–793.

Pennebaker, J. W., Kiecolt-Glaser, J. K., & Glaser, R. (1988). Disclosure of traumas and immune function: Health implications for psychotherapy. *Journal of Consulting and Clinical Psychology* 56, 239–245.

Pennebaker, J. W., & Susman, J. R. (1988). Disclosure of traumas and psychosomatic processes. *Social Science and Medicine* 26, 327–332.

Petrie, K. J., Booth, R. J., Pennebaker, J. W., Davison, K. P., & Thomas, M. G. (1995). Disclosure of trauma and immune response to a hepatitis B vaccination program. *Journal of Consulting and Clinical Psychology* 63, 787–792.

Phillips, R. L., Kuzma, J. W., Benson, W. L., & Lotz, T. (1980). Influence of selection versus lifestyle on risk of fatal cancer and cardiovascular disease among Seventh-Day Adventist men. *Journal of the American Medical Association* 198, 137–146.

Seeman, T. E., Kaplan, G. A., Knudsen, L., Cohen, R., & Guralnik, J. (1987). Social network ties and mortality among the elderly in the Alameda County study. *American Journal of Epidemiology* 126, 714–723.

Strawbridge, W. J., Cohe,n, R. D., Shema, S. J., & Kaplan, G. (1997). Frequent attendance at religious services and mortality over 28 years. *American Journal of Public Health* 87, 957–961.

Walton, C. G., Shultz, C. M., Beck, C. M., & Walls, R. C. (1991). Psychological correlates of loneliness in the older adult. *Archives of Psychiatric Nursing* 5, 165–170.

Wingard, D. L. (1982). The sex differential in mortality rates: Demographic and behavioral factors. *American Journal of Epidemiology* 115, 205–216.

14

Psychoneuroimmunology and Religion: Implications for Society and Culture

Howard L. Kaye

What if ongoing research in the new discipline of psychoneuroimmunology (PNI)—research of the sort discussed in this volume—succeeds in identifying the biochemical pathways by which spirituality and religious practice may exert a powerful influence on our health and longevity? What might the "implications" be for the practice of medicine and for the culture at large? How might a responsible physician use such knowledge and the mounting evidence of positive links between religiosity and health to benefit his or her patients? How might a health care system, hemorrhaging money yet leaving millions of citizens with inadequate access to care, respond to such an inexpensive therapeutic intervention, whose potential health benefits might be vast and whose costs and side effects are minimal?

At first glance, the "implications" would seem to be enormous. Just as responsible physicians properly concern themselves with the diet, lifestyle, and psychological well-being of their patients, it would seem to be only good medicine to examine the religious lifestyles of patients as well, encouraging them to increase their level of spiritual exercise and to improve the nutrition of their souls. As Gregg Easterbrook has argued in the *New Republic*, "Recommending religion . . . is quite pragmatic advice. Anyone can join a faith; attending services is a lot easier than quitting smoking" (1999, p. 23). But to successfully incorporate religion into the arsenal of medicine would seem to require considerable change in the prevailing attitudes and orientation of physicians toward the body and its infirmities. Rather than a purely technological approach to malfunctioning components in the body machine, physicians would have to be trained and encouraged to diagnose and treat the whole person: body, mind, and spirit. This, in turn, would necessitate the appropriate changes in medical education, the medical school selection process, the organization of health care, and the system of reimbursement, thereby altering fundamentally the practice and profession of medicine.

Beyond the sphere of medicine, the "implications" of scientific proof of the power of faith would seem to be no less profound for the broader culture. To the religiously committed, for example, such research findings would appear to be a godsend. After centuries of scientific assault on the reality and value of religious faith, here is rigorous scientific research offering evidence of its effectiveness, thereby returning to religion a certain legitimacy and worth long denied. After decades in which "the tremendous advances in the biomedical approach to disease" has encouraged a reductionistic view of human behavior and experience, characterized by "a near complete denial of the existence or relevance of man's soul or spirit" (Koenig, 1994, pp. 14–15), here is powerful evidence of the mind's, and perhaps even the soul's, impact upon the body.

Although the medical, philosophical, and cultural implications of psychoneuroimmunological research into the "faith factor's" impact on health would appear to be vast and wholly beneficial, there are two important reasons for being cautious whenever we speak of science's human implications. First, to speak of the implications of any scientific or technological development is seriously misleading, because it suggests that an unambiguous and univocal relation exists between a particular scientific claim and a particular social, ethical, or political outcome, so that the latter is presented as a logical and necessary consequence of the former. Yet, this is rarely the case. Instead, what are touted as implications are more properly viewed as speculative "interpretations" of the meaning of science and of its possible impact on other spheres of life. As such, a variety of interpretations are possible, no one of which is logically or culturally compelling. Second, the attempts to extract implications from scientific developments, prompted by the weakening hold of religion and tradition and by our growing faith in science, too often have produced regrettable, even malignant results, very different from those proclaimed by their champions. Both problems are amply demonstrated by the contentious debates surrounding the implications of modern biology and particularly Darwinism, which for nearly 140 years has been mined for its social, religious, and philosophical significance.

Historical Overview

According to the clichés of cultural history, the publication of Darwin's *Origin of Species* in 1859 set in motion a profound revolution in the Western worldview and self-conception, as its antireligious implications were immediately grasped. If Darwin's theory of evolution by natural selection was correct, then the biblical account of creation must be false. No longer could the marvelous adaptation of organism to environment be used as proof of God's existence and benevolence, nor could *Homo sapiens* continue to think itself special in nature, status, and purpose. With God a victim of "structural unemployment," the species created in "his" image was reduced in stature to its proper position: a rather plebeian primate species descended from other, even less remarkable primates. As such, the "higher" aspirations and responsibilities claimed for humans must have appeared illusory in light of Darwin's theory.

When Darwin finally turned to human evolution explicitly in *The Descent of Man* (1871), he expanded the scope of evolution to include human moral and spiritual traits, and not simply physical ones. By underscoring human physiological, psychological, and even moral similarities with the great apes, Darwin hoped both to shatter the belief in the biblical account of creation and to convey a moral message of greater humility and compassion toward other species and races as well.

The last of Darwin's sequels to the *Origin, The Expression of the Emotions in Man and Animals* (1872), continued to emphasize the continuity between human and nonhuman animals, now by arguing that the expression of such feelings as suffering, anxiety, grief, joy, love, devotion, hatred, and anger is not unique to human beings. Darwin connected studies of facial muscles and the emission of sounds with the corresponding emotional states in humans and then argued that the same facial movements and sounds in nonhuman animals express similar emotional states. Once again, Darwin hoped that the appropriate metaphysical and moral implications would be drawn: "Man in his arrogance thinks himself a great work, worthy the interposition of a deity. More humble and I believe true to consider him created from animals" (quoted in Himmelfarb, 1967, p. 153).

However self-evident such antireligious and culturally transformative implications may appear to be, historical reality was far more complex than many standard accounts allow. Most believers, then and now, have been able to find satisfactory ways to reconcile their faith in both biology and the Bible and to reassert their belief in humans' special status. "Man is indeed an animal," it is often said, "but he is an animal with a difference; he is a 'political' animal, a 'rational' animal, an 'ethical' animal, a 'cultural' animal. The qualities of mind and conscience which make us so may have emerged in the course of evolution, but they have long since taken on a certain independence and life of their own which frees us from the tyranny of natural selection and renews our faith in a higher life for man."

Equally widespread and misleading is the view that the social implications derived from Darwinism and Mendelian genetics emphasized the necessity of brutal, competitive struggle among individuals, nations, and races as the engine of human progress, thereby contributing to two devastating world wars. In reality, however, every conceivable social lesson was ostensibly drawn from biological teaching. Capitalists and socialists, liberals and reactionaries, pacifists and militarists, racists and antiracists, nationalists and internationalists—all appealed to biology to buttress their positions or attack their opponents (see Bannister, 1979; Crook, 1994; Greene, 1981; Kaye, 1986/1997; Moore, 1979). Although the "conservative" uses of Darwinism may be better known in the Anglo-American world, "social Darwinism" for many has meant *socialist* Darwinism. Karl Marx and Friedrich Engels, for example, greatly admired Darwin's work because they believed it provided a natural-scientific justification for their own social theory, which was itself a "scientific" study of the evolving "social organism" as a "process of natural history" (Marx, 1867/1906, pp. 14–16).

Even those arch villains of "social Darwinism," British philosopher Herbert Spencer and American sociologist William Graham Sumner, were not as brutal and reactionary in their appeals to evolutionary theory as they have often been made to appear. Similar to Darwin himself, they balked at taking natural selection as a model for human social conduct. A world ruled by natural selection of random variations seemed to call into question both the beneficence of God, nature, and the historical process and the status of humans and their highest aspirations. Instead of a brutal competitive struggle among men, they emphasized the dominant role of intelligence, cooperation, and virtue—cultivated through education and experience, not biological elimination—in order to preserve their faith in human progress.

However contentious the debates surrounding Darwinism's implications were, the source of such diverse opinions lay not simply in the ambiguities of the theory. Of far greater importance was the fundamental fact that what passed as implications was essentially wishful thinking. Theo-

rists of all persuasions turned to biology not to *discover* its human significance, but to lend pseudoscientific support to their preconceived moral,
political, and metaphysical positions. But one person's wishful fantasies
need not be compelling to others. Darwin himself may have claimed that
his theory sanctioned human cooperation and brotherhood, but despite
his scientific authority, others had no trouble appealing to his ideas to justify the opposite conclusions. Much to Darwin's discomfort, even his own
cousin, Francis Galton, read the *Origin* as sanctioning eugenics (i.e., the
idea of ameliorating human social life through selective breeding). In the
hope of correcting such a "misreading," Darwin emphasized, in *The Descent of Man*, that future progress would be achieved "much more through
the effects of habit, the reasoning powers, instruction, religion, etc., than
through natural selection" (1871/1981, 1:168–169, 2:404).

Unfortunately, eugenics, as proposed by Galton and expounded upon
by him until his death in 1911, had widespread appeal, particularly in the
United States, where it was seized upon by a WASP establishment feeling
increasingly threatened in a rapidly changing and ever more heterogeneous American society. Based both on their belief that social success,
immorality, and social failure were determined by heredity and on their
fear that under civilized conditions the genetically weak were outrepro-
ducing the genetically strong, American eugenicists supported restrictions
on immigration from nations they believed were of "inferior" genetic
stock, such as Italy, Greece, and the countries of Eastern Europe. Furthermore, this movement succeeded in pushing for and winning passage of
laws in 30 states that by the early 1930s had allowed for the compulsory
sterilization of 12,000 of the allegedly "feeble minded," the insane, and the
criminal (Degler, 1991, pp. 45–46, 52–53).

The most horrific eugenic laws, justified as applied biology, were passed
in Nazi Germany in the 1930s, where efforts to "purify" the German race
led to the eventual sterilization of as many as 400,000 people deemed unworthy of propagating and the extermination of millions more deemed
unworthy of life. Because of the association of eugenics and militant social
Darwinism with the horrors of the Nazi regime, intellectuals in the immediate post–World War II era arrived at a consensus that biological concepts
and analogies were of virtually no use as an aid to understanding human
social life and that the very quest for biology's human implications was
simply too dangerous to be tolerated. Remarkably, this consensus proved
to be short-lived, for with the dramatic rise of molecular biology, the quest
for biology's implications was renewed. In 1953, James Watson and

Francis Crick successfully elucidated the double helix structure of the DNA molecule, a structure that immediately suggested how it could perform its genetic and biological functions and how mutations could arise. By the late 1950s, French researchers Jacques Monod and François Jacob had begun to explain the direct role played by DNA in the regulation and coordination of chemical activity within the living organism. Within a few short years, the genetic code was broken, thereby making it possible for us to ultimately decipher the "book of life."

In light of the stunning triumph of molecular biology and its extraordinary promise, some of the leading molecular biologists felt inspired to educate the lay public about what they believed were the transformative social implications of their work. In 1966, Crick announced in *Of Molecules and Men* that "the development of biology is going to destroy to some extent our traditional grounds for ethical belief" and replace our culture's "particular prejudice about the sanctity of life" with a new culture based on "science in general, and natural selection in particular" (Crick, 1966, pp. xii, 7, 93–95). Monod's 1971 best-seller, *Chance and Necessity*, presented molecular biology's revolutionary implications even more forcefully. The knowledge that all life is the product of meaningless chance and mindless genetic replication, Monod asserted, would at last destroy the "disgusting farrago of Judeo-Christian religiosity, scientistic progressism, belief in the 'natural' rights of man and utilitarian pragmatism" with which we have deluded ourselves for centuries (Monod, 1971, p. 171). Monod argued that by destroying the "anthropocentric illusion" that is the main ingredient in this noxious mixture, we will at last be able to create a truly scientific culture built on a proper understanding of human nature and biological processes. The essence of this new conception of life was clearly expressed in Jacob's *The Logic of Life*: "The organism thus becomes the realization of a programme prescribed by its heredity. . . . An organism is merely a transition, a stage between what was and what will be. Reproduction [of its constituent molecules] represents both the beginning and the end, the cause and the aim" (Jacob, 1973, p. 102).

The writings of Crick, Monod, Jacob, and others of similar mind helped inspire the development of the field of sociobiology (now called "evolutionary psychology")—that is, the study of the genetic basis of the social behavior of all animals, including humans. Indeed, sociobiology's foremost proponent, E. O. Wilson, often has acknowledged his debt to the molecular revolution and to the philosophical writings that it spawned. In his

seminal text, *Sociobiology: The New Synthesis* (1975), Wilson first presented to a broader public his theories about the biological basis of all social behavior and began to explore its "revolutionary implications" for our
understanding of human nature and social organization. From a Darwinian point of view, he proclaimed, an organism "is only DNA's way of making more DNA," and all characteristics of all organisms—anatomical,
physiological, behavioral, mental, social, and even cultural—are merely
the genes' "devices" and "techniques for replicating themselves" (Wilson,
1975, p. 3). In subsequent works, such as his Pulitzer Prize–winning *On
Human Nature* (1978), *Genes, Mind, and Culture* (1981), and, most recently, *Consilience* (1998), Wilson has presented his reductionistic account
of all things human with ever greater boldness and certainty.

Following Wilson's lead, over the last 25 years other scientists (e.g.,
Richard Dawkins, David Barash, Steven Pinker, and David Buss), philosophers (e.g., David Dennett), and journalists (e.g., Robert Wright) have
joined in the effort to popularize the new biology and to proclaim the implications of the new Darwinian viewpoint. Although influential critics
such as biologists Richard Lewontin and Stephen Jay Gould have denounced such literature as potentially racist, sexist, and classist in its message, proponents of the "selfish gene" perspective have painted a far rosier
picture. What they have promised is a broad array of psychological, moral,
and social benefits sanctioned by biology: universal human rights, democ-
racy, "scientific socialist humanism," altruism, the brotherhood of man, "a
genetically accurate and hence completely fair code of ethics," and a renewed sense of awe and wonder toward the world (Kaye, 1997).

In spite of such wishful thinking, to date the impact of this ever-grow-
ing body of literature has not been so beneficial. Evolutionary accounts of
such moral abominations as rape (Thornhill & Palmer, 2000), infanticide
(Pinker, 1997), and adultery (Wright, 1994) have come dangerously close
to justifying such behaviors as natural, adaptive, and genetically programmed. In addition, rampant speculation about the genetic origins of a
broad range of human behaviors has led to increasing attempts to identify
biological markers and genes for socially destructive forms of human behavior, such as violence. In the minds of many, such efforts are inherently
racist, particularly in the United States, where African Americans, for example, account for a little over 12% of the population but almost 40% of
arrests for violent crime (Gibbs, 1995, p. 106; FBI, 1999; U.S. Bureau of the
Census, 2000). Despite such criticisms, the abuses of the past, and the

overwhelming evidence that the roots of violent behavior can be found in other factors such as drug use and family dysfunction, research on biological markers for undesirable behavior continues to grow.

Implications of PNI for Medicine and Religion

After decades of such militant reductionism, supplemented by the latest news in genetics, neurology, and endocrinology, the public at large is getting the sense that "biochemistry governs all" and "that we are all machines [constructed by natural selection to serve genetic self-interest], pushed and pulled by forces we can't discern but that science can" (Wright, 1994, pp. 351, 353). In such a cultural climate, psychoneuroimmunology and research into the impact of religion on health might prove to be particularly attractive as a counterweight to such an extreme, mechanistic reductionism, because it suggests a more complex understanding of the mind-body connection and grants to human longings for meaning, coherence, control, fellowship, and forgiveness a certain reality and significance that is scientifically demonstrable.

Nevertheless, the implications of PNI and the "faith factor" are ambiguous enough to warrant caution on the part of both the medical and faith communities. Certainly medical personnel need to demonstrate greater sensitivity to and support of the religious lives of patients. Beyond that, however, a whole host of problems are foreseeable. For example, the well-intentioned inquiries by physicians, particularly when made to patients from a different religious background, may easily be perceived as a violation of privacy, thereby increasing mistrust and tension between patient and doctor. In addition, imparting information to patients about the potential health benefits of religious participation and spiritual practice may unwittingly do them psychological harm by adding a burden of guilt to their physical suffering. If faith heals, but their own illness persists, might they not view this as punishment for a lack of faith (Sloan et al., 1999)? And what if some denominations, spiritual beliefs, or conceptions of God are healthier than others? Does the responsible physician inform patients of this, so that they can make medically sound religious choices? Might this not encourage religious "shopping" and a religiosity of the most superficial sort?

Similarly, faith communities must be extremely careful in how they interpret and attempt to use the findings of PNI. To encourage religious practice and greater spirituality for its putative health benefits on the order of physical exercise, a low-fat diet, and relaxation training runs the risk of trivializing religion into little more than magic. Ironically, such religiosity may be too extrinsic, too utilitarian, to produce the desired medical result. But if this proves to be the case, what then? Might not bitterness, spiritual anguish, and even loss of faith ensue?

Rather than stimulating the reintegration of religion back into medical practice, research on PNI and the faith factor may well encourage the "medicalization of religion," not the "spiritualizing of medicine," by fostering a purely "therapeutic" attitude toward religion. But if religion is practiced essentially for its therapeutic benefits, what happens to religious practice if scientists discover that some other psychotherapeutic technique, such as meditation or self-hypnosis, is more effective as a source of stress reduction, or if scientists identify the biochemical pathways by which prayer strengthens the body's immune system and then develops a more potent pharmacological means of doing so? Might religion then become medically obsolete, similar to the early antidepressants?

Over the last four decades, the adoption of a therapeutic attitude toward marriage has produced devastating effects on that social institution, for once marriage was conceived as a means of enhancing the psychological well-being of the individuals involved, it was no longer stabile enough, enduring enough, or emotionally powerful enough to achieve this end (Bellah, 1985; Lasch, 1977; Rieff, 1987). Religious life—especially among those Protestant denominations that have turned to the therapeutic attitude in order to compete for congregants in the spiritual marketplace by offering them a friendly, nonjudgmental God and a feel-good faith—might be next.

By demonstrating the biological pathways by which religion may produce beneficial health effects, one may wish to lend scientific support to religious practice, thereby serving God and human well-being in the process. But those who attempt to make such a case must remember that appeals to biology always cut both ways and thus may well prove to be self-defeating, both medically and spiritually.

REFERENCES

Bannister, R. C. (1979). *Social Darwinism: Science and myth in Anglo-American social thought.* Philadelphia: Temple University Press.

Bellah, R. N. (1985). *Habits of the heart.* New York: Harper and Row.

Crick, F. (1966). *Of molecules and men.* Seattle: University of Washington Press.

Crook, P. (1994). *Darwinism, war and history: The debate over the biology of war and the "Origin of Species" to the First World War.* New York: Cambridge University Press.

Darwin, C. (1859). *On the origin of species by natural selection.* London: John Murray.

Darwin, C. (1871). *The descent of man and selection in relation to sex.* Reprint (1981). Princeton, NJ: Princeton University Press.

Degler, C. N. (1991). *In search of human nature: The decline and revival of Darwinism in American social thought.* New York: Oxford University Press.

Easterbrook, G. (1999, July 19). Faith healers: Is religion good for your health? *New Republic,* 20–23.

Federal Bureau of Investigation (1999). *Uniform Crime Reports 1999.* Accessed online at www.fbi.gov/ucr/99cius.html.

Gibbs, W. W. (1995). Seeking the criminal element. *Scientific American* 273(3), 100–107.

Greene, J. C. (1981). *Science, ideology, and world view.* Berkeley: University of California Press.

Himmelfarb, G. (1967). *Darwin and the Darwinian revolution.* Gloucester, MA: Peter Smith.

Jacob, F. (1973). *The logic of life: A history of heredity.* Trans. Betty E. Spillman. New York: Pantheon.

Kaye, H. L. (1997). *The social meaning of modern biology: From social Darwinism to sociobiology.* New Brunswick, NJ: Transaction.

Koenig, H. G. (1994). *Aging and God: Spiritual pathways to mental health in midlife and later years.* New York: Haworth Pastoral Press.

Lasch, C. (1977). *Haven in a heartless world: The family besieged.* New York: Harper and Row.

Marx, K. ([1897] 1906). *Capital: A critique of political economy.* Trans. Samuel Moore and Edward Aveling. New York: Charles H. Kerr & Co.

Monod, J. (1971). *Chance and necessity: An essay on the natural philosophy of modern biology.* Trans. Austryn Wainhouse. New York: Knopf.

Moore, J. R. (1979). *The post-Darwinian controversies.* Cambridge: Cambridge University Press.

Pinker, S. (1997). Why they kill their newborns. *New York Times Magazine,* November 2, 52–54.

Rieff, P. (1987). *The triumph of the therapeutic.* Chicago: University of Chicago Press.

Sloan, R. P., Bagiella, E., & Powell, T. (1999). Religion, spirituality, and medicine. *Lancet* 353, 664–667.

Thornhill, R., & Palmer, C. (2000). *A natural history of rape: Biological bases of sexual coercion.* Cambridge: MIT Press.

U.S. Bureau of the Census (2000). *Census 2000.* Accessed online at
www.census.gov/population/cen2000/html.

Wilson, E. O. (1975). *Sociobiology: The new synthesis.* Cambridge: Harvard University Press.

Wright, R. (1994). *The moral animal: The new science of evolutionary psychology.*
New York: Pantheon.

15

Avenues for Future Research

HARVEY JAY COHEN & HAROLD G. KOENIG

In this final chapter, we summarize and prioritize research studies that are needed to further elucidate the relationships between religion, immunity, and illness. This information is based on both the chapters in this book and a recent conference at Duke University Medical Center that brought together the world's leading experts in psychoneuroimmunology (mentioned earlier) to discuss the future of research on religion and immune function. We now briefly describe what went on during that conference and then discuss areas of research that conference participants and chapter authors felt should have the highest priority.

The conference to explore psychoneuroimmunology and faith in human health was organized to allow each participant to describe briefly his or her area of research and to comment on the potential for future studies relating psychoneuroimmunology to spiritual and religious factors. An attempt was made to prioritize studies from the standpoint of both importance and practicality at this time. Though each conference participant approached the topic from his or her own research and personal point of view, a number of recurring themes and potential approaches did arise.

Because the immune response is part of the "stress response," one recurring theme was the need to study spirituality or religion as a potential moderator of the stress response in *situations of high stress*. This could include populations at risk for negative outcome from stress—for example, Scandinavians at high risk for suicide, Irish Catholics at high risk for alcoholism, HIV patients at risk for progression of their disease, the recently bereaved, the medically ill elderly, caregiver spouses of Alzheimer's patients and others. Assessment of both immune function and health out-comes in such groups, comparing them across members with varying degrees of spiritual or religious participation and belief, would be informative. This approach is analogous to using a cognitive-behavioral stress management intervention, except that it could be difficult to "administer" spirituality or religion; thus, at least the initial studies would need to be observational and descriptive. Such studies might start with simply defining any differences in immune function observed among people with different levels of religious participation, belief, or commitment. Challenges could then be either experimentally induced (for example, randomly assigning subjects to a supportive prayer group intervention or to a control group) or observed as experiments of nature, examining for differential effects within groups based on levels of religious practice.

Other specific health effects might be studied as well, such as wound healing, responses to viral illness, or immune responses following administration of vaccines such as Pneumovax, influenza, or hepatitis A and B. In these situations (in a sense, experiments of nature), one could assess whether groups with different clusters of characteristics, such as religious participation, have different responses to immune manipulations or different immune responses to diseases known to affect immune functioning.

Studies of this type need to take into account the *social context of the observations*, because religion and spirituality effects might differ in different contexts, such as location (e.g., rural vs. urban), culture (Eastern vs. Western), or race (African American vs. European American). Relationships between immune function and intensity of religious belief or practice also could be examined to determine whether these relations are always linear or have positive (or negative) effects at opposite ends of the spectrum.

Several cautions, however, are necessary, including recognition of the extreme degree of heterogeneity of religious practices and beliefs that exist in the population and the need to account for this in any research study design. There is also a need to account for the difference between external practice (extrinsic) and true belief and commitment (intrinsic) if we are to accurately determine what aspects of religion are most active in modifying neuroendocrine and immunological responses. Also, from a theological perceptive—as Kaye and Griffiths point out—it is important to remember that health effects of religion are by-products of, not necessarily the rationale for, religious or spiritual beliefs and practices.

In general, then, a substantial and meaningful agenda of future research appears possible, and many aspects of such studies could be begun now if appropriate support is forthcoming. Continued open dialogue and free-flowing discussion among those from multiple disciplines, as exemplified in our recent conference, are necessary to begin to understand the complexity of such research and its far-reaching implications.

High-Priority Research Projects

Based on what we already know from research completed and based on the consensus of experts contributing to this book, we have come up with a list of research projects that are most likely to advance the field. These are listed here, not necessarily in order of importance.

- Conduct observational studies. Do people with different religious practices or degree of practice differ in immune functions? Simple descriptive studies are needed first. Those studies, however, may show no immunological differences not because they are not there, but because baseline differences do not necessarily tell what is happening in the face of a challenge. The lack of a difference is not necessarily informative; thus, it is important to have challenges to immune function—either naturally or experimentally induced.
- Study the immune system's response to challenge, whether this is a biologically induced challenge (immunization), a physical stress (injury or trauma), or a psychological stress (bereavement or loss). These challenges should be studied in different populations based on age, ethnicity, disease type, and level of immune system compromise.
- Piggyback religious variables on other major epidemiological studies now under way or in the planning phase, and assess immunological, endocrine, and health outcomes by degree of religious involvement. Offer investigators a "supplement" to an ongoing grant to examine religious or spiritual influences. This is a cost-effective way of stimulating research in a particular area.
- Examine the physiological aspects of people who are religious (self-reported and perhaps observed), both at the biochemical level (catecholamine, cortisol, serotonin, endorphins, etc.) and at the organ system level (cardiovascular, central and peripheral nervous systems, etc.).
- Look at relationships between individual components of religiosity and emotional responses (negative affect/depression, anger/hostility,

positive affect/happiness). By influencing affect, meaning and purpose, optimism and hope, self-efficacy, and mastery and sense of
control, religion may affect immune function in diverse ways. Develop a model in which religion is seen as a multidimensional concept, possibly leading to better mental health and social functioning,
possibly leading to better endocrine and immune functioning. Test
each part of this model separately.

- Study the neurobiological underpinnings of trait clusters such as high
religious activities/beliefs, low hostility, and high well-being. What is
the hormonal milieu that bathes the central nervous system of such
persons? The central nervous system will affect mediator substances
such as catecholamines and cortisol levels, which in turn will affect
immune functioning and health. For example, we might hypothesize
that the cluster of traits just described is driven by high serotonin in
the brain or low serotonin turnover in the hippocampus.

- Study the effects of cognitive-behavioral stress management
(CBSM) on hostility, depression, and, consequently, biochemical
markers. We might hypothesize that CBSM training as a secular intervention could be used with low-religious people to make the hormonal milieu more like that of those who are religious. Might the
CBSM intervention have a sustained effect over time—even though
it is less *meaningful* to the individual than religion is? These are research questions that can be tested.

- Conduct studies of wound healing by experimentally inducing
wounds (punch biopsies, for example) during various stressful set-
tings in subjects of varying levels of religious belief and commitment
or by conducting clinical trials of patients undergoing surgery with
and without religious interventions (assessing immune parameters,
along with speed of wound healing).

- Conduct studies of susceptibility to viral infections or of progression
of viral illnesses (herpes zoster, influenza, HIV, etc.) among persons
of varying degrees of religious belief or commitment; alternatively,
subjects could be a randomized to receive a religious intervention
prior to being challenged by the virus. Conduct the studies in subjects with different clusters of characteristics (high religious, low
hostility, high well-being).

- Conduct studies that examine immune function before and after
religious practices. Examine both the short-term and long-term
temporal course of immune changes. For example, assess immune

and biochemical parameters before and after a person attends a worship service or before and after a person attends a religious retreat. Such studies would be far superior to simple cross-sectional assessments that provide no information concerning the temporal course of changes necessary for determining the causal nature and direction of relationships.

- Study similar practices in different contexts. Social context may affect outcomes of interventions, particularly religious interventions. In a rural setting, religion may be protective against depression, whereas in the city of London it may not be protective. Studies must be sophisticated at the sociocultural level in the same way as at the neurobiological level.

- Identify intrinsically versus extrinsically religious subjects, induce a stressor, and measure immune responses; conducting such a study in high-risk, stressed populations would be particularly revealing.

- Conduct studies in subjects under a variety of conditions of vulnerability and resilience. When examining the impact of religion on immune function and disease progression, use a vulnerable population. Until a subject is challenged by some kind of stressor, religion may not matter much with regard to immune functioning.

- Study the effects of religion on immune functioning in the context of personal relationships. Does it make a difference if subjects believe that "someone" is listening to their prayers (i.e., God)? This follows the same logic as studying whether it makes a difference (in terms of biochemical and immune changes) if a stressed individual simply writes down what is bothering him or her and then tears it up, compared with the stressed individual writing to someone who will actually read the letter. This may be an indirect way of assessing the effect of God-centered religious belief systems such as the Judeo-Christian and Muslim faith traditions, compared with Buddhism and related practices (which do not focus on a personal God relationship). In other words, are PNI effects similar when assessed in the context of interpersonal relationships both with God and in the context of religious community, compared with religious belief systems that are more individually oriented? The cultural setting in which such studies are conducted may also be very important (e.g., compare Buddhists in Tibet with Christians in Texas).

- Study situations in which there is a loss of religious faith, and examine the effects on immune system functioning. For example, a religious family loses several children in a fire. This event causes family members to lose their faith in God as well, because they attributed the fire and the loss of their children to God. They experience future decline in mental and physical health. Studies are needed to examine the effects on immune functioning of positive or negative attributions to God in the face of a severe psychosocial stressor.

- Studies should be conducted in well-defined religious groups, isolating a specific aspect of religious practice and then looking at immune and other biochemical parameters. One example is Buddhist meditation among Buddhists; another example might be religious attendance among Catholics in Chicago or Boston.

- In conducting these studies, immune components should be examined that are relevant to the particular disease outcome being studied. For example, do religious people have higher natural killer cell activity (compared with nonreligious people) during the month after they are diagnosed with cancer? We know that natural killer cell activity may be related to speed of cancer metastasis, so this is an appropriate immune parameter to study when examining the effects of religious involvement or religious interventions on cancer prognosis.

- Studies are needed of immune function changes during the course of training of clergy. As clergy become more mature in their religious faith, do immune parameters change? Studies of immune function among agnostics who undergo religious training and ultimately experience conversion might also be interesting.

Most Practical Studies

Besides identifying high-priority studies, we also must consider the order in which such studies should be accomplished from a practical standpoint. Some studies may be too expensive. Other studies, although less important, may need to be done first simply because they will provide the research base necessary for conducting more substantial research in the future. For that reason, we have listed the following studies in order of when they should be conducted.

- Study existing data sets that have religious measures and assessments of immune function. Alternatively, an epidemiological study could be designed to collect such data from a large population base sample. If a relationship is found between an indicator of religious involvement and immune functioning, then researchers should develop path models to identify mediating variables that could help explain the mechanism (including the examination of partial variances so that the relative contributions of different variables in the model can be examined).

- Take a study already planned with defined health outcome and immunological impact (for example, effects of stress on wound healing or on antibody response to vaccination), and piggyback religious assessments or interventions onto the study.

- Design a study to test the immune system's ability to respond to vaccine. We would recommend a trial involving hepatitis B vaccine, because administration involves both cross-sectional and longitudinal components with three separate injections given over a 6-month period. The population to test might involve health care workers (especially those in highly stressed positions) who are required to get the hepatitis B vaccine anyway. Time for seroconversion, plus antibody T cell responses over time, could be examined as outcome variables among persons with greater or lesser religious belief or involvement (or following a religious intervention).

- Examine postsurgical recovery and wound healing, assessing both religious measures and immune function. Such a study could be either observational (looking at the effects of different levels of religious involvement) or interventional (a chaplain visit or other religious intervention prior to surgery). Such a project could be piggybacked onto an existing study that is examining health outcomes in subjects undergoing surgery. The type of surgery selected should be one with well-known base rates concerning recovery and speed of wound healing. Avoid choosing surgery for pathology that is immune mediated.

- Short-term and long-term changes in immune functioning should both be examined, in that changes may be time dependent. For example, stress in the short term results in an increase in T cells or NK cells, whereas chronic stress results in a decrease. A study could be designed to assess pre- and postevent immune and endocrine functioning in persons who attend a 2-week religious retreat. By focusing on the effects of an experience that occurs over time, this will provide more useful information than simply measuring immune changes at one point in time following a prayer or other religious activity.

- Study a group of religious cancer patients. Try to increase religiousness (support and encourage religion; increase prayer, scripture study, or religious attendance) in half of the group and not in the other half (control group). Immune functioning and health outcomes could be compared between testing and control groups. Such a study might get around some of the ethical problems involved in seeking to make nonreligious subjects more religious, although institutional review boards may still see this as coercive.

- A study is needed to determine whether religious people are "hardwired" differently (have different genetic susceptibility) than those who are not religious. This hardwiring could determine low hostility, high sociability levels, extraversion, and the like, lead to religion —rather than the other way around (i.e., religious activity causing these positive character traits conducive to health). This could be accomplished by measuring serotonin transporter genotype, salivary cortisols, or salivary prolactin (which correlates well with cerebrospinal fluid serotonin and is relatively inexpensive to assess).

- A religious intervention could be applied to subjects with an immunologically mediated condition like psoriasis that is easy to visually assess for disease activity. Alternatively, an observational study could be designed in which subjects are categorized into groups with different levels of religious activity and disease outcomes measured over time. In studying immune-mediated diseases (autoimmune disorders), immune regulation is the key goal, rather than increasing or decreasing immune function. Stress may cause a decrease in the balance of certain immune factors, reducing one factor that then allows another factor to become overactive.

- There are many clinical trials currently going on to assess the effects of various types of chemotherapy in cancer patients. Adding religious variables and immune measures to these clinical trials, or even adding a religious intervention, may provide useful information at low cost.

In this book, leaders in the field of psychoneuroimmunology have reviewed their particular areas of expertise and thoughtfully considered how religion may affect health through neuroendocrine and immunological processes. The area of religion-spirituality and psychoneuroimmunology remains wide open for study. We have tried to point out projects that might help to advance knowledge in this field, equip readers with the tools and resources necessary to carry out such studies, and direct funding agencies to areas that are likely to have the highest payoff.

Conclusions

HAROLD G. KOENIG

There is growing epidemiological evidence that religious beliefs and behaviors are correlated with mental health and predict both better physical health outcomes and longer survival. Exactly how religions influence physical health, however, remains an enigma. Establishing plausible biochemical and physiological mechanisms by which religion conveys its health effects is of utmost importance for advancing our knowledge about the religion-health relationship. Given the strong associations between religious involvement, social support, and stress reduction, it seems almost natural that religious beliefs and practices might affect health through neuroendocrine and immune pathways.

Studies in psychoneuroimmunology recently have shed light on the delicate and finely balanced interactions between the mind and physical body. Psychological stress, anxiety, depression, hopelessness, social isolation, and negative health behaviors such as cigarette smoking, excessive alcohol intake, and illicit drug use all have been shown to adversely affect neuroendocrine and immune system functioning. By impairing immune function, psychosocial and behavioral factors may increase susceptibility to disease or affect the course of disease once present.

Religious beliefs and practices are associated with improved coping, reduced anxiety, less depression, faster recovery from depression, greater hope and optimism, greater meaning and purpose, greater social support, and fewer negative health behaviors. Consequently, they are highly likely to influence neuroendocrine and immune function, thereby affecting physical health outcomes. Preliminary studies, although few in number and limited in sophistication, appear to support this hypothesis.

295

In *The Link between Religion and Health*, we have explored the many possible connections between religion, immune functioning, and physical illness. We also have discussed future avenues for research in this exciting, largely unexplored area. The next steps are to carefully design studies of this relationship and obtain research funding to carry them out. The results of such research are likely to have enormous public health impact, given the wide prevalence of religious beliefs and practices in the United States and around the world and the importance that many adherents ascribe to these practices.

We recognize that religion has its own intrinsic value separate and apart from the health benefits that it may convey and that those health benefits probably result only as a by-product of religious faith that has the sacred as its ultimate concern, not health. *Because religion and science both search for the truth, neither should fear the other*. It is our hope that each of these disciplines, rather than competing or conflicting, will add to each other's richness and depth. According to Albert Einstein, "Science without religion is lame; religion without science is blind." Likewise, medical research on the religion-health relationship, we believe, will ultimately yield benefits for both our faith and our health.

Index